Dr. Bernstein's
Diabetes Solution

Theories, no matter how pertinent,
Cannot eradicate the existence of facts.

— *Jean Martin Charcot*

Dedicated to the Memory of
My Dear Friends Heinz I. Lippmann, MD,
Ephraim Friedman, MD,
and
Samuel M. Rosen, MD,
who fervently believed that people with diabetes are
entitled to the same blood sugars as nondiabetics

Preface to the Newly Revised and Updated Edition

Since the publication of the previous edition of *Dr. Bernstein's Diabetes Solution* in 2007, many new developments have occurred in the field of diabetes research, and as each significant one has come along, I have further refined my techniques for normalizing blood sugars. This newly revised and updated edition discusses new medications, new insulins, new dietary supplements, new hardware (tools for the diabetic), and other new products. It also explores new methods that I have developed for more elegantly controlling blood sugars.

Exciting new approaches to weight loss will be found here, including the use of new, injectable medications (incretin mimetics) that are wonderfully effective for alleviating carbohydrate craving and overeating.

This newly revised and updated edition builds upon the prior three editions of this book and upon my three earlier books about diabetes. It is designed as a tool for patients to be used under the guidance of their physicians or diabetes educators. It covers, in a step-by-step fashion, virtually everything that must be done to keep blood sugars in the normal range.

In these pages I attempt to present nearly everything I know about blood sugar normalization, how it can be accomplished and maintained. With this book, and with the help of your physician or diabetes educator, I hope that you will learn to take control of your diabetes, whether it's type 1 (juvenile-onset), as mine is, or the much more common type 2 (maturity-onset) diabetes. To my knowledge, there is no other book in print addressed strictly to blood sugar control for both types of diabetes.

This volume contains much material that may be new to many physicians treating diabetes. It is my hope that doctors and health care professionals will use it, learn from it, and do their best to help their patients take control of this potentially deadly but controllable disease.

Although this book contains considerable background information on diet and nutrition, it is intended primarily as a comprehensive how-to guide to blood sugar control, including detailed instructions on techniques for painless insulin injection and so on. It must, therefore, leave out other related issues (such as pregnancy), some of which require their own volumes. My office telephone number is listed several times in this book, and we are always happy to hear from readers who seek our latest recommendation for a blood sugar meter, other equipment, or new medications.

I urge you to visit the website for this book, www.diabetes-book .com. The site contains some of my recent articles, a history of blood sugar self-monitoring, links to other sites, testimonials from readers who have tried the program, an opportunity to share your own experiences in an ongoing chat group for diabetics and their loved ones,* and more. The site also permits you to forward information by e-mail to anyone you think could benefit from this book.

Recent news releases and advertisements have described "developments" and products that are not mentioned here, and you may be curious about them. If a medication is not discussed here, then it is likely I have deliberately omitted it as either useless or potentially harmful, or it was not available when this volume was written. There are many drugs, old and new, used in the treatment of diabetes. Some, like metformin, or Glucophage, are truly wonderful, but others, such as the sulfonylureas, are insidious and can impair your body's remaining insulin-producing capability, if it has any. I have omitted anything I think is either too far into the future to be of near-term consequence or is simply not going to be effective at getting you on track. I have neither the time nor the space to attempt to debunk every "miracle cure" that comes along, most of which are neither miraculous nor cures.

Should you become pregnant while on this program, of all the medications mentioned in this book, metformin, aspirin, and insulin

---

* At least two members of this group have married each other.

Dr. Bernstein's
Diabetes Solution

Newly Revised and Updated

THE COMPLETE GUIDE TO ACHIEVING NORMAL BLOOD SUGARS

Richard K. Bernstein, MD, FACE, FACN, FCCWS

Foreword by Frank Vinicor, MD, MPH

Recipes by Karen A. Weinstock and Timothy J. Aubert, CWC

LITTLE, BROWN AND COMPANY

NEW YORK   BOSTON   LONDON

Little, Brown and Company
Hachette Book Group
237 Park Avenue, New York, NY 10017
littlebrown.com

Originally published in hardcover by Little, Brown and Company, 1997
Newly revised and updated edition, November 2011

Little, Brown and Company is a division of Hachette Book Group, Inc.
The Little, Brown name and logo are trademarks of Hachette Book Group, Inc.

Illustrations by Terry Eppridge

AUTHOR'S NOTE
This book is not intended as a substitute for professional medical care. The reader should regularly consult a physician for all health-related problems and routine care.

The author is grateful for permission to include the following previously copyrighted material:

Figure 1-3. Reproduced from the *Journal of Clinical Investigation*, 1967; 46:1549–1557. By permission of The American Society for Clinical Investigation.
Figure 9-1. Reproduced from the *Journal of the American Dietetic Association*, 1995; 45:417–420. Copyright © by The American Dietetic Association. Reprinted by permission of The American Dietetic Association.
Figure 19-1. Reproduced from Humalog PI. Reprinted by permission of Eli Lilly and Company.

The publisher is not responsible for websites (or their content) that are not owned by the publisher.

Library of Congress Cataloging-in-Publication Data

Bernstein, Richard K.
    Dr. Bernstein's diabetes solution : the complete guide to achieving normal blood sugars / Richard K. Bernstein ; foreword by Frank Vinicor ; recipes by Karen A. Weinstock and Timothy J. Aubert. —Newly rev. and updated.
        p. cm.
    Includes bibliographical references and index.
    ISBN 978-0-316-18269-0
  1. Diabetes—Popular works. 2. Blood sugar monitoring—Popular works. I. Title. II. Title: Diabetes solution.
    RC660.4.B464 2011
    616.4'62—dc23   2011023064

10 9 8 7 6 5 4

RRD-C

Printed in the United States of America

Contents

PART THREE

Your Diabetic Cookbook

Appendices

Foreword

by Frank Vinicor, MD, MPH
Former Director, Division of Diabetes Translation
National Center for Chronic Disease Prevention and
    Health Promotion
Centers for Disease Control and Prevention
Atlanta, Georgia

We are learning a lot about diabetes — especially during the past five years. This accumulation of new knowledge is both encouraging and at the same time *very* challenging. On the "challenging" side:

- Diabetes seems to be everywhere and steadily increasing in its presence. Think about it — 1 in 3 babies born in 2000 will develop diabetes in their lifetimes. Every day, about 1,400 people are diagnosed with diabetes in the United States. And now no country in the world is free from diabetes, and its growth.
- We now do know how to prevent type 2 diabetes, but today for type 1 diabetes, neither prevention nor a long-lasting cure is available.
- Once diabetes is present, good care based on solid science now can prevent much of the devastation formerly caused by elevated blood sugars. But there remains a sizable gap between what we know to do and how well and widely we are doing it. In other words, the "translation" of diabetes science into daily practice still has a way to go.

Nonetheless, in spite of these and other important challenges, we are all better prepared to deal with diabetes in 2011 than we were even a few years ago, let alone decades ago. Remarkable progress has occurred. For example, many people at high risk for type 2 diabetes do not develop it. Modest weight loss and increased physical activity have been shown to eliminate or at least delay the development of this type of diabetes by 60–70 percent — *regardless* of race, ethnicity, or age.

In addition, for both types 1 and 2 diabetes, we now have many more effective medications which, when taken appropriately and in combination with proper nutrition and activity, will result in controlled plasma glucose, blood pressure, and blood fats — with *definite* reduction in the likelihood of eye, kidney, nerve, and heart problems. In other words, while the goals of diabetes research still in large part should be prevention or cure, even now the devastation formerly caused by this condition *does not have to happen*!

Nowadays, too, we have better ways to follow and keep track of diabetes — with improved health care systems, better educational programs, less painful self-monitoring of blood sugars, more quickly available and accurate glycated hemoglobin levels, ways to identify kidney problems early, and so forth. We can know what is going on!

So, in fact, we are actually seeing an improvement in diabetes care in the United States, although not with all people and not yet to an adequate level or fast enough.

What does all this have to do with Dr. Bernstein and this edition of *Diabetes Solution*? As mentioned earlier, the rate of accumulation of new diabetes knowledge is quite remarkable and daunting. Yet Dr. Bernstein stays on top of it all. The care pattern for diabetes has become much more complex and demanding, and Dr. Bernstein and his approach have proved equal to the challenge. In essence, diabetes is in many ways "less easy" than in the past — for the patient and for his or her health care professional. There are lots of nutritional approaches to consider, lots of medications to be used in varying combination, and often less time within a busy office practice to make all these wonderful advances real and meaningful for people facing diabetes. This newly revised edition presents the advances in diabetes thinking and management with passion, compassion, caring, and conviction. Certainly, for some people, his approaches are not easy! But they do reflect evolving medical science as well as his personal experiences in managing his own diabetes. He does not ask anyone to do anything that he himself would not do, and for this I have respect and admiration. He is offering to persons challenged by the presence or risk of diabetes a way to be in charge of the disease. And he is ensuring that important advances in diabetes science get out there *now* to make a difference in people's lives. Take a look! Think about the ideas and suggestions — they can further our mutual and ongoing effort to prevent, capture, and control this disease called diabetes.

are the only ones that have been tested in pregnant women. Nevertheless, check out all your medications with your obstetrician and pharmacist — ideally before you become pregnant.

Many thousands of diabetics have successfully used this program. Like them, if you, with your physician's help, seriously follow these guidelines, you should be able to avoid the discomfort of inappropriate blood sugar swings. You may even be able to prevent or reverse the development of many of the grave complications long associated with chronically high blood sugars.

Finally, much of what I will cover in this book is in direct opposition to the recommendations of the American Diabetes Association (ADA) and other national diabetes associations. Why? Because if I had followed those guidelines, they would have killed me long ago. Such conflicts include the low-carbohydrate diet I recommend; the avoidance of certain oral agents (such as sulfonylureas) that impair surviving insulin-producing beta cells in type 2 diabetics; my preference for certain insulins over others, which I avoid; my desire to preserve remaining beta cells (an alien concept to traditional practice); and my insistence that *diabetics are entitled to the same normal blood sugars that nondiabetics enjoy,* rather than the ADA's current insistence upon higher levels.

Most important, unlike the ADA guidelines, ours work.

My Life with Diabetes

BEYOND SIXTY-FIVE YEARS AND COUNTING

I do not know of many diabetics who developed the illness around the time I did, in 1946, who are still alive. I know of none who do not suffer from long-term complications of this disease. The reality is, had I not taken charge of my diabetes, it's very unlikely that I'd be alive and active today. Many myths surround diet and diabetes, and much of what is still considered by the average physician to be sensible nutritional advice for diabetics can, over the long run, be fatal.

I know, because conventional "wisdom" about diabetes almost killed me.

I developed diabetes in 1946 at the age of twelve, and for more than two decades I was an "ordinary" diabetic, dutifully following doctor's orders and leading the most normal life I could, given the limitations of my disease.

Over the years, the complications from my diabetes became worse and worse, and like many diabetics in similar circumstances, I faced a very early death. I was still alive, but the quality of my life wasn't particularly good. I have what is known as type 1, or insulin-dependent, diabetes, which usually begins in childhood (it's also called juvenile-onset diabetes). Type 1 diabetics must take daily insulin injections just to stay alive.

Back in the 1940s, which were very much still the dark ages of diabetes treatment, I had to sterilize my needles and glass syringes by boiling them every day, and sharpen my needles with an abrasive stone. I used a test tube and an alcohol lamp (flame) to test my urine for sugar. Many of the tools the diabetic can take for granted today were scarcely dreamed of back then—there was no such thing as a rapid, finger-stick blood sugar–measuring device, nor disposable insulin syringes. Still, even today, parents of type 1 diabetics have to live with the same fear my parents lived with — that something could go disastrously wrong and they could try to wake up their child and discover him comatose, or worse. For any parent of a type 1 diabetic, this has been a real and constant possibility.

Because of my chronically elevated blood sugar levels, and the inability to control them, my growth was stunted, as it is for many juvenile-onset diabetics even to this day.

Back then, the medical community had just started to speculate about the relationship between high blood cholesterol and vascular (blood vessel and heart) disease. It was then widely believed that the cause of high blood cholesterol was consumption of large amounts of fat. Since many diabetics, even children, have high cholesterol levels, physicians were beginning to assume that the vascular complications of diabetes — heart disease, kidney failure, blindness, et cetera — were caused by the fat that diabetics were eating. As a result, I was put on a low-saturated-fat, high-carbohydrate diet (45 percent of calories were to be carbohydrates) before such diets were advocated by the American Diabetes Association or the American Heart Association. Because carbohydrate raises blood sugar, I had to compensate with very large doses of insulin, which I injected with a 10 cc "horse" syringe. These injections were slow and painful, and eventually they destroyed all the fatty tissue under the skin of my thighs. In spite of the low-fat diet, my blood cholesterol and triglycerides became very high. I developed visible signs of this state — fatty growths on my eyelids and gray deposits around the iris of each eye.

During my twenties and thirties, the prime of life for most people, many of my body's systems began to deteriorate. I had severe midchest burning all day long (diabetic gastroparesis), "frozen" shoulders, a progressive deformity of my feet with impaired sensation, and more. I would point these out to my diabetologist (who was then president of the American Diabetes Association), but I was inevitably told, "Don't worry, it has nothing to do with your diabetes. You're doing fine." But I wasn't doing fine. I now know that most of these problems are commonplace among those whose diabetes is poorly controlled, but then I was forced to accept my condition as "normal."

By this time I was married. I had gone to college and trained as an engineer. I had small children, and even though I was not much more than a kid myself, I felt like an old man. I had lost the hair on the lower parts of my legs, a sign that I had developed peripheral arterial disease — a complication of diabetes that can eventually lead to amputation. During a routine exercise stress test, I was diagnosed with cardiomyopathy, which is a replacement of muscle tissue in the heart with fibrous (scar) tissue—a common cause of heart failure and death among those with type 1 diabetes.

Even though I was "doing fine," I suffered a host of other complications. My vision deteriorated: I suffered night blindness, microaneurysms (ballooning of the blood vessels in my eyes), and early cataracts. Just lying in bed caused pain in my thighs, due to a common but rarely diagnosed and barely pronounceable diabetic complication called iliotibial band/tensor fascialata syndrome. Putting on a T-shirt was agonizing because of my frozen shoulders.

I had begun testing my urine for protein and found substantial amounts of it, a sign, I had read, of advanced kidney disease. In those days—the middle and late 1960s—the life expectancy of a type 1 diabetic with severe proteinuria was five years. Back in engineering school, a classmate had told me how his nondiabetic sister had died of kidney disease. Before her death she had ballooned with retained water, and after I discovered my own proteinuria, I began to have nightmares of blowing up like a balloon.

By 1967 I had these and other diabetic complications and clearly appeared chronically ill and prematurely aged. I had three small children, the oldest only six years old, and with good reason was certain I wouldn't live to see them grown.

At my father's suggestion, I started working out daily at a local gym. He thought that if I were to engage in vigorous exercise, I might feel better. Perhaps exercise would help my body help itself. I did feel slightly less depressed about my condition—at least I felt I was doing something—but I couldn't build muscles or get much stronger.

After two years of pumping iron, I remained a 115-pound weakling, no matter how strenuously I worked out. It was at about this time, in 1969, that my wife, a physician, pointed out to me that I had spent much of my life going into, experiencing, or recovering from hypoglycemia, which is a state of excessively low blood sugar. It was usually accompanied by fatigue and headaches, and was caused by the unpredictable action of the large doses of insulin I was taking to cover my high-carbohydrate diet. During such episodes, I became confused and unruly and snapped at people. These frequent hypoglycemic episodes had earlier taken their toll upon my parents, and were now taking their toll upon my wife and children. The strain on my family was clearly becoming untenable.

Suddenly, in October of 1969, my life turned around.

I had been the research director of a company that made equipment for hospital laboratories, but recently I had taken a new job as an officer of a housewares corporation. I was still receiving trade journals from my old field, and one day I opened the latest issue of a publication called *Lab World*. I came upon an advertisement for a new device to help hospital emergency rooms distinguish between unconscious diabetics and unconscious drunks during the night, when laboratories were closed. Knowing that an unconscious person was a diabetic and not drunk could easily help hospital personnel save his or her life. What I stumbled upon was an ad for a blood sugar meter that would give a reading in 1 minute, using a single drop of blood.

Since I'd been experiencing many blood sugars that were too low, and since the tests I had been performing on my urine were wholly inadequate (sugar that shows up in the urine is already on its way out of the bloodstream), I figured that if I knew what my blood sugars were, perhaps I could catch and correct my hypoglycemic episodes before they made me disoriented and irrational.

I marveled over the instrument. It had a 4-inch galvanometer with a jeweled bearing, weighed 3 pounds, and cost $650. I tried to order one, but the manufacturer wouldn't sell it to patients, only to doctors and hospitals.

Fortunately, because my wife, as I've said, was a physician, I could order one in her name. I started to measure my blood sugar about 5 times each day, and soon saw that the levels were on a roller coaster. Engineers are accustomed to solving problems mathematically, but you have to have information to work with. You have to know the mechanics of a problem in order to solve it, and now, for the first time, I was gaining insight into the mechanics and mathematics of my disease. What I learned from my frequent testing was that my own blood sugars swung from lows of under 40 mg/dl to highs of over 400 mg/dl about twice daily. A normal blood sugar level is about 83 mg/dl.* Small wonder I was subject to such vast mood swings.

---

* Although most medical journals and textbooks throughout the world measure blood glucose in mmol/l (millimoles per liter), most physicians, laboratories, and blood glucose meters in the United States measure blood glucose in mg/dl (milligrams per deciliter). Blood glucose values in this book are as a rule given in mg/dl. If you should need to translate from one to the other, 1 mmol/l = 18 mg/dl.

In an effort to level my blood sugars, I began to adjust my insulin regimen, and went from one injection a day to two. I made some experimental modifications to my diet, cutting down on the carbohydrates to permit me to take less insulin. The very high and low blood sugar levels became less frequent, but few were normal.

Three years after I started measuring my blood sugar levels, my diabetic complications were still progressing, and I was still a 115-pound weakling. My sense of gaining insight into the long-term complications of my diabetes had diminished, and so I ordered a search of the scientific literature to see if exercise could prevent diabetic complications. In those days, literature searches were not the simple, almost instant computer searches they are today. In 1972 you made your request to the local medical library, which mailed it to Washington, DC, where it was processed. It took about two weeks for my $75 list to arrive.

There were quite a few entries of interest, and I ordered copies of the original articles. For the most part these were from esoteric journals and dealt with animal experiments. The information I had hoped to find didn't exist. I didn't find a single article pertaining to the prevention of diabetic complications by exercise.

What I did find was that such complications had repeatedly been prevented, and even reversed, in animals. Not through exercise, but by normalizing blood sugars! To me, this was a total surprise. All diabetes treatment was heavily focused in other directions, such as low-fat diets, preventing severe hypoglycemia, and preventing a potentially fatal extreme high blood sugar condition called ketoacidosis. Thus, it had not occurred to me that keeping blood sugar levels as close to normal as possible for as much of the time as possible would make a difference.

Excited by my discovery, I showed these reports to my physician, who was not impressed. "Animals aren't humans," he said, "and besides, it's impossible to normalize human blood sugars." Since I had been trained as an engineer, not as a physician, I knew nothing of such impossibilities, and since I was desperate, I had no choice but to pretend I was an animal.

I spent the next year checking my blood sugars 5–8 times each day. Every few days, I'd make a small, experimental change in my diet or insulin regimen to see what the effect would be on my blood sugar. If a change brought an improvement, I'd retain it. If it made my blood sugars worse, I'd discard it. I discovered that 1 gram of carbohydrate raised my blood sugar by 5 mg/dl, and ½ unit of the old beef/pork insulin lowered it by 15 mg/dl.

Within a year, I had refined my insulin and diet regimen to the point that I had essentially normal blood sugars around the clock. After years of chronic fatigue and debilitating complications, almost overnight I was no longer continually tired or feeling washed-out. People commented that my gray complexion was gone. After years of sky-high readings, my serum cholesterol and triglyceride levels had now not only dropped, but were at the low end of the normal ranges.

I started to gain weight, and at last I was able to build muscle as readily as nondiabetics. My insulin requirements dropped to about one-third of what they had been a year earlier. With the subsequent development of human insulin, my dosage dropped to less than one-sixth of the original. The painful, slow-healing lumps the injections of large doses of insulin left under my skin disappeared. The fatty growths on my eyelids from high cholesterol vanished. My digestive problems (chronic burning in my chest and belching after meals) and the proteinuria that had so worried me eventually vanished. Today, my results from even the most sensitive kidney function tests are all normal. I recently discovered that even the calcified muscle lining the arteries in my legs has normalized. As chief of the peripheral vascular disease clinic of a major medical school, I had been teaching physicians that a cure for this Monckeberg's atherosclerosis was impossible. I proved myself wrong. My deformed feet, droopy eyelids, and loss of hair on my lower legs are not reversible and still remain. When I was seventy-three years old (four years ago), my coronary artery calcium score was only 1, less than that of most teenagers.

I had the new sensation of being the boss of my own metabolic state, and began to feel the same sense of accomplishment and reward I had in engineering when I solved a difficult problem. I had taught myself how to make my blood sugars whatever I wanted them to be and was no longer on the roller coaster. Things were finally under my control.

Back in 1973, I felt quite exhilarated by my success, and I felt that I was onto something big. Since getting the results of my literature search, I had been a subscriber to all of the English-language diabetes journals, and none of them had mentioned the need for normalizing blood sugars in humans.

In fact, every few months I'd read another article saying that blood sugar normalization wasn't even remotely possible. How was it that I, an engineer, had figured out how to do what was impossible for medical professionals? I was deeply grateful for the fortuitous combination of events that had turned my life, my health, and my family around and put me on the right path. At the very least, I felt, I was obliged to share my newfound knowledge with others. Millions of "ordinary" diabetics were no doubt suffering needlessly, as I had. I was sure that all physicians treating diabetes would be thrilled to learn how to so easily prevent and possibly reverse the grave complications of this disease.

I hoped that if I could tell the world about the techniques I had stumbled upon, physicians would adopt them for their patients. So I wrote an article detailing my discoveries. I sent a copy to Charles Suther, who was then in charge of marketing diabetes products for the Ames Division of Miles Laboratories, the company that made my blood glucose meter. He gave me the only encouragement I received in this new venture, and arranged for one of his company's medical writers to edit the article for me.

I submitted it and its revisions to many medical journals over a period of years—a period during which I was continually improving in health, and continually proving to myself and my family, if to no one else, that my methods were correct. The rejection letters I received are testimony that people tend to ignore the obvious if it conflicts with the orthodoxy of their early training. Typical rejection letters read in part: "Studies are not unanimous in demonstrating a need for 'fine control'" (*New England Journal of Medicine*), or "How many patients would use the electric device for measurement of glucose, insulin, urine, etc.?" (*Journal of the American Medical Association*). As a matter of fact, since 1980, when these "electric devices" finally were made available to patients, the worldwide market for blood glucose self-monitoring supplies has come to exceed $4 billion annually. Look at the array of blood glucose meters in any pharmacy and you can get an idea of just how many patients use, and will use, the "electric device."

Trying to cover several routes simultaneously, I joined the major lay diabetes organizations, in the hope of moving up through the ranks, where I could get to know physicians and researchers specializing in the disease. This met with mediocre success. I attended conventions, worked on committees, and became acquainted with many prominent diabetologists. In this country, I met only three physicians who were willing to offer their patients the opportunity to put these new methods to the test.

Meanwhile, Charlie Suther was traveling around the country to university research centers with copies of my unpublished article, which by now had been typeset and privately printed at my expense. The rejection by physicians specializing in diabetes of the concept of blood sugar self-monitoring, even though essential to blood sugar control, was so intense, however, that the management of his company had to turn down the idea of making meters available to patients until many years later. His company and others could clearly have profited from the sale of blood glucose meters and test strips. However, the backlash from the medical establishment prevented it on a number of counts. It was unthinkable that patients be allowed to "doctor" themselves. They knew nothing of medicine—and if they could, how would doctors earn a living? In those days, patients visited their doctors once a month to "get a blood sugar." If they could do it at home for 25 cents (in those days), why pay a physician? But almost no one believed there was any value to normal blood sugars anyway. In some respects, blood glucose self-monitoring still remains a serious threat to the incomes of many physicians who specialize in the treatment of the *symptoms* of diabetes and not the disease. Drop into your neighborhood ophthalmologist's office and you will find the waiting room three-quarters filled with diabetics, many of whom are waiting for expensive fluorescein angiography, ocular computer tomography, or laser treatment.

With Suther's backing in the form of free supplies, by 1977 I was able to get the first of two university-sponsored studies started in the New York City area. These both succeeded in reversing early complications in diabetic patients. As a result of our successes, the two universities separately sponsored the world's first two symposia on blood glucose self-monitoring. By this time I was being invited to speak at international diabetes conferences, but rarely at meetings in the United States. My very first medical publication appeared in the abstracts of one of those meetings. It was titled "Protein as the Principal Source of Carbohydrate in the Treatment of Diabetes." Curiously, more physicians outside the United States seemed interested in controlling blood sugar than did their American colleagues. Some of the earliest converts to blood glucose self-monitoring were from Israel and England.

By 1978, perhaps as a result of Charlie Suther's efforts, a few additional American investigators were trying our regimen or variations of it. Finally, in 1980, manufacturers began to release blood glucose meters for use by patients.

This "progress" was entirely too slow for my liking. I knew that while the medical establishment was dallying, there were diabetics dying whose lives could have been saved. I knew also that there were millions of diabetics whose quality of life could be vastly improved. So in 1977 I decided to give up my job and become a physician—I couldn't beat 'em, so I had to join 'em. This way, with an MD after my name, my writings might be published, and I could pass on what I had learned about controlling blood sugar.

After a year of premed courses and another year of waiting, I entered the Albert Einstein College of Medicine in 1979. I was forty-five years old. During my first year of medical school I wrote my first book, *Diabetes: The Glucograf Method for Normalizing Blood Sugar*, enumerating the full details of my treatment for type 1, or insulin-dependent, diabetes. I subsequently succeeded in getting eight more books and many articles in scientific and popular journals published. For the past five years, I have been giving free teleseminars to thousands of medical professionals and patients. These question-and-answer sessions are available in the last week of every month at www.askdrbernstein.net. One thousand of these questions and answers are available in two new electronic books, *Beating Diabetes: Type 1 Diabetes* and *Beating Diabetes: Type 2 Diabetes*. Both of these can be found on the Internet.

In 1983 I finally opened my own medical practice near my home in Mamaroneck, New York. By that time, I had well outlived the life expectancy of an "ordinary" type 1 diabetic. Now, by sharing my simple observations, I was convinced I was in a position to help both type 1 and type 2 diabetics who still had the best years of their lives ahead of them. I could help others take control of their diabetes as I had mine, and live long, healthy, fruitful lives.

The goal of this book is to share the techniques and treatments I have taught my patients and used on myself, including the very latest developments. If you or a loved one suffers from diabetes, I hope this book will give you the tools to turn your life around as I did mine.

Acknowledgments

I would like to thank the following people, whose aid and guidance made this book possible:

Frank Vinicor, MD, MPH, past president of the American Diabetes Association, who took time from his overwhelming schedule to write the foreword.

Stephen Stark, novelist, critic, and essayist, whose suggestions about tone, clarity, and structure were of immeasurable value.

Pharmacists Stephen Freed, David Joffee, and George E. Jackson, who wrote the important appendix "Drugs That Can Affect Blood Glucose Levels." Patricia A. Gian, dear friend and director of my medical office, who shared the stresses of this endeavor and gave me invaluable aid and guidance all along the way. Three top-of-the-line professionals, Tracy Behar, editor of the current version of this book, and Channa Taub and Carol Mann, my literary agents, whose efforts made this undertaking possible. Barbara Jatkola, copyeditor, and Michael Pietsch, publisher, whose whisper can make things happen. Karen A. Weinstock and Timothy J. Aubert, for the recipes.

Finally, my love and thanks to my wife, Professor Anne E. Bernstein, MD, FAPA, FABPN, who allowed me to steal so much time that really belonged to her and who probably saved my life during many hypoglycemic episodes.

Dr. Bernstein's
Diabetes Solution

Before and After

Y ou're the only person who can be responsible for normalizing your blood sugars. Although your physician may guide you, the ultimate responsibility is in your hands. This task will require significant changes in lifestyle that may involve some sacrifice. The question naturally arises, "Is it really worth the effort?" As you will see in this chapter, others have already answered this question for themselves. Perhaps their experiences will give you the incentive to find out whether you can reap similar benefits. If these reminiscences are not adequately convincing, visit the page for this book at www .amazon.com or www.amazon.co.uk and select "Reader Reviews." You'll find well over one hundred stories similar to these.

J.L.F. is seventy-one years old and has three grandchildren. He still works as a financial consultant, and was a naval aviator in World War II. His blood sugars are currently controlled by diet, exercise, and pills called insulin-sensitizing agents. Thanks to the diet described in this book, his cholesterol/HDL ratio, an index of heart disease risk (see page 60), has dropped from a very high risk level of 7.9 to a below-average level of 3.0. His hemoglobin A_{IC} test, which reflects average blood sugar for the prior four months, has dropped from 10.1 percent (very high) to 5.6 percent (nearly in the nondiabetic range). His R-R interval study (see Chapter 2, "Tests: Baseline Measures of Your Disease and Risk Profile"), an indicator of injury to nerves that control heart rate, has progressed from an initial value of 9 percent variation (very abnormal) to a current value of 33 percent, which is normal for his age.

"I probably had mild diabetes for most of my adult life without realizing it. It first appeared as lethargy, later as fainting, stumbling, or falling, but as rare occurrences. I also had difficulty attaining full erection of my penis.

"In early 1980, I began to experience dizziness, sweating, arm pains, tendencies to fainting, and the symptoms usually associated with heart problems. An angiogram revealed severe disease of the arteries that supplied my heart. I therefore had surgery to open up these arteries. All was well for the next seven years, and I again enjoyed good health.

"In late 1985, I began to notice a loss of feeling in my toes. My internist diagnosed it as neuropathy probably due to high blood sugar. He did the usual blood test, and my blood sugar was 400. His advice was to watch my diet, especially to avoid sweets. I returned for another checkup in 30 days. My blood sugar was 350. Meanwhile, my neuropathy was increasing, along with the frequency of visits. My blood test results were consistently at the 350 level, my feet were growing more numb, and I was becoming alarmed.

"I felt okay physically, walked at least two miles a day, worked out in the gym once or twice a week, worked a full schedule as a business consultant, and didn't worry a great deal about it. But I did begin to inquire of friends and acquaintances about any knowledge or experience they might have relative to neuropathy or diabetes.

"My first jolt came from a story from one of my friends who had diabetes, foot neuropathy, deep nerve pain in his feet, and a nonhealing ulcer on a toe. He told me that as the neuropathy progressed, amputation of the feet was likely, elaborating by describing the gruesome 'salami surgery' of unchecked diabetes.

"That's when I became emotionally unglued, as they say. One thing about aging and disease, you think a great deal about the utter horror of becoming a cripple, dependent upon others for your mobility. Suddenly foot numbness is no longer a casual matter, more like a head-on crash into reality.

"Then I met a wealthy car dealer at the golf club, with his legs cut off as high as legs go, who explained he hadn't paid too much attention to his diabetes at the time and his doctor couldn't help him. He could never leave his chair, except for relief and sleep, and he had to be lifted for that. Oh, he was cheerful enough. He joked that they would cut him off at the middle of his butt the next time, that is, if he didn't die first. A display of courage to others was a macabre nightmare to me. I got serious about getting someone, somewhere, to tell me what to do about my ever-worsening numbness, which by now had spread to my penis. My condition became an ever-present, gnawing anxiety with me, a creeping presence I couldn't fight against because I simply didn't know how to fight it.

"Then, in early April 1986, my wife and I went to visit Dr. Bernstein. The first visit lasted 7½ hours. Each detail of diagnosis and treatment was discussed. Each symptom of the disease, however minute, was described in great detail, the importance of each balanced with another, with specific remedies for managing them. Take the seemingly insignificant matter of scaly feet, a common, dangerous symptom of diabetes. Dr. B. prescribed mink oil, rubbed into the feet morning and night. Practiced as directed, instead of split skin and running foot sores, you have skin as soft and smooth as velvet. Consider the alternative—feet split, painful, and slow (if at all) to heal—which can change your entire life. Special shoes, debilitating gait, not to mention the horrible possibility of progressive amputation—all things that really can happen if your diabetes is not treated properly.

"What is of highest importance, I believe, is the in-depth explanation of diabetes, its causes, symptoms, and treatment. He gives you the rationale for treatment, so that you have a comprehensive understanding of what is wrong and how it can be corrected.

"First, through frequent finger-stick blood testing, we came to an understanding as to the specifics of how to attack my diabetes. We started with diet. It wasn't just eat this, don't eat that, but eat this for these reasons and eat that for other reasons. Know the reasons and the differences. Knowing the how and why of diet keeps you on track, and the discipline of that knowledge makes control easy. For without continuous diet observance, you will surely worsen your diabetes. He explains that the effect of uncontrolled diabetes on the heart can be much more deleterious than the other popular demons—cholesterol, fat in the diet, stress, tension, et cetera—demons not to be ignored, obviously, but merely put into proper perspective to the main villain—diabetes.

"Well, the results for me are the numbness of my feet and penis have regressed, and my erections have improved. My feet are now beautifully supple and healthy. The severe belching, flatulence, and heartburn after meals have disappeared. The other ills of diabetes have apparently not greatly affected me, and now that I know that controlling my diabetes is the key to a healthy heart, I expect to reduce greatly any future risk of heart attacks.

"One great result of my ability to normalize my blood sugars has been the stabilizing of my emotional attitude toward the disease. I no longer have a sense of helplessness in the face of it; no longer wonder what to do; no longer feel hopelessly dependent on people who have no answers to my problems. I feel free to exercise, walk vigorously, enjoy good health without worry, enjoy my precious eyesight without fear of diabetic blindness, yes, even have a new confidence in normal sexual activities.

"All of the enjoyments of health that were slowly ebbing away are now within my control, and for that I thank my new knowledge and skills."

Thomas G. Watkins is a forty-year-old journalist. His diabetes was diagnosed twenty-three years ago. For the past nine years he's been following one of the treatment protocols described in this book for people who require insulin.

"Following the instructions of several diabetologists over a period of years, I had the illness 'under control.' At least that's what they told me. After all, I was taking two shots a day, and adjusting my insulin doses depending on urine test results, and later on blood sugar measurements. I was also following the common recommendation that carbohydrates fill at least 60 percent of my caloric intake.

"But something was not right; my life was not 'relatively normal' enough. I was avoiding heavy exercise for fear of my blood sugar dropping too low. My meal schedule was inflexible. I still had to eat breakfast, lunch, and dinner even when I wasn't hungry. Aware that recent research seemed to associate high blood sugars with an increased risk of long-term complications, I tried to keep blood sugars normal, but wound up seesawing daily between lows and highs. By the end of 1986, I had ballooned to 189 pounds and was at a loss for how to lose weight. My 'good control' regimen had left me feeling out of control. Clearly, something had to be done.

"In that year, I attended a meeting of medical writers at which Dr. Bernstein spoke. It became clear that his credentials were impressive. He himself at that time had lived with the disease for four decades and was nearly free of complications. His approach had been formulated largely through self-experimentation. His knowledge of the medical literature was encyclopedic. Some of his proposals were heretical; he attacked the usual dietary recommendations and challenged dogma surrounding such basics as how insulin ought to be injected. But it seemed like he was doing something right. During his talk, I had to use the bathroom twice; he didn't.*

"I decided to spend a day at his office to gather material for an article to be published in the *Medical Tribune*. There, his independence of thought became clear. 'Brittle' diabetes [entailing an endless sequence of wide blood sugar fluctuations] was a misnomer that usually indicated an inadequate treatment plan or poor training, more than any inherent physical deficit, he said. Normal blood sugars around-the-clock were not just an elusive goal but were frequently achievable, if the diabetic had been taught the proper techniques. Beyond treatment goals, he armed his patients with straightforward methods to attain them. His secret: small doses of medication resulted in small mistakes that were easily correctable.

"By then, my interest had become more personal than journalistic. In early 1987, still wary, I decided to give it a try. The first thing I noticed was that this doctor visit was unlike any previous ones. Most had lasted about 15 minutes. This took 8 hours. Others said I had no complications; Dr. Bernstein found several. Most said my blood sugars were just fine; Dr. Bernstein recommended I make changes to flatten them out and to lower my weight. Those hours were spent detailing the intricacies involved in controlling blood sugar. His whole approach blasted the theory espoused by my first doctor—that I should depend on him to dole out whatever information I needed. Dr. Bernstein made it clear that for diabetics to control their disease, they needed to know as much as their doctors did about the disease.

"Two arguments commonly rendered against tight-control regimens are that they increase the incidence of low blood sugar reactions and that they cause subjects to gain weight. I have found the opposite to be true: I shed about 9 pounds within four months after my first visit, and, years later, I have kept them off. And once the guesswork of how much to inject was replaced by simple calculations, my blood sugar levels became more predictable.

"For the first time since I was diagnosed, I felt truly in control. I no

---

* Very high blood sugars cause frequent urination.

longer am at the mercy of wide mood swings that mirror wide swings in blood sugar. Though I remain dependent on insulin and all the paraphernalia that accompany its use, I feel more independent than ever. I am comfortable traveling to isolated areas of the world, spending an hour scuba diving, or hiking in the wilderness, without fear of being sidetracked by diabetes. Now if I feel like skipping breakfast, or lunch, or dinner, I do so without hesitation.

"I no longer have delayed stomach-emptying, which can cause very low blood sugars right after a meal followed by high blood sugars many hours later. My cardiac neuropathy, which is associated with an increased risk for early death, has reversed. Though I eat more fat and protein than before, my blood lipids have improved and are now well within normal ranges. My glycated hemoglobin measurements, used by life insurance companies to detect diabetics among applicants, no longer give me away. Most important, I now feel well.

"Many doctors will not embrace Dr. Bernstein's work, for the simple reason that Dr. Bernstein demands a commitment of time, energy, and knowledge not only from patients, but from physicians. Diabetics are the bread and butter of many practices. For decades, the usual treatment scenario has been a blood test, a short interview, a prescription for a one-month supply of needles, a handshake, and a bill. But that is changing. In the past few years, evidence has been amassing in support of Dr. Bernstein's modus operandi. No longer is the old high-carbohydrate diet unquestioned; more and more doctors are espousing a multiple-shot regimen controlled by the patients themselves. Most important, though, tight control is being associated with fewer of the diabetic complications that can ravage every major organ system in the body. Dr. Bernstein's scheme provided me with the tools not only to obtain normal blood sugars, but to regain a feeling of control I had not had since before I was diagnosed."

Frank Purcell is a seventy-six-year-old retiree who, like many of my married patients, works closely with his wife to keep his diabetes on track. Eileen, who goes by the nickname Ike, tells the first part of his story.

IKE: "Frank had been treated for many years for diabetes, and had been treated orally because he was a type 2. As far as we were aware, he had a functioning pancreas. The thing was, as a younger man, he'd been told that he had high blood sugar, but it was ignored. This was going back to his army days, in 1953 or so. No one suggested medication, no one called it diabetes, and nothing more was done. They just said he had high blood sugar. They called it 'chemical' diabetes. It showed up on blood tests, but not on urinalysis. I guess in those days, having it show up on a urinalysis was some sort of determinant. He did modify his diet—he stopped eating so much candy, and he took off weight—he lost about 30 pounds in those days.

"In about 1983, Frank had a mild heart attack. He began to see a cardiologist, who has been monitoring his health care very carefully since then. For about two to three years, he took beta blockers and maybe one or two heart medications. As far as we could tell, his heart problems were very much in resolution—I mean he'd had a heart attack, he'd had no surgery, and seemed to be doing okay. But when he started working with the cardiologist, the doctor noted that his blood sugar thing was ongoing, and he began to feel it was of concern. He prescribed Diabinese, which was the oral medication of choice of the time, I guess, and he monitored Frank's blood sugar about every four months.

"I might say that I never even knew what a normal blood sugar was. No one ever talked about it. I had no idea whether it was 1,000 or 12. The only thing we were ever told was that it was high or wasn't high. This went on and on for close to seven or eight years. If he had seen Dr. Bernstein back then, who knows what could have been different? But eventually, the cardiologist said he thought Frank ought to see an endocrinologist. He didn't feel he was able to control Frank's blood sugar well enough himself with medication, and so he felt the condition warranted closer attention.

"We went to see a gentleman who was chief of the diabetes clinic at a major hospital here in upstate New York, where we live. Now, this is a very well-thought-of medical facility. The doctor met with us, and he kept Frank on the Diabinese, and monitored him every three months or s . His blood sugars were 253, 240, and he would say, 'Let's try another pill.' It was always medication. Glyburide, Glucophage—the whole bit. But trying to get his blood sugar down was very difficult. No one ever mentioned diet, really. And rarely was it ever below 200 when we went in. Rarely. When I finally found out what the numbers meant, I said to the doctor, 'Don't you think we ought to see a dietitian? I mean, we're eating the same food we always have.' We were on the normal diet that anybody's on. I have friends who are diabetics who watch certain things that they eat, and so I thought it made a certain amount of sense. He said, 'Sure. That's a really good idea.'

"He gave us the name of a young woman, and we saw her three times. She said, 'Eat eleven carbohydrates every day,' and she gave us the food pyramid—we didn't need her for that—and nothing changed, except Frank stopped eating dessert. He would have the occasional bowl of ice cream, or a piece of cake when he felt like it, or a cookie. I always bought the newest foods that came out—low-fat, low-sugar. I was more concerned about fat during that stage, as I recall.

"This went on until God intervened. I mean that. What happened was, Frank had an attack of serious hypoglycemia [low blood sugar]. No one had warned us that this could happen. No one had told us what hypoglycemia looked like. I thought it was a stroke. He was out of his head. He couldn't answer questions. The only thing that gave me some smidgen of doubt was that he got up and walked to the bathroom and put on his trousers. I called 911. When the medic got here, he hooked him up to some glucose, put him on a gurney and trundled him out of here, and headed for the medical center. In the middle of the ride, Frank woke up and said, 'What the hell am I doing here?' The young man said he certainly seemed to be coming out of his stroke well. By the time we got to the hospital, he was virtually himself. When they decided to do a finger stick, his blood sugar was 26—26 mg/dl. I didn't have the education in diabetes that I've gotten with Dr. Bernstein, but I knew enough to know that this was not good. Who knows what it was before he got the intravenous?

"Now, we'll never know if he accidentally took his oral medication twice the night before—it's very possible—but I tell you, however it happened, it was the Lord who was watching over Frank and said, 'Now it's time to do something.' As scary as it was, it was also a blessing.

"I have a doctor friend who's a close colleague of Dick Bernstein's. My friend had had an uncle who'd been very ill with diabetes and its complications, but his life had been prolonged in a much more comfortable fashion by Dick Bernstein. I would talk to my friend about Frank's diabetes, and he'd say to me, 'Nothing's really going to change. You're not going to get his blood sugars down until you see Dick Bernstein.' Even though my friend is a doctor, I brushed off his advice. Frank was seeing a doctor. Why would some private doctor be any more capable than the head of the diabetes clinic at a major medical center? But after this episode with hypoglycemia, Frank went to my friend's office with me, and my friend laid it out for him, told us in grinding detail what we could expect from Dr. Bernstein, what it would be like, and how he hoped we would relate to Dick, because he's rather controversial, and how hard it was going to be — how much of a commitment it was going to take. We went away thinking, 'Let's give it a try.'"

FRANK: "To be honest, when I first met Dr. Bernstein, I felt he was somewhat of a flake. I had worked with doctors in the army, and I was used to a particular kind of guy. Dr. Bernstein — now, he's a horse of another color. Until I came across him, I never met a doctor who was so focused on one thing. He is so completely directed toward this one failing of the human body that I kind of thought that maybe it was a little too intense. But the results have been rather spectacular, and I'm very happy with him. He has specific programs, he has direction, he has goals, and he is not sidetracked by anything other than tending to diabetes. He's given me a regimen. I keep track of my blood sugar, and it's pretty much under control. Instead of blood sugar counts of over 200, I now get them in the range of 85 to 105, which was the goal he set for me. I take insulin in the morning and before my midday and evening meals, and before I go to bed. I don't eat ice cream, and I don't do a lot of things I used to do routinely. When I first came to Dr. B., I was looking very pale and wan, and now I'm looking much ruddier and healthier. I'm a little irritated with this constant puncturing of my fingers, but I just do it automatically now, like second nature.

"When I found out I was going to have to inject insulin, I just broke down and cried. It was like the final straw, and I thought, 'My life is over.' Now I hardly think about it. I use Dr. Bernstein's painless injection method and it doesn't bother me at all. It only takes a split second. The needle is so tiny, I can barely feel the shots of minute doses of insulin. I use the 'love handles' on the sides of my waist. Now, I'm a pretty skinny guy, so there isn't much there, but I can hardly feel it. He made me do it in the office. He showed me — did it to himself — and then he made me do it. Since then, I just do it routinely, all on my own. If I'm out, I do it wherever I am — at a table in a restaurant, in the men's room, et cetera — I'm not the least bit ashamed and no one seems much to notice."

IKE: "About the insulin, I had the feeling that it was going to be inevitable, and when Frank got the news he just broke into tears and really felt that this was the final insult. He'd had many physical problems, and insulin seemed like a very low blow for him. But he did it, stayed with the program, and within a month to six weeks, we began to feel that we were on top of this, knew what was going on. He can manage his blood sugar when it's a little low, when it's a little high. He knows just what to do. His overall health has improved since the beginning. Dr. Bernstein really gave us an education."

Joan Delaney is a fifty-three-year-old mother and financial editor. Her story is not unusual.

"I must admit that the prospect of following this new regimen for diabetes control seemed daunting at first. My life, I thought, would be dominated by needles, testing, and confusion. However, after a few weeks, the program became a simple part of my day's routine, like putting on makeup.

"Before I became a patient of Dr. Bernstein, I was somewhat resigned to the probability of suffering complications from diabetes. Although I took insulin, I in no way felt I had control of the disease. I had leg pains at night. My hands and feet tingled. I had gained weight, having no understanding of the exchange diet my previous doctor had thrust into my hands. I became chronically depressed and was usually hungry.

"Now that I follow a blood sugar–normalizing program, I know I am in control of my diabetes, especially when I see that number normal most of the time on the glucose meter. Best of all, I feel good, both physically and emotionally. I am now thin. I eat healthful, satisfying meals and am never hungry. My leg pains have disappeared, as has the tingling in my hands and feet. And now that I am in control of the disease, I no longer find the need to hide from friends the fact that I have diabetes."

About 65 percent of diabetic men are unable to have sexual intercourse, because high blood sugars have impaired the mechanisms involved in attaining erection of the penis. Frequently partial, albeit inadequate, erections are still possible; such "borderline" men may still be able to enjoy adequate erections for intercourse after extended periods of nor-

mal blood sugars. We have seen such improvements in a number of patients—but only in those whose problem was caused mainly by neuropathy (nerve damage), as opposed to blockages of the blood vessels that supply the penis. When we initially saw L.D., in the pre-Viagra era, he asked me to evaluate his erectile dysfunction. I found that the blood pressures in his penis and his feet were normal, but that the nerve reflexes in the pelvic region were grossly impaired. L.D.'s comments refer in part to this problem.

"I'm a fifty-nine-year-old male, married, with three children. Approximately four years ago, after being afflicted with type 2 diabetes for about ten years, I noticed that I was always tired. In addition, I was quite irritable, short-tempered, and had difficulty maintaining concentration for extended periods of time. Otherwise I was feeling well, with the exception that I was becoming impotent, having difficulty maintaining an erection during sexual intercourse. At the time, I had no knowledge whether these conditions were interrelated.

"After Dr. Bernstein taught me to measure my blood sugars, I discovered that they averaged about 375 mg/dl, which is very high. With my new diet and small doses of insulin, they are now essentially normal all the time.

"I began to feel better than I had in years, both physically and mentally. The problem with impotency has improved. I maintain a daily check of my blood sugars and feel that my overall improvement has also helped me recuperate quickly from a total hip replacement without any complications."

R.J.N, MD, is board certified in orthopedic surgery. He has been following one of the regimens described in this book for the past three years.

"I am fifty-four years old and have had diabetes since the age of twelve. For thirty-nine years I had been treated with a traditional diet and insulin regimen. I developed severe retinopathy, glaucoma, high blood pressure, and neuropathy that required me to wear a leg brace. Both of my kidneys ceased functioning, and I was placed on kidney dialysis for many months until I received a kidney transplant. The dialysis treatments required me to be in the hospital for about 5 hours per visit, 3 times a week. They were very debilitating and left me totally exhausted.

"Years of widely fluctuating blood sugars affected my mental and physical stability, with great injury to my family life as a result. The resultant disability also forced me to give up my surgical practice, and to suffer almost total loss of income.

"Frequent low blood sugars would cause me to exhibit bizarre behavior, so that people unaware of my diabetes would think I was taking drugs or alcohol. I was hostile, anxious, irritable, or angry, and had extreme mood changes. I would experience severe physical reactions that included fatigue, twitching of limbs, clouding of vision, headaches, and blunted mental activity. I suffered many convulsions from low blood sugars and was placed in hospital intensive care units. When my blood sugars were high, I had no energy and was always sleepy. My vision was blurred and I was usually thirsty and urinating a lot.

"For the past three years, I have been meticulously following the lessons that Dr. Bernstein taught me. I measure my blood sugars a number of times each day and know how to rapidly correct slight variations from my target range. I follow a very low carbohydrate diet, which makes blood sugar control much easier.

"In return for my conscientious attention to controlling blood sugars, I've reaped a number of rewards. My neuropathy is gone, and I no longer require a leg brace. My retinopathy, which was deteriorating, has now actually reversed. I no longer suffer from glaucoma, which had required that I use special eyedrops twice each day for more than ten years. My severe digestive problems have markedly improved. My mental confusion, depression, and fatigue have resolved so that I am now able to work full-time and productively. My blood sugar control has been excellent.

"I now deal with my diabetes in a realistic, organized manner, and as a result I feel stronger, healthier, happier, and more positive about my life."

LeVerne Watkins is a sixty-eight-year-old grandmother and associate executive director of a social service agency. When we first met, she had been taking insulin for two years, after developing type 2 diabetes thirteen years earlier. Her comments relate in part to the effects of large amounts of dietary carbohydrate, covered by large amounts of insulin, while she was following a conventional treatment plan.

"In less than two years, my weight had increased from 125 to 155 pounds; my appetite was always ready for the next snack or the next meal. All my waking hours were focused on eating. I always carried a bag of goodies—unsalted saltine crackers, regular Coca-Cola, and glucose tablets. I always had to eat 'on time.' If I was a half-hour late at mealtime, my hands would begin sweating, I would become very jittery, and if in a social gathering or a conference or meeting at work, I would have to force myself to concentrate on what was taking place. During a meeting that I was chairing, the last thing I remember saying was, 'Oh, I'm so sorry,' before I toppled out of the chair to wake up and find myself in the emergency room of a local hospital.

"During a subway ride which generally took about 25 minutes, the train was delayed for close to 2 hours and—to my utter dismay—I had forgotten my bag of goodies. As I felt myself 'going bananas,' sweating profusely and perhaps acting a little strange, a man sitting across from me recognized my MedicAlert bracelet, grabbed my arm, and screamed, 'She has diabetes!'

"Food, juice, candy bars, cookies, and fruit came from all directions. It was a cold, wintry day, but people fanned and fed me. And I was so grateful and so very embarrassed. I stopped riding the subway, and rescheduled as many meetings and conferences as I could to take place directly after lunch so that I would have more time before the next snack or meal would be necessary.

"I felt that I had no control over my life; I was constantly eating, I outgrew all my clothing, shoes and underwear included. I had been a rather stylish dresser since college days. Now I felt rather frumpy, to say the least. Once, I tried to discuss with my diabetologist how I was feeling about gaining weight and eating all the time. I was told, 'You just don't have any willpower,' and 'If you put your mind to it, you wouldn't eat so much.' I was very, very angry, so much so that I never consulted him again.

"On my own, I tried Weight Watchers, but the diet I had been given by the dietitian to whom the diabetologist had referred me did not mesh with the Weight Watchers diet. So along I limped, trying to accept that I was getting fatter each day, was always hungry, had no willpower, and most of the time was feeling unhappy.

"My husband was my constant support through all this. He would say, 'You look good with a few more pounds. . . . Go buy yourself some new clothes,' especially when I would ask him to zip something that I was trying to squeeze into. He always clipped newspaper and magazine articles about diabetes and would remind me to watch specials on TV. He encouraged me to be active in the local diabetes association, and would accompany me to lectures and various workshops. Then, on Sunday, April 3, 1988—Easter Sunday—he clipped an article from the *New York Times* entitled 'Diabetic Doctor Offers a New Treatment.' Little did I realize that this thin news article would be a new beginning of my life with diabetes. I must have read it several dozen times before I finally met with Dr. Bernstein. Since that first meeting, I haven't had one single episode of hypoglycemia, which I had formerly experienced very often. Following the regimen of correcting my high and low blood sugars, taking small doses and different kinds of insulin, and eating meals calibrated for specific amounts of carbohydrates and protein, my outlook brightened and I began to feel more energetic and more in charge of myself and my life. I could now hop on the train, ride the subway, drive several hours, and not fear one of those low blood sugar episodes. I started once again to exercise every day. My stamina seemed to increase. I didn't have to push hard to accomplish my daily goals at work and at home. Within a couple of months, I was back to 129 pounds, had gone from size 14 to size 10, and ten months later to size 8 and 120 pounds. Even the swelling and pain in my right knee—arthritis, I was told—abated. I feel great. My self-esteem and self-worth are whole again. I now take only 8 units of insulin each day, where I had previously been taking 31 units.

"I am also conquering my uneasy and frightening feelings about the long-term consequences of having diabetes. While I once thought that heart disease, kidney failure, blindness, amputations, and many other health problems were what the future probably held for me, I now believe that they are not necessarily outcomes of living with diabetes.

"But my life is not perfect. I still occasionally throw caution to the wind by eating too much and eating foods I know are taboo. Sticking with my diet of no bread, no fruit, no pasta, no milk, seemed easy when it was new, but now it is not easy, and loads of my efforts go into making salads, meat, fish, or poultry interesting and varied. My fantasies are almost always of some forbidden food—a hot fudge sundae with nuts, or my mother's blueberry cobbler topped with homemade ice cream. But when all is told, I feel that I am really lucky. All my efforts have really paid off."

A.D. is a fifty-five-year-old former typesetter whose diabetes was diagnosed fourteen years ago. As with many other people who use our regi-

men, his test of average blood sugar (hemoglobin A_{1C}) and his tests for cardiac disease risk (cholesterol/HDL ratio) simultaneously dropped from high levels to essentially normal values.

"I watched my mother deteriorate in front of me from the complications of diabetes, finally resulting in an amputation of the leg above the knee, and a sorrowful existence until death claimed her. My oldest brother, who was also diabetic, was plagued with circulatory complications that resulted in the amputation of both feet, with unsightly stumps. Diabetes robbed him of a normal existence.

"When I began to experience the all-too-familiar diabetes symptoms, my future looked bleak and I feared the same fate. I immediately searched for help, but for two years floundered around getting much medical advice but not improving. In fact, I was getting sicker. My doctor had said, 'Watch your weight,' and prescribed a single daily oral hypoglycemic pill for my type 2 diabetes. It sounded easy, but it wasn't working. My glucose levels were in the 200 range all too often, and occasionally reached 400. I was constantly exhausted.

"I started Dr. Bernstein's program in 1985. Since then I have recovered my former vitality and zest for life. At my first visit, he switched me to another approach—a fast-acting blood sugar–lowering pill 3 times a day, before meals, along with a slower-acting pill in the morning and at bedtime. My regimen was totally overhauled to eliminate foods that raised blood sugar, and to reduce greatly my consumption of carbohydrates in general. Macaroni and ravioli had been important parts of my diet since birth. I had to give these up. I didn't mind a greater emphasis on protein. I even began to include fresh fish in my diet.

"My initial reaction was that these restrictions were too high a price to pay, and that I would be unable to continue them for long. Also, I was asked to check my blood with a blood sugar meter for a week prior to every visit to Dr. Bernstein. That meant sticking my finger several times a day. I was willing to discipline myself for a short period in order to be able to return to a more active, vigorous life and to put my malaise to rest. At the beach, I was sorely tempted to give up the diet, while watching family and friends eat without restrictions. But since my body was feeling healthier, I continued with the program. After about two months, with many dietary slips on my part, I managed to better discipline myself because I sensed it made me feel better. My glucose level started to descend to 140, 130, and finally to 100 or less on a consistent basis.

"Dr. Bernstein also encouraged me to purchase a pedometer, a device that clipped to my belt and measured the distance that I walked each day. I began to walk daily, holding 3-pound weights and swinging my arms. This was yet another thing to bother with, and I felt it would cut into my free time. But the result was an invigorating high. By this time, I didn't mind pricking my fingers several times each day, as it showed me the way to better blood sugars. Fortunately for me, New Rochelle has many beautiful parks. I chose Glen Island Park because it is near Long Island Sound and nicely kept. This meant getting up earlier in the morning to walk during the week, but that was no problem since I am an early riser. I bought some cast-iron dumbbells for additional exercise. I learned about arm curls, overhead raises, arm circles, and chest pulls. I didn't realize that there were so many different exercises that you could do at home to benefit your health.

"My glucose levels are now consistently within or near the normal range, not at the sorry levels which nearly put me in the hospital. That all-consuming fatigue is gone, and I feel that now I'm in control of my diabetes instead of the reverse. With adherence to the program, I know that I don't have to suffer the same debilitating effects that afflict so many other diabetics."

Harvey Kent is fifty-one. He has known about his diabetes for approximately six years, and we suspect that he probably had it for three to four years prior to his diagnosis. He has a family history of diabetes, and his story is fairly typical.

"I went in for a routine physical. I've always had high risk factors—both my parents had diabetes, my brother had diabetes, and my sister has diabetes. My brother, who was forty-nine, passed away from diabetic complications. My sister, who is fifty-nine, is on dialysis. When I found out I had it, I felt I was going down the same slippery slope. I'd been trying to lose weight, but not very successfully. The doctor I was seeing, an endocrinologist, kept upping my medication. Every time I went to see him, I wound up taking more and more, and my blood sugars weren't going anywhere but up.

"I kept having the feeling that as far as treatment went, nothing was happening. I wasn't in bad shape, but then I watched my brother pass away, and I thought, 'I've got to do something.'

"I happen to live in Mamaroneck, New York, near Dr. Bernstein, and my wife suggested that I see him for a second opinion. I kept wondering, 'Is there another approach?' That's really how it started. The standard approach was always to tell me to lose weight, to exercise, and to take medication. I was trying to do all those things, but I wasn't having much success at any of them except the taking of medication. As it turned out, Dr. Bernstein still said the same three things, but his approach to each of the categories was radical, especially on the diet. The diet has been a major factor — I've lost a lot of weight.

"Once I started getting a sense of what Dr. B. was talking about — which was really right from the first visit; he's very thorough in his explanations — I kind of figured it out. Just to demonstrate the effects of diet, he told me to stay on my same diet and measure my blood sugars, but I started cutting back on the carbohydrates, so by the time we sat down to negotiate a meal plan, which was maybe the third or fourth session, he just confirmed what I'd already started about a month before.

"Before I met Dr. Bernstein, I'd been under treatment for diabetes by three different doctors. The guy I was seeing before Dr. B. is an endocrinologist/diabetes doctor with a fairly large practice. He never once said to me, 'You know, by controlling your blood sugars, most of these complications are reversible.' When Dr. B. told me that — well, for a diabetic who's stuck with this disease for the rest of his life, that's nice to hear. Nobody ever tells you this. At least I don't remember anyone ever explaining this to me. I've been a member of the ADA [American Diabetes Association] for several years, and no one ever said anything like that to me, anywhere. I was lucky. I hadn't developed that many complications — not like my brother and sister — but I knew how fast they could get you.

"With my old doctor, I'd been told to monitor my blood sugars and then come in every three months. What it was supposed to do, I wasn't sure — keep you honest, maybe, but I couldn't figure that out. I was checking my fasting blood sugars in the mornings. They were averaging somewhere about 140 mg/dl. And when I'd go in, the doctor would do blood work, scratch the bottoms of my feet, and check my eyes, then say, 'See me in three months.' The whole thing would take maybe half an hour and then I'd see him again in three months. I wasn't sure what the whole thing was about. The thing is — and I found this out with my sister and my brother — it's a slippery slope.

You start out as a type 2 and you get this kind of treatment, and you burn out your pancreas, and before long, you're insulin-dependent.

"When I saw Dr. B., he did a very extensive medical exam and uncovered everything there was to uncover. He checked everything. He found that I had an anemia, and so we started doing things to deal with that. I had not had retinopathy or neuropathy. I had some protein in my urine, a potential sign of kidney disease. But he said that could be from my old kidney stone, or it could be from the diabetes. He said we'd wait awhile until my blood sugars were normalized, then test again and find out, because if it was the diabetes, it should clear up.

"The first thing he did was get me off Micronase and onto Glucophage. Micronase is one of those oral hypoglycemic agents that stimulate your pancreas, and he said, 'Why are you doing this? You're burning your pancreas out quick.' He looked at my blood sugars carefully and told me I was low at particular times of the day and told me what I had to do to cover the valleys as well as the peaks. Insulin. I never wanted to take insulin. My father did it, and the idea just brought back horrible memories. My other doctor would say, 'All else is failing; now you have to go on insulin.' What Bernstein says is, 'I want you to take insulin in order to cover your peaks and to keep your pancreas from burning out.' This seems to me a much more sensible approach.

"My wife is very perceptive about the whole thing, and she said what I really needed was a coach, and Bernstein is very much like a coach. Having read up about him and knowing that he was an engineer, you can see the difference in his approach. You can see less of the medical model and more of an engineering model: he's putting you back together, taking your components and manipulating them in order to accomplish something. He's a diabetic himself, he knows the thing inside and out, and so you get the sense that he's much more actively involved. Now I measure my blood sugars 5 times a day, but instead of just jotting them down and saying come back in three months, he adjusts the medication, using it to tweak the peaks and valleys, to get the most optimum response. Now I have excellent control.

"The diet takes some getting used to. Most diabetics, I would surmise, love to eat. Especially if you come from a culture where food is the coin of the realm. People ask me now, 'What do you eat?' I say, 'I have turkey, some salad, and a Diet Coke.' I used to be a big pancake eater. Talk about your carbohydrate! Every Saturday and Sunday morning for years I would make pancakes for my wife. Now I make them for her and for my daughter and don't have any—or occasionally steal just a bite—and I miss it, but I am so much more in control now, and I feel so much better. I've seen so much of my family go down the slippery slope, it seems a small sacrifice for good health.

"Since the time I started seeing Dr. Bernstein, I've lost close to 30 pounds. My blood sugars have dropped by about 35 percent, but my weight loss was not on a weight-loss diet, just on Dr. Bernstein's meal plan. I still have a way to go, but for the first time I feel like I'm in control."

J.A.K. is a sixty-seven-year-old business executive who had had type 2 diabetes for twenty-four years, and had been taking insulin for twenty, when he started on our regimen. He writes the following:

"I visited Dr. Bernstein on the recommendation of some good friends, as I had just lost the central vision in my right eye due to subretinal bleeding.

"It took hours of instruction, counseling, and explanation to make me clearly understand the relationships between diet, blood sugar control, and physical well-being. I was hoping for the possibility that I might experience an improvement in my already deteriorated physical condition. I have diligently followed up on what I was taught, and the results are obvious:

- I no longer have cramps in my calves and toes.
- The neuropathy in my feet has normalized.
- Various skin conditions have cleared up.
- Tests for autonomic neuropathy (R-R interval study) totally normalized in only two years.
- The difficulty I had with digestion has cleared up completely.
- My weight dropped from 188 to 172 pounds in six months.
- My original cholesterol/HDL ratio of 5.3 put me at increased risk for a heart attack. With a low-carbohydrate diet and improved blood sugars, this value has dropped to 3.2, which puts me at a lower cardiac risk than most nondiabetics of my age.
- My daily insulin dose has dropped from 52 units to 31 units, and I no longer have frequent episodes of severe hypoglycemia.
- My overall physical condition and stamina have improved considerably.

"All these improvements occurred because I learned how to control my blood sugars. As a matter of fact, my glycated hemoglobin (a test that correlates with average blood sugar during the prior four months) dropped from 7.1 percent to 4.6 percent, so that I am now in the same range as nondiabetics. I have developed full confidence in my ability to manage my own diabetes. I understand what is happening. I can adjust and compensate my medications as the need arises.

"If I have to miss a meal, for whatever reason, I can adjust accordingly and am not tied to a clock, as I was before I learned these new approaches to blood sugar control.

"I would say that not only has my physical condition improved, but my mental attitude is far better today than it was ten or fifteen years ago. My only regret is that I did not learn how to be in charge of my diabetes years earlier."

Lorraine Candido has had type 1 diabetes for more than twenty years and has been my patient for ten. She is in her sixties, and she and her husband, Lou, her "copilot," work together to keep her blood sugars normal. Like a lot of happily married couples, Lorraine and Lou sometimes almost speak as one. When Lorraine comes in for treatment, Lou is with her. When she calls on the phone, Lou is on the other line. They talk about how starting the program changed their lives.

LORRAINE: "I had a lot of complications. Bladder infections, kidney infections—and then my eyes. My feet were numb up to my heels. As a matter of fact, one day I was walking barefoot and I wasn't aware of it but I had a thumbtack in my foot all day long. I had neuropathy of the vagus nerve. I had an ulcer from medication. My mother had had eye problems, and so when I went to an ophthalmologist, he said, 'You have some of your mother's problems. We'll keep an eye on you; come back in a year.' And I thought, 'Uh-oh.' When Dr. Bernstein examined my eyes, he said, 'Oh, I'll make an appointment for you.' Right away I had laser surgery."

LOU: "I firmly believe that if she hadn't gone to Dr. Bernstein, she would've been blind. Her last two visits to the eye doctor she got excellent reports. As a matter of fact, he said he had no idea where the fluid in one eye had gone, but it was all gone."

LORRAINE: "I was elated. He said my left eye had made great progress and I was doing well.

"When I first met Dr. Bernstein, I had no idea what I was getting into. All I knew was that I wasn't feeling well and I was going nowhere. I was kind of scared, didn't know what I was getting into, and didn't know if I wanted to. It was plain and simple. I liked Snickers candy bars. He said, 'No.' I couldn't have anything I liked and wanted, and we kind of butted heads—but then I realized, 'Hey, come on, is there really a candy bar worth dying for?'

"He's a very gentle gentleman. I think he's extremely caring; you're not treated like cattle, you're treated as a person, and he answers all your questions. Between the two of us, at the beginning we had a lot of questions. Really, I don't know if I could live without him.

"We found him—it's kind of embarrassing, but our son used to have a newsstand, and Lou would go help him out on Sundays, and Lou would bring me home the papers to read. Well, in one of those horrible tabloids—you know, when they run out of weird stuff, they run unusual medical stories reprinted from somewhere else—the headline on this was 'Diabetic Heals Himself,' and you know, we didn't think that much about it. But I wasn't feeling well, and so we made some inquiries. Now of course we're in a different state and nobody I knew had ever heard of him, but we called his office. I didn't talk to a nurse or someone, he got on the phone himself and he offered us references. Well, that settled it right there. I mean, how many doctors do you know of who'd offer you references? So Lou said, 'Pack up, honey, we're going.'"

Lou: "She had a doctor up here in Springfield, Massachusetts, she was seeing and I was getting pretty concerned about it. Her feet were getting numb, she had kidney problems. I don't have diabetes, but I happened to have the same doctor as my internist, and I said to him, 'Isn't there something you can do for my wife?' He had a son who worked at the Joslin Clinic, which we had heard was very good. 'Can we take her to the Joslin Clinic?' But he said, 'What can he do for her up there that we can't do for her here?' We got sort of scared. They were running her the standard way they treat diabetics—standard but safe. Safe for them, but not much help for Lorraine.

"At Dr. Bernstein's, to start, it was a 10-hour training period—two 5-hour sessions that she had to take at the start."

LORRAINE: "It was my husband, me, and the doctor. No waiting room for hours. Now, to be honest, when we walked out of there—it's a 2-hour drive between our house and there—I didn't want to do it. But on the drive back home after the first session, we talked. We talked constantly, and I knew I didn't want to do it, but I also knew I was going to do it. Common sense just dictated it. I wanted to live, and I wanted both feet and both eyes. It was plain and simple. The feeling in my feet has come back almost 100 percent, by the way."

Lou: "We found out about the diet on the first visit, and it took about a month to get her blood sugars into the target range. She had been running 300, 400 mg/dl blood sugars pretty regularly."

Lorraine: "I was kind of reluctant to start with. It was clear that Dr. Bernstein's program wasn't a ride in an amusement park. In some respects, it was a whole new way of living, and we had to change all our grocery lists—but I had a supportive friend here in Lou. When I started on the diet, we pretty much ate the same food. He didn't have to, but he did. He would have a few extras here and there and I wouldn't, but it was years before I could go into the supermarket, because it felt like I couldn't have anything there. It was very hard to get used to. I resented being told what to do and how to do it."

Lou: "It's very difficult. You have to understand something. When she started the program she was close to sixty years old, and we were accustomed to living in a particular way."

Lorraine: "We have grandkids—we've been married forty-five years—we have six kids and seven grandkids, and they come over for chocolate chip cookies and ice cream."

Lou: "The program works—"

Lorraine: "Because I'm still here."

Lou: "—but it's difficult to do, because you really have to be dedicated."

Lorraine: "Let's put it this way. There are no hot fudge sundaes here. Ever. Not for Thanksgiving, not for Christmas, birthdays, anniversaries—there are no deviations from the program. The first week, because of the change in diet, I lost 15 pounds. You looked at what you were eating, measured it—"

Lou: "It was a combination of things. The amount of insulin changed a lot. She was taking sometimes 80 to 90 units of insulin on a daily basis, and now she's taking 13½ units. Insulin is the fat-building hormone, so reducing your dosage changes things substantially. And you're changing the amount of carbohydrate you're taking in, and so she lost all this weight."

Lorraine: "Altogether, I lost 85 pounds. I wear junior size clothes. Call me stubborn, but I still resent being told what to eat."

Lou: "Let me put it this way. You live a quality of life and give up what you have to—"

LORRAINE: "Like fudge."

LOU: "Or potatoes. The point is, you have to decide somewhere along the line. Are you going to live and enjoy the rest of your life without problems, or are you going to fight the reality of the situation and go down the tubes? It's a choice."

LORRAINE: "It's an attitude. I don't like his program, but it works. I'm still here. I miss the goodies I give my grandkids, all the cookies, candy bars, ice cream. And the holidays. Everything's kind of restricted."

LOU: "The irony of this is, my wife, since she lost all the weight, she dresses in very sporty clothes. Now, I'm a racewalker. She doesn't exercise, but because of heredity or whatever, she has beautiful, strong legs, and so she wears these spandex tights and such, and people ask her, 'How much do you run?'"

LORRAINE: "He's a champion racewalker, very self-disciplined. Not me. I had a conversation with God, and He said, 'Don't sweat.' I'm Lou's cheerleader. I stay home and read books."

LOU: "She walks with me sometimes. But I laugh my ass off."

LORRAINE: "It's fun to go shopping and buy junior sizes with my granddaughters—but I don't let them borrow my clothes. Before I started the program, I never thought about how I looked, how I felt—all I know is, the clothes I was buying were one size fits all."

LOU: "Now look at her."

By the way, Lorraine's cholesterol/HDL ratio has dropped from a high cardiac risk 5.9 to a very low risk 3.3.

It isn't unusual for people with diabetes to make major changes in other aspects of their lives once their blood sugars have been restored to normal after years of poor control. The changes that we see include marriages, pregnancies, and reentry into the workforce. The story of Elaine L. falls into the last category. She also points out the disabling fatigue that she experienced when her blood sugars were high. This problem has led other diabetics, desperate to retain their abilities to function productively, to abuse amphetamines. Elaine is a sixty-year-old mother and artist. Her story is not unusual.

"When I developed diabetes twenty-one years ago, I began a fruitless odyssey to learn all I could about this disease and to have the tools to be able to deal with the psychological and physical roller coaster that I was experiencing.

"The hardest thing to cope with was the total loss of control over my life. I was told that I was a 'brittle' diabetic and that I would just have to endure the very high and very low blood sugars that were totally exhausting me. I feared that my eyes would be damaged. I'm an artist, and this frightened me the most. I knew that this disease was destroying my body every day and that I was helpless.

"We went from doctor to doctor and to major diabetes centers around the country. I never could get a handle on how to become 'controlled.' I was given a gold star for 'good' blood sugar by one doctor; told I 'had imbued the number 150 with mystical significance' by another; informed that if my blood sugars were high after lunch today, I could correct them before lunch tomorrow. All the while, I was feeling worse and worse. I stopped painting. I was just too tired. I was so scared to read any more of the diabetes magazines, because I kept learning more and more about what was in store for me.

"I'd been diabetic about five years when an uncle in Florida advised me to read Dr. Bernstein's first book. It made a lot of sense, but when I read it, I thought, 'Diabetes has robbed me of so much already, I don't have any more time or effort to give to it—and who wants to be a professional diabetic?' Of course, there was a lot of anger and denial and even attempts to forget about being diabetic. Maybe I could forget about it for a while, but it never forgot about me.

"A seed was now planted, however, in spite of myself. I knew that no matter what happened down the road, I needed to feel that I had tried everything possible, so that I would never have to say, 'I wish I had done more.'

"I was very wary of my first visit to Dr. Bernstein's office. I really thought I would hate having to change my diet yet again. I did not relish the idea of multiple daily injections, testing my blood so often, and keeping records. The fact is that I did hate all of that until I found I was recording better and better blood sugars. The diet wasn't any more restrictive than the American Diabetes Association diet I had been following, and most important, I was feeling better and much less tired. In fact, I began to paint again and soon rented a studio. I now paint full-time, but this time I actually sell my work.

"The regimen that I feared has, in the end, given me the freedom of which I had dreamed."

Although Elaine does not mention it in her story, her cholesterol/HDL ratio dropped from an elevated cardiac risk level of 4.74 to the "cardioprotective" level of 3.4 as her long-term blood sugars approached normal.

Furthermore, her weight has dropped from 143 pounds to 134 pounds, and her hemoglobin A_{1C} has dropped from a very high 10.7 percent to a nearly normal 6.0 percent.

Carmine DeLuca is in his early sixties and has had type 2 diabetes since about age forty-five. Like many of my patients, he had been in "standard" treatment and found his condition getting progressively worse.

"I was taking pills, tried some diet changes, but after about ten years my diabetes just got worse. Through the years, as a diabetic, I had seen some articles about Dr. Bernstein, and he had appeared several times in the local newspaper. A colleague at work mentioned this Dr. Bernstein to me, the same guy who had been in the paper. She said, 'If you ever want to go to someone, go to this guy.' And I heard from a few other people around the area who said, 'He's excellent.'

"Over the years, I've had trouble with my eyes, my feet, and my hands, but that was before Dr. Bernstein saw me. I had tried to watch my diet, but being Italian, you know, you're always involved with the pasta, the bread, and so forth, and so I really didn't do very well on dieting. Apparently the pill that I was taking was literally burning me out. I was just going to a general doctor, an internist, and what did he know? I used to keep blood sugar about 140 to 160, and then all of a sudden it started hitting the 200 mark, and it was starting to hit it consistently, and then close to 300, and then over 300, and the nerve endings in my feet were gone, and the feeling in my hands. I did have, at age fifty, two cataracts. I don't know if you want to blame it on diabetes, but I guess you can. Finally, when it was so high, I said, 'Well, something has to be done. What have I got to lose?'

"And so when the time came, I thought, *Let me go to the best.* Everybody talks about how excellent he is, so I made an appointment. My blood sugars were very high, in the high 300s, like 375. When I saw Dr. Bernstein, I had no idea what I was getting myself into. I had just heard that he was one of the best, and so I said, 'Lemme do it.' He struck me as very, very knowledgeable. I learned an awful lot—he told me things about diabetes that I just never heard about, even from people with diabetes. He made you feel good, because he literally grew up with it. He was very professional, yet you could sit down and talk to him. He said he was always available, available 24 hours a day, and he has been, no matter what. You go into that, and you feel pretty good.

"I've lost weight since I started seeing him. A few pounds here and there, but the thing is, even though I haven't taken off a lot of weight yet, everybody says, 'Hey, you look great.' But you could see, prior to seeing Dr. Bernstein, that it was tearing me down; people could see I wasn't looking that good.

"Starting the program was tough, but it was carbohydrates that were killing me. He put me on the diet. I never had a problem with cholesterol, but for some reason, every time you turn around, people are talking about high cholesterol this, high cholesterol that, so I thought about it. But I didn't give a damn about carbohydrates; nobody talks about carbohydrates and cholesterol. At least until Dr. Bernstein said, 'You don't eat this, you don't eat that,' and I said, 'These are all carbohydrates.' And so I'm on the diet and, boom, I start losing a little weight.

"The thing was to get used to doing without the carbohydrates, but it's okay, because I like meat, I like salad, I like vegetables. I can eat all the cheese I want — I mean, within reason. My blood sugar has been good, averaging under 100, and I feel like a million.

"I'm strictly on insulin and one pill, and we've reduced the insulin, and as my blood sugar improves, I think we'll reduce it even more. I see him now every two months or so, and for a week prior, I measure my sugars 4 times a day and bring the chart to him. He really analyzes it — you know, 'All right, take this, don't do this. We'll reduce this. Don't eat that.' He's got a system all his own and it's great. It works. It can be a pain in the neck, but hey. He tells me I'm a good patient. I'm here to prove that it's not impossible to change, and the results are there."

Mark Wade, MD, is one of many physicians with diabetes. He is board certified in pediatric medicine. He and his lovely wife not long ago had their third child. His story has a number of parallels with my own.

"Dr. Bernstein's program turned my life around. Prior to meeting Dick Bernstein at age thirty-four, I had spent twenty-two years of my life as what I then considered a well-controlled insulin-dependent, juvenile-onset diabetic. I'd never been hospitalized for ketoacidosis [a serious condition caused by high blood sugar in combination with dehydration] or severe hypoglycemia, had what I considered good circulation and nerve function, exercised daily, and ate pretty much whatever I felt like eating.

"However, cuts and lacerations took months or years to heal instead of days, and always left ugly scars. Once or twice each year, I would develop pneumonia that typically lasted four months and had me, without fail, out of school or work for two and a half months per episode. My mood swings went from kind and lovable to short-tempered, hotheaded, and uncaring four to five times daily, congruent with my routine blood sugar swings from high blood sugars (300 to 500) after meals to hypoglycemia (less than 50) before meals. This Dr. Jekyll/ Mr. Hyde personality made me very unpredictable and unpleasant to be around, and came close to causing me to lose my wife and the closeness of family and friends. I was forced to eat my meals at exactly the same times each day in order to avoid life-threatening episodes of low blood sugar. Even so, I had to adjust my life around the inevitable periods of hypoglycemia. If I didn't eat, my life was in trouble, and unfortunately so were the people who had to interact with me when I was hypoglycemic. Most of the times those were the ones I loved most.

"My training as a physician, as an intern and resident, averaging 110 hours a week of work, was at times a nightmare, though I did it, trying to balance rounds, clinics, emergency room and ICU schedules, screening patients, long hours of reading, and an unreal demand on physical tolerance, emotional stability, and consistency that almost drove me to the breaking point. My mission was to be an excellent doctor, and I was, with a calm, cool demeanor which I presented externally. But inside I was a mess, and my interactions with my loved ones and close friends were horrible. I was an avid basketball player, jogger, and weight lifter, but despite doing these activities daily, I found my performance and endurance were usually modulated by my blood sugar — and I was never really sure whether I would be able to perform for 10 minutes or 2 hours. In addition, despite my high level of exercise, 1 to 1½ hours daily for twelve years, I was never able to develop a muscular or athletic body type, even though I worked hard at it.

"I was always extremely conscientious about testing and exercising and eating and doctor visits, to the point that my friends thought I was neurotic. I was consistently following the conventional guidelines recommended to diabetics, and I thought I was a rather model patient.

The problems that I described above, I had been led to believe, were a natural part of life for a diabetic. No one showed me that my life could be better, that I could control my diabetes rather than let my diabetes control me, that with recognition of a few principles that are really just common sense, a few extra finger sticks and a few extra injections and better control of my dietary intake—I could be in charge for real!

"Nine years ago, I met Dick Bernstein. Dr. Bernstein not only gave me the most complete, comprehensive, logical, reasonable, and informative teaching on diabetes that I have ever encountered, but his uniquely expert and comprehensive physical examination and testing illuminated for me the most accurate picture of my overall health and the subtle tolls that the previous management of my diabetes had permitted. Then with a personalized, comprehensive, tightly controlled but reasonable diet, exercise, and a blood sugar–monitoring plan, he put me in control of my diabetes for the first time. Sure, the diet plan, finger sticks, and 5 to 8 painless insulin injections a day for my program require a high degree of discipline and self-control, but it's doable, it works, and this comparatively small sacrifice brings me the freedom of lifestyle, quality of life, and longevity that nondiabetics take for granted.

"The results have been as follows: I can eat or fast whenever I choose. I plan my day around my activities rather than around my meals, have the ability to be much more flexible in my schedule and participation in activities, and now have the ability to adjust my daily activities easily to accommodate 'emergencies' or sudden changes in schedule—activities and adjustments that nondiabetics take for granted. Best of all, the wild mood swings have been eliminated and I'm sick much less often and less seriously."

All of these people have been patients of mine and have seen wonderful improvements in their health. If you're curious about how people have fared using the prior three editions of this book, I urge you to look at the testimonials on the website for this book, www.diabetes-book.com/testimonials/testimonials.shtml, and those in reader reviews of the prior editions at www.amazon.com to see similar reactions from people who have tried the program but have never been under my direct care. For some reason, readers in the United Kingdom present more complete and more impassioned reviews. Many of these can be seen at www.amazon .co.uk. It is well worth a visit. These people have been successful in spite of the major obstacles imposed by their National Health Service.

For my monthly free teleseminar, where I answer questions from medical professionals and patients, visit www.askdrbernstein.net.

PART ONE

Before You Start

1

Diabetes

THE BASICS

Diabetes is so common in this country that it touches nearly everyone's life—or will. The statistics on diabetes are staggering, and a diagnosis can be frightening: diabetes is the third leading cause of death in the United States. According to the most recent statistics compiled by the National Institutes of Health (NIH), as of 2007, a staggering 10.7 percent of the U.S. population over nineteen years old, or 23.5 million people, have diabetes, with about 350 million diabetics worldwide. About 25 percent of those people do not know they have diabetes. About 88 percent have blood sugars in excess of the very high levels recommended by professional diabetes associations. This number will no doubt increase. It is estimated that 66 million U.S. citizens already have "pre-diabetes," which I would treat as diabetes. Most death certificates of diabetics do not list diabetes as the underlying cause of their heart attacks, strokes, kidney failure, hypoglycemia, ketoacidosis, or fatal infections. If it were included, it might well be the leading cause of death in the United States. On top of this, there is growing evidence that the incidence of many forms of cancer goes up considerably for people with elevated blood sugars. According to the American Diabetes Association, more than 1.6 million new diabetics will be diagnosed each year—more than double the number predicted in the 2007 edition of this book.

Even more alarming, the incidence of type 2—or what was once known as maturity-onset diabetes—among children eighteen years old and younger has skyrocketed. A Yale University study of obese children between ages four and eighteen appeared in the March 14, 2002, issue of the *New England Journal of Medicine.* The study found that nearly a quarter had a condition that's often a precursor to diabetes. According to *USA Today*'s story on the report the same day, "The incidence of type 2 diabetes, the form that usually occurs in adults, has increased in young people, especially Hispanics, blacks, and Native Americans. Some studies suggest that in some regions, the incidence of type 2 in children has jumped from less than 5%, before 1994, to up to 50%." That children are increasingly getting a disease that once targeted fifty- to sixty-year-olds presents a new and frightening potential public health disaster.

A huge portion of U.S. health care costs ($218 billion in 2007) is spent on the treatment of diabetes (mostly for long-term complications).

Each year, tens of thousands of Americans lose their eyesight because of diabetes, the leading cause of new blindness for people ages twenty to seventy-four. Ninety to ninety-five percent of diabetics have type 2 diabetes. Because 80 percent of type 2 diabetics are overweight, many inappropriately feel that the disease is their own fault, the result of some failure of character that causes them to overeat.

Since you are reading this book, you or a loved one may have been diagnosed recently with diabetes. Perhaps you have long-standing diabetes and are not satisfied with treatment that has left you plagued with complications such as encroaching blindness, foot pain, frozen shoulder, inability to achieve or maintain a penile erection, restrictive lung disease, hip and leg pain, or heart or kidney disease.

Although diabetes is still an incurable, chronic disease, it is very treatable, and the long-term "complications" are fully preventable. For sixty-five years, I've had type 1 diabetes, also called juvenile-onset or insulin-dependent diabetes mellitus (IDDM). This form of diabetes is generally far more serious than type 2, or non-insulin-dependent diabetes mellitus (NIDDM), although both have the potential to be fatal.* Most type 1 diabetics who were diagnosed back about the same time I was are now dead from one or more of the serious complica-

_____

* For a period of time, many people considered the designations type 1 and type 2 out-of-date, replacing them with the terms IDDM and NIDDM, which are slightly misleading and are losing credence. While it is true that most of those with type 2 can stay alive without injecting insulin, many patients who suffer from type 2, or so-called NIDDM, do inject insulin to preserve their health. The terms "autoimmune diabetes" for type 1 and "insulin-resistant diabetes" for type 2 are more precise, but are unlikely to take over for the much-easier-to-say type 1 and type 2. The situation is further complicated by the recent discovery that most type 2 diabetes also has an autoimmune component.

tions of the disease. Yet after living with diabetes for all these years, instead of being bedridden or out sick from work (or dead, the most likely scenario), I am more fit than most nondiabetics who are considerably younger than I. I regularly work 12-hour days, travel, sail, and pursue a vigorous exercise routine.

I am not special in this regard. If I can take control of my disease, you can take control of yours.

In the next several pages I'll give you a general overview of diabetes, how the body's system for controlling blood sugar (glucose) works in the nondiabetic, and how it works — and doesn't work — for diabetics. In subsequent chapters we'll discuss diet, exercise, and medication, and how you can use them to control your diabetes. If discussion of diet and exercise sounds like "the same old thing" you've heard again and again, read on, because you'll find that what I've espoused is almost exactly the opposite of "the same old thing," which is what you've probably been taught. The tricks you'll learn can help you arrest the diabetic complications you may now be suffering, may reverse many of them, and should prevent the onset of new ones. We'll also explore new medical treatments and new drugs that are now available to help manage blood sugar levels and curtail obesity and even overeating.

THE BODY IN AND OUT OF BALANCE

Diabetes is the breakdown or partial breakdown of one of the more important of the body's autonomic (self-regulating) mechanisms, and its breakdown throws many other self-regulating systems into imbalance. There is probably not a tissue in the body that escapes the effects of the high blood sugars of diabetes. People with high blood sugars tend to have osteoporosis, or fragile bones; they tend to have tight skin; they tend to have inflammation and tightness at their joints; they tend to have many other complications that affect every part of their body, including the brain, with impaired short-term memory and even depression.

Insulin: What It Is, What It Does
At the center of diabetes is the pancreas, a large gland about the size of your hand, which is located toward the back of the abdominal cavity and is responsible for manufacturing, storing, and releasing the hormone insulin. The pancreas also makes several other hormones, as well as digestive enzymes. Even if you don't know much about

diabetes, in all likelihood you've heard of insulin and probably know that we all have to have insulin to survive. What you might not realize is that many diabetics may not need insulin shots.

Insulin is a hormone produced by the beta cells of the pancreas. Insulin's major function is to regulate the level of glucose in the bloodstream, which it does primarily by facilitating the transport of blood glucose into most of the billions of cells that make up the body. The presence of insulin stimulates glucose transporters to move to the surface of cells to facilitate glucose entry into the cells. Insulin also stimulates centers in the hypothalamus of the brain responsible for hunger and satiety. Indeed, there is some insulin production even as one begins to eat, before glucose hits the bloodstream. Insulin also instructs fat cells to convert glucose and fatty acids from the blood into fat, which the fat cells then store until needed. Insulin is an anabolic hormone, which is to say that it is essential for the growth of many tissues and organs.* Too much and it can cause excessive growth — as, for example, of body fat and of cells that line blood vessels. Finally, insulin helps to regulate, or counterregulate, the balance of certain other hormones in the body. More about those later.

One of the ways insulin maintains the narrow range of normal levels of glucose in the blood is by regulation of the liver and muscles, directing them to manufacture and store glycogen, a starchy substance the body uses when blood sugar falls too low. If blood sugar does fall even slightly too low — as may occur after strenuous exercise or fasting — the alpha cells of the pancreas release glucagon, another hormone involved in the regulation of blood sugar levels. Glucagon signals the muscles and liver to convert their stored glycogen back into glucose (a process called glycogenolysis), which raises blood sugar. When the body's stores of glucose and glycogen have been exhausted, the liver, and to a lesser extent the kidneys and small intestines, can transform some of the body's protein stores — muscle mass and vital organs — into glucose.

Insulin and Type 1 Diabetes

As recently as ninety years ago, before the clinical availability of insulin, the diagnosis of type 1 diabetes — which involves a severely

---

* Anabolic and catabolic hormones normally work in harmony, building up and breaking down tissues, respectively.

diminished or absent ability to produce insulin—was a death sentence. Most people died within a few months of diagnosis. Without insulin, glucose accumulates in the blood to extremely high toxic levels; yet since it cannot be utilized by the cells, many cell types will starve. Absent or lowered fasting (basal) levels of insulin also lead the liver, kidneys, and intestines to perform gluconeogenesis, turning the body's protein store—the muscles and vital organs—into even more glucose that the body cannot utilize. Meanwhile, the kidneys, the filters of the blood, try to rid the body of inappropriately high levels of sugar. Frequent urination causes insatiable thirst and dehydration. Eventually, the starving body turns more and more protein to sugar.

The ancient Greeks described diabetes as a disease that causes the body to melt into sugar water. When tissues cannot utilize glucose, they will metabolize fat for energy, generating by-products called ketones, which are toxic at very high levels and cause further water loss as the kidneys try to eliminate them (see the discussion of ketoacidosis and hyperosmolar coma in Chapter 21, "How to Cope with Dehydration, Dehydrating Illness, and Infection").

Today type 1 diabetes is still a very serious disease, and still eventually fatal if not properly treated with insulin. It can kill you rapidly when your blood glucose level is too low—through impaired judgment or loss of consciousness while driving, for example—or it can kill you slowly, by heart or kidney disease, which are commonly associated with long-term blood sugar elevation. Until I brought my blood sugars under control, I had numerous automobile accidents due to hypoglycemia, and it's only through sheer luck that I'm here to relate this.

The causes of type 1 diabetes have not yet been fully unraveled. Research indicates that it's an autoimmune disorder in which the body's immune system attacks the pancreatic beta cells that produce insulin. Whatever causes type 1 diabetes, its deleterious effects can absolutely be prevented. The earlier it's diagnosed, and the earlier blood sugars are normalized, the better off you will be.

At the time they are diagnosed, many type 1 diabetics still produce a small amount of insulin. It's important to recognize that *if they are treated early enough and treated properly, what's left of their insulin-producing capability frequently can be preserved.* Type 1 diabetes typically occurs before the age of forty-five and usually makes itself apparent quite suddenly, with such symptoms as dramatic weight loss and frequent thirst and urination. We now know, however, that as sudden as its appearance may be, its onset is actually quite slow. Routine commercial laboratory studies are available that can detect it earlier, and it may be possible to arrest it in these early stages by aggressive treatment. My own body no longer produces any detectable insulin at all. The high blood sugars I experienced during my first year with diabetes burned out, or exhausted, the ability of my pancreas to produce insulin. I must have insulin shots or I will rapidly die. I firmly believe—and know from experience with my patients—that if the kind of diet and medical regimen I prescribe for my patients had been utilized when I was diagnosed, the insulin-producing capability left to me at diagnosis would likely have been preserved. My requirements for injected insulin would have been lessened, and it would have been much easier for me to keep my blood sugars normal.

Blood Sugar Normalization: Restoring the Balance

According to the NIH, approximately 233,600 people died in 2005 from diabetes, but it is likely that most deaths due to diabetes are underreported. (Is a diabetic's death from heart disease, kidney disease, or stroke, for example, really a death from diabetes?) It is the NIH's contention that "the risk for death among people with diabetes is about twice that of people without diabetes of a similar age."

Certainly everyone has to die of something, but you needn't die the slow, torturous death of diabetic complications, which often include blindness and amputations. My history and that of my patients support this.

The Diabetes Control and Complication Trial (DCCT), conducted by the NIH's National Institute of Diabetes and Digestive and Kidney Diseases (NIDDK), began in 1983 as a ten-year study of type 1 diabetics to gauge the effects of improved control of blood sugar levels. Patients whose blood sugars were nearly "normalized" (my patients' blood sugars are usually much closer to normal than were those in the intensive care arm of the trial because of our low-carbohydrate diet) had dramatic reductions of long-term complications. Researchers began the DCCT trying to see if they could, for example, lessen the frequency of diabetic retinopathy by at least 33.5 percent.

Instead of a one-third reduction in retinopathy, they found *more than a 75 percent reduction* in the progression of early retinopathy. They found similarly dramatic results in other diabetic complications and announced the results of the study early in order to make the good news immediately available to all. They found a 50 percent reduction of risk for kidney disease, a 60 percent reduction of risk for nerve damage, and a 35 percent reduction of risk for cardiovascular disease. This reduction continues to this day, many years after the study was terminated. I was present at the meeting where the results were announced and was congratulated by many of the physicians who had previously endured my long-term insistance that diabetics were entitled to the same blood sugars as nondiabetics.

I believe that with truly normal blood sugars, which many of my patients have, these reductions can be 100 percent.

The patients followed in the DCCT averaged twenty-seven years of age at the beginning of the trial, so reductions could easily have been greater in areas such as cardiovascular disease if they had been older or followed for a longer period of time. The implication is that full normalization of blood sugar could totally prevent these complications. In any case, the results of the DCCT are good reason to begin aggressively to monitor and normalize blood sugar levels. The effort and dollar cost of doing so do not have to be remotely as high as the DCCT's findings suggested.

The Insulin-Resistant Diabetic: Type 2

Different from type 1 diabetes is what is officially known as type 2. This is by far the more prevalent form of the disease. According to statistics from the American Diabetes Association, 90–95 percent of diabetics are type 2. Furthermore, as many as a quarter of Americans between the ages of sixty-five and seventy-four have type 2 diabetes. A study published by Yale University in 2002 found that 25 percent of obese teenagers had type 2 diabetes.

(A new category of "pre-diabetes" has been recently called latent autoimmune diabetes, or LADA. This category applies to mild diabetes with onset after the age of thirty-five, in which the patient has been found to produce an antibody to the pancreatic beta cell protein called GADA, just as in type 1 diabetes. Eventually these people may develop overt diabetes and require insulin. When the symptoms of diabetes finally occur, they are often more severe than at the "onset" of type 1 diabetes.)

Approximately 80 percent of those with type 2 diabetes are overweight and are affected by a particular form of obesity variously known as abdominal, truncal, or visceral obesity. It is quite possible that the 20 percent of the so-called type 2 diabetics who do not have visceral obesity actually suffer from a mild form of type 1 diabetes that causes only partial loss of the pancreatic beta cells that produce insulin.* If this proves to be the case, then fully all of those who have true type 2 diabetes may be overweight. (Obesity is usually defined as being at least 20 percent over the ideal body weight for one's height, build, and sex.)

While the cause of type 1 diabetes may still be somewhat mysterious, the cause of type 2 is less so. As noted previously, another designation for type 2 diabetes is insulin-resistant diabetes. Obesity, particularly visceral obesity, and insulin resistance — the inability to fully utilize the glucose-transporting effects of insulin — are interlinked. For reasons related to genetics (see Chapter 12, "Weight Loss — If You're Overweight"), a substantial portion of the population has the potential when overweight to become sufficiently insulin-resistant that the increased demands on the pancreas burn out the beta cells that produce insulin. These people enter the vicious circle depicted in Figure 1-1. Note in the figure the crucial role of dietary carbohydrate in the development and progression of this disease. This is discussed in detail in Chapter 12.

Insulin resistance appears to be caused at least in part by inheritance and in part by high levels of fat — in the form of triglycerides released from abdominal fat — in the branch of the bloodstream that feeds the liver. (Transient insulin resistance can be created in laboratory animals by injecting triglycerides — fat — directly into their liver's blood supply.)† Abdominal fat is associated with systemic inflammation, another cause of insulin resistance, as are infections. Insulin resistance by its very nature increases the body's need for insulin, which therefore causes the pancreas to work harder to produce elevated insulin levels (hyperinsulinemia), which can indirectly cause high blood pressure and damage the circulatory system. Excessive levels of insulin in the blood down-regulate the affinity for insulin that insulin receptors all over the body have naturally. This "tolerance" to insulin causes even greater insulin resistance.

So, to simplify somewhat, inheritance plus inflammation plus fat

---

* Recent studies show that even type 2 diabetics experience some degree of immune attack on their beta cells.
† New evidence demonstrates a role for fat contained in muscle cells (intramyocyte fat) as another important factor in causing insulin resistance.

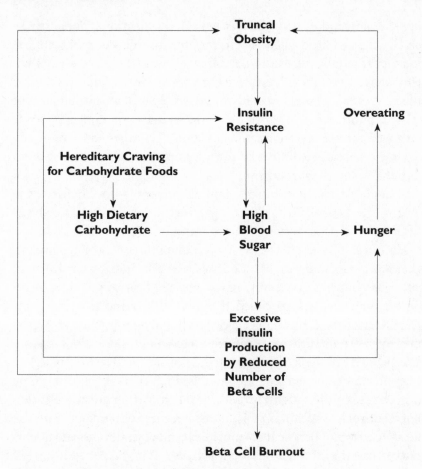

Fig. 1-1. *The vicious circle of insulin resistance.*

in the blood feeding the liver causes insulin resistance, which causes elevated serum insulin levels, which cause the fat cells to build even more abdominal fat, which raises triglycerides in the liver's blood supply and enhances inflammation, which causes insulin levels to increase because of increased resistance to insulin.

If that sounds circular, it is. But note that the fat that is the culprit here is not *dietary* fat.

Triglycerides are in circulation at some level in the bloodstream at all times. High triglyceride levels are not so much the result of intake of dietary fat as they are of carbohydrate consumption and existing body fat. (We will discuss carbohydrates, fat, and insulin resistance more in Chapter 9, "The Basic Food Groups.") The culprit is actually a particular kind of *body* fat. Visceral obesity is a type of obesity in which a special kind of fat is concentrated around the middle of the body, particularly surrounding the intestines (the viscera). A man who is viscerally obese has a waist of greater circumference than his hips. A woman who is viscerally obese has a waist at least 80 percent as big around as her hips. All obese individuals and especially those with visceral obesity are insulin-resistant. The ones who eventually become diabetic are those who cannot make enough extra insulin to keep their blood sugars normal.

Though treatment has many similar elements—and many of the adverse effects of elevated blood sugar are the same—type 2 diabetes differs from type 1 in several important ways.

The onset of type 2 diabetes is slower and more stealthy, but even in its earliest stages abnormal blood sugar levels, though not sky-high, can cause damage to nerves, blood vessels, heart, eyes, and more. Type 2 diabetes is often called the silent killer, and it is quite frequently discovered through one of its complications, such as hypertension, visual changes, or recurrent infections.*

Type 2 diabetes is, at the beginning, a less serious disease—patients don't melt away into sugar water and die in a few months' time. Type 2, however, can through chronically but less dramatically elevated blood sugars be much more insidious. Because so many more people are affected, it probably causes more heart attacks, strokes, and amputations than the more serious type 1 disease. Type 2 is a major cause of hypertension, heart disease, kidney failure, blindness, and erectile dysfunction. That these serious complications of type 2 diabetes can progress is no doubt because it is initially milder and is often left untreated or treated more poorly.

Individuals with type 2 still make insulin, and many will never require injected insulin to survive, though if the disease is treated poorly, they can eventually burn out their pancreatic beta cells and require insulin shots. Because of their resistance to the blood sugar–lowering effects of insulin (though not its fat-building effects), many overweight type 2 diabetics actually make more insulin than slim nondiabetics.

---

* A common early sign of mild chronic blood sugar elevation in women is recurrent vaginal yeast infections that cause itching or burning.

BLOOD SUGARS: THE NONDIABETIC VERSUS THE DIABETIC

Since high blood sugar is the hallmark of diabetes, and the cause of every long-term complication of the disease, it makes sense to discuss where blood sugar comes from and how it is used and not used.

Our dietary sources of blood sugar are carbohydrates and proteins. One reason the taste of sugar—a simple form of carbohydrate—delights us is that it fosters the production of neurotransmitters (principally serotonin) in the brain that relieve anxiety and can create a sense of well-being or even euphoria. This makes carbohydrate quite addictive to certain people whose brains may have inadequate levels of or sensitivity to these neurotransmitters, the chemical messengers with which the brain communicates with itself and the rest of the body. When blood sugar levels are low, the liver, kidneys, and intestines can, through a process we will discuss shortly, convert proteins into glucose, but very slowly and inefficiently. The body cannot convert glucose back into protein, nor can it convert fat into sugar. Fat cells, however, with the help of insulin, do transform glucose into saturated fat.

The taste of protein doesn't excite us as much as that of carbohydrate—it would be the very unusual child who'd jump up and down in the grocery store and beg his mother for steak or fish instead of cookies. Dietary protein gives us a much slower and smaller blood sugar effect, which, as you will see, we diabetics can use to our advantage in normalizing blood sugars.

The Nondiabetic
In the fasting nondiabetic, and even in most type 2 diabetics, the pancreas constantly releases a steady, low level of insulin. This baseline, or basal, insulin level prevents the liver, kidneys, and intestines from inappropriately converting bodily proteins (muscle, vital organs) into glucose and thereby raising blood sugar, a process known as gluconeogenesis. The nondiabetic ordinarily maintains blood sugar immaculately within a narrow range—usually between 70 and 95 mg/dl (milligrams per deciliter),*

---

* A deciliter is one-tenth of a liter, or a little over 3 ounces. A milligram is one one-thousandth of a gram, or about one three-thousandth of the weight of sugar in a level teaspoon.

with most people hovering near 83 mg/dl. There are times when that range can briefly stretch up or down—as high as 160 mg/dl and as low as 65—but generally, for the nondiabetic, such swings are rare.

You will note that in some literature on diabetes, "normal" may be defined as 60–120 mg/dl, or even as high as 140 mg/dl. This "normal" is entirely relative. No nondiabetic will have blood sugar levels as high as 140 mg/dl except after consuming a lot of carbohydrate. "Normal" in this case has more to do with what is considered "cost-effective" for the average physician to treat. Since a postmeal (postprandial) blood sugar under 140 mg/dl is not classified as diabetes, and since the individual who experiences such a value will usually still have adequate insulin production eventually to bring it down to reasonable levels, many physicians would see no reason for spending their valuable time on treatment. Such an individual may be sent off with the admonition to watch his weight or her sugar intake. Despite the designation "normal," an individual frequently displaying a blood sugar of 140 mg/dl is a good candidate for full-blown type 2 diabetes. I have seen "nondiabetics" with sustained blood sugars averaging 120 mg/dl develop diabetic complications.

Let's take a look at how the average nondiabetic body makes and uses insulin. Suppose that Alice, a nondiabetic, arises in the morning and has a mixed breakfast, that is, one that contains both carbohydrate and protein. On the carbohydrate side, she has toast with jelly and a glass of orange juice; on the protein side, she has a boiled egg. Her basal (i.e., before-meals) insulin secretion has kept her blood sugar steady during the night, inhibiting gluconeogenesis. Shortly after the sugar in the juice or jelly hits her mouth, or the starchy carbohydrates in the toast reach certain enzymes in her saliva and intestines, glucose begins to enter her bloodstream. The mere presence of food in her gut as well as the rise in her blood sugar signal her pancreas to release the granules of insulin it has stored in order to offset a jump in blood sugar (see Figure 1-2). This rapid release of stored insulin is called phase I insulin response. It quickly corrects the initial blood sugar increase and can prevent further increase from the ingested carbohydrate. As the pancreas runs out of stored insulin, it manufactures more, but it has to do so from scratch. The insulin released now is known as the phase II insulin response, and it's secreted much more slowly. As she eats her boiled egg, the small amount of insulin of phase II can cover the glucose that, over a period of hours, is slowly produced from the protein of the egg.

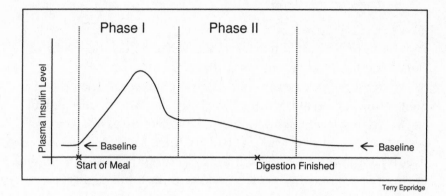

Fig. 1-2. *Phase I and phase II insulin response in a normal, nondiabetic person.*

Insulin acts in the nondiabetic as the means to admit glucose—fuel—into the cells. It does this by activating the movement of glucose "transporters" within the cells. These specialized protein molecules protrude from the cytoplasm of the cells and their outer surfaces to grab glucose from the blood and bring it to the interiors of the cells. Once inside the cells, glucose can be utilized to power energy-requiring functions. Without insulin, the cells can absorb only a very small amount of glucose, not enough to sustain the body.

As glucose continues to enter Alice's blood, and the beta cells in her pancreas continue to release insulin, some of her blood sugar is transformed to glycogen, a starchy substance stored in the muscles and liver. Once glycogen storage sites in the muscles and liver are filled, excess glucose remaining in the bloodstream is converted to and stored as saturated fat. Later, as lunchtime nears but before Alice eats, if her blood sugar drops slightly low, the alpha cells of her pancreas will release another pancreatic hormone, glucagon, which will "instruct" her liver and muscles to begin converting glycogen to glucose, to raise blood sugar. When she eats again, her store of glycogen will be replenished.

This pattern of basal, phase I, then phase II insulin secretion is perfect for keeping Alice's blood glucose levels in a safe range. Her body is nourished, and things work according to design. Her mixed meal is handled beautifully. This is not, however, how things work for either the type 1 or type 2 diabetic.

The Type 1 Diabetic

Let's look at what would happen to me, a type 1 diabetic, if I had the same breakfast as Alice, our nondiabetic.

Unlike Alice, because of a condition peculiar to diabetics, if I take a long-acting insulin at bedtime, I might awaken with a normal blood sugar, but if I spend some time awake before breakfast, my blood sugar may rise, even if I haven't had anything to eat. Ordinarily, the liver is constantly removing some insulin from the bloodstream, but during the first few hours after waking from a full night's sleep, it clears insulin out of the blood at an accelerated rate. This dip in the level of my previously injected insulin is called the dawn phenomenon (see page 97). Because of it, my blood glucose can rise even though I haven't eaten. A nondiabetic just makes more insulin to offset the increased insulin clearance. Those of us who are severely diabetic have to track the dawn phenomenon carefully by monitoring blood glucose levels, and can learn how to use injected insulin to prevent its effect upon blood sugar.

As with Alice, the minute the meal hits my mouth, the enzymes in my saliva begin to break down the sugars in the toast and juice, and almost immediately my blood sugar would begin to rise. Even if the toast had no jelly, the enzymes in my saliva and intestines and acid in my stomach would begin to transform the toast rapidly into glucose shortly after ingestion.

Since my beta cells no longer produce detectable amounts of insulin, there is no stored insulin to be released by my pancreas, so I have no phase I insulin response. My blood sugar (in the absence of injected insulin) will rise while I digest my meal. None of the glucose will be converted to fat, nor will any be converted to glycogen. Eventually much will be filtered out by my kidneys and passed out through the urine, but not before my body has endured damagingly high blood sugar levels — which won't kill me on the spot but will do so over a period of days if I don't inject insulin. The natural question is, wouldn't injected insulin "cover" the carbohydrate in such a breakfast? Not adequately! This is a common misconception — even by those in the health care professions. Injected insulin — even with an insulin pump — doesn't work the same as insulin created naturally in the body. Conventional insulin/diet therapy resulting in high blood sugar after meals is a guaranteed slow, incremental, "silent" death from the ravages of diabetic complications.

Normal phase I insulin is almost instantly in the bloodstream. Rapidly it begins to hustle blood sugar off to where it's needed. Injected insulin, on the other hand, is injected either into fat or muscle (not usually into a vein) and absorbed slowly. The fastest insulin we have starts to work in about 20 minutes, but its full effect is drawn out over a number of hours, not nearly fast enough to prevent a damaging upswing in blood sugars if fast-acting carbohydrate, like bread, is consumed.

This is the central problem for type 1 diabetics — the carbohydrate and the drastic surge it causes in blood sugar. Because I know my body produces essentially no insulin, I have a shot of insulin before every meal. But I no longer eat meals with fast-acting or large amounts of carbohydrate, because the blood sugar swings they caused were what brought about my long-term complications. Even injection by means of an insulin pump (see the discussion near the end of Chapter 19, "Intensive Insulin Regimens") cannot automatically fine-tune the level of glucose in my blood the way a nondiabetic's body does naturally.

Now, if I ate only the protein portion of the meal, my blood sugar wouldn't have the huge, and potentially toxic, surge that carbohydrates cause. It would rise less rapidly, and a small dose of insulin could act quickly enough to cover the glucose that's slowly derived from the protein. My body would not have to endure wide swings in blood sugar levels. (Dietary fat, by the way, has no direct effect on blood sugar levels, except that it can slightly slow the digestion of carbohydrate.)

In a sense, you could look at my insulin shot before eating only the protein portion of the meal as mimicking the nondiabetic's phase II response. This is much easier to accomplish than trying to mimic phase I, because of the much lower levels of dietary carbohydrate (only the slow-acting kind) and injected insulin that I use.

The Type 2 Diabetic

Let's say Bob, a type 2 diabetic, is 6 feet tall and weighs 300 pounds, much of which is centered around his midsection. Remember, at least 80 percent of type 2 diabetics are overweight. If Bob weighed only 170 pounds, he might well be nondiabetic, but because he's insulin-resistant, Bob's body no longer produces enough excess insulin to keep his blood sugar levels normal.

The overweight tend to be insulin-resistant as a group, a condition that's not only hereditary but also directly related to the ratio of visceral and total body fat to lean body mass (muscle). The higher this ratio, the more insulin-resistant a person will be. Whether or not an overweight individual is diabetic, his weight, intake of carbohydrates, and insulin resistance all tend to make him produce considerably more insulin than a slender person of similar age and height (see Figure 1-3).

Many athletes, because of their low fat mass and high percentage of muscle, tend as a group to require and make less insulin than nonathletes. An overweight type 2 diabetic like Bob, on the other hand, typically makes two to three times as much insulin as the slender nondiabetic. In Bob's case, from many years of having to overcompensate, his pancreas has partially burned out, his ability to store insulin is diminished or gone, and his phase I insulin response is attenuated. Despite his huge output of insulin, he no longer can keep his blood sugars within normal ranges. (In my medical practice, a number of patients come to me for treatment of their obesity, not diabetes. On examination, however, most of these very obese "nondiabetics" have slight elevations of their hemoglobin A_{1C} (HgbA$_{1C}$) test for average blood sugar.)

Let's take another look at that mixed breakfast and see how it affects a type 2 diabetic. Bob has the same toast and jelly and juice

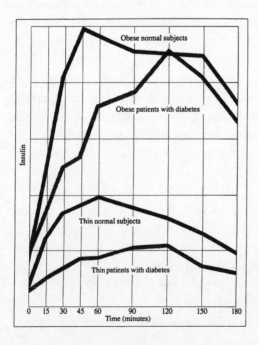

Fig. 1-3. *Serum insulin response to glucose consumption of individuals with and without type 2 diabetes.*

and boiled egg that Alice, our nondiabetic, and I had. Bob's blood sugar levels at waking may be normal.* Since he has a bigger appetite than either Alice or I, he has two glasses of juice, four pieces of toast, and two eggs. Almost as soon as the toast and juice hit his mouth, his blood sugar begins to rise. Unlike mine, Bob's pancreas eventually releases insulin, but he has very little or no stored insulin (his pancreas works hard just to keep up his basal insulin level), so he has impaired phase I secretion. His phase II insulin response, however, may be partially intact. So, very slowly, his pancreas will struggle to produce enough insulin to bring his blood sugar down toward the normal range. Eventually it may get there, but not until hours after his meal, and hours after his body has been exposed to high blood sugars. Insulin is not only the major fat-building hormone; it also serves to stimulate the centers in the brain responsible for feeding behavior. Thus, in all likelihood, Bob will grow even more overweight, as demonstrated by the cycle illustrated in Figure 1-1.

Since he's resistant to insulin, his pancreas has to work that much harder to produce insulin to enable him to utilize the carbohydrate he consumes. Because of insulin's fat-building properties, his body stores away some of his blood sugar as fat and glycogen; but his blood sugar continues to rise, since his cells are unable to utilize all of the glucose derived from his meal. Bob, therefore, still feels hungry. As he eats more, his beta cells work harder to produce more insulin. The excess insulin and the "hungry" cells in his brain prompt him to want yet more food. He has just one more piece of toast with a little more jelly on it, hoping that it will be enough to get him through until lunch. Meanwhile, his blood sugar goes even higher, his beta cells work harder, and perhaps a few burn out.† Even after all this food, he still may feel many of the symptoms of hunger. His blood sugar, however, will probably not go anywhere near as high as mine would if I took no insulin. In addition, his phase II insulin response could even bring his blood sugar down to normal after many hours without more food.

Postprandial (after-eating) blood sugar levels that I would call

---

* Waking, or fasting, blood sugars are frequently normal in mild type 2 diabetics. After they eat carbohydrate, however, their postprandial blood sugars are usually elevated.
† Beta cell burnout can be caused both by overactivity of the cells and by the toxicity of high glucose levels.

unacceptably high — 140 mg/dl, or even 200 mg/dl — may be considered by other physicians to be unworthy of treatment because the patient still produces adequate insulin to bring them periodically down to normal, or "acceptable," ranges. If Bob, our type 2 diabetic, had received intensive medical intervention before the beta cells of his pancreas began to burn out, he would have slimmed down, brought his blood sugars into line, and eased the burden on his pancreas. He might even have "cured" his diabetes by slimming down, as I've seen in several patients. But many doctors might decide such "mildly" abnormal blood sugars are only impaired glucose tolerance (IGT) and do little more than "watch" them. Again, it's my belief that aggressive treatment at an early stage can save most patients considerable lost time and personal agony by preventing complications that will occur if blood sugar levels are left unchecked. Such intervention can make subsequent treatment of what can remain — a mild disease — elegantly simple.

ON THE HORIZON

I include some hopeful forecasts of future treatments in this first chapter because as you're learning how to control your diabetes, hope is a valuable asset. But your hope should be realistic. Your best hope for controlling your diabetes is normalizing your blood sugars now. That does not mean that the future will not bring great things. Diabetes research progresses on a daily basis, and I hope as much as you do for a cure, but it's still on the horizon.

Researchers are currently trying to perfect methods for replicating insulin-producing pancreatic beta cells in the laboratory. Doing this in a fashion that's comparatively easy and cost-effective should not be an insurmountable task, and indeed the preliminary results are quite encouraging. Once patients' cells are replicated, they can be transplanted back into patients to actually cure their diabetes. After such treatment, unless you were to have another autoimmune event that would destroy these new beta cells, you would, at least in theory, remain nondiabetic for the rest of your life. If you had another autoimmune attack, you would simply have to receive more of your replicated cells. Another very hopeful approach currently undergoing clinical trials in humans is the transformation of the precursors of beta cells (the cells that line the ducts of the pancreas) into actual beta cells without even removing them from your body. This may be achieved by the simple intramuscular injection of a special protein and is now being tested for efficacy and possible adverse effects at several centers.

Another potential approach might be to insert the genes for insulin production into liver or kidney cells. These are potential opportunities for a cure, and have successfully cured diabetes in rats, but there are still obstacles to overcome.

Yet another approach to replacing lost beta cells has been used by two competing companies to cure diabetes in animals. The technique involves a series of ordinary injections of proteins that stimulate the remaining beta cells to replicate until the lost ones have been replaced.

One problem with all of these "solutions" is that the immune systems of diabetics are still capable of destroying the new beta cells. The following paragraph describes a way around this problem.

A very promising new approach relies on the fact that most diabetics, even most type 1s, have a few beta cells that still replicate. Their immune systems, however, make white blood cells that destroy the new beta cells as fast as they are made—or faster. If the culprit white cells can be isolated, they can be replicated and used to create vaccines that can be injected into diabetics, stimulating their immune systems to destroy all of their culprit cells. A diabetic's few remaining beta cells would then be able to replicate, eventually curing the diabetes. It's possible that these new "former diabetics" would require antibody injections every few years to prevent the appearance of more culprit cells. I have applied for a patent on a method for isolating these culprit cells.

With respect to the replication of beta cells, the catch for me and other diabetics who no longer have any insulin-producing capacity is that the cells from which new beta cells would be replicated ideally should be your own, and after more than six decades I may have none. Had my diabetes been diagnosed, say, a year earlier, and had my blood sugars been immaculately controlled immediately upon diagnosis, the injected insulin might have taken much of the strain off my remaining beta cells and allowed them to survive.

Many people (including the parents of diabetic children) view having to use insulin as a last straw, a final admission that they are (or their child is) diabetic and seriously ill. Therefore they will try anything else—including things that will burn out their remaining beta cells—before using insulin. Many people in our culture have the notion that you cannot be well if you are using medication. This is nonsense, but some patients are so convinced that they must do things the "natural" way that I practically have to beg them to use insulin, which is as "natural" as one can go. In reality, nothing could be *more* natural. Diabetics who still have beta cell function left may well be carrying their own cure around with them—provided they don't burn it out with high blood sugars and the refusal to use insulin.

> I will personally answer questions from readers for
> one hour every month. This free service is available by
> visiting www.askdrbernstein.net.

2

Tests

BASELINE MEASURES OF YOUR
DISEASE AND RISK PROFILE

The goal in the treatment program laid out in this book is to give you the tools and the knowledge to take control of your disease by normalizing blood sugars. My interest is not just in treating the symptoms of diabetes, but in preventing or reversing its consequences and preserving pancreatic beta cell function. Essential to treatment is learning to monitor your own blood sugars.

Before you begin to monitor and then normalize your blood sugars, you should ideally have a baseline analysis of your disease. How much have your beta cells "burned out" in part from high blood sugars? Have you already developed some easily measured long-term complications of diabetes? What are your risks for other diabetic complications?

Answering these questions will aid you and your doctor in learning the extent and the consequences of the disease. Your test results will also serve as valuable baseline data to which you will be able to compare the effects of blood sugar normalization. Once your blood sugars have been normalized, such tests can be repeated from time to time, to show what you're achieving. Your improvements will give both you and your physician ongoing incentive for sticking to the program.

The remainder of this chapter describes a number of tests your doctor's laboratory can perform in order to give both of you a picture of your diabetic condition. I have laid these out *not* because it's necessary for you to memorize them, research them, and know all the ins and outs of them, but so that you may be more likely to get the treatment you deserve. By outlining these tests, I'm giving you a "shopping list" of tests I perform on myself and on my patients.

Generally, I recommend as many as you can afford or your insurance or health maintenance organization (HMO) will pay for. Completing more of the tests will add more dimensions to the picture you gain of your disease. As some of these tests are costly, any or all may be skipped if you cannot afford them or if your insurance or HMO won't pay for them.

It is your physician's obligation to provide you with copies of all your test results, whether from laboratory tests or from physical examinations. This is your right; however, you must request them. The laws governing medical records vary state by state, and legislatures are listening to health care consumers and making changes regularly. At this writing, however, it is most often the case that medical records are the property of the provider, so do not neglect to request copies of any results. Such results can be potentially of great value when you visit another physician or specialist for treatment of any problems.

BLOOD AND URINE TESTS

Glycated Hemoglobin (HgbA$_{1C}$)

Glucose binds to hemoglobin (the pigment of red blood cells) when new red cells are manufactured. Since the average red cell survives about four months, the percentage of hemoglobin molecules that contain glucose (HgbA$_{1C}$) provides an estimate of average blood sugar over this time frame. One of the benefits of this test is that it gives your physician an index by which to test the accuracy of your own blood glucose self-monitoring results. If your measurements are strictly normal but your HgbA$_{1C}$ is elevated, then your doctor has a clue that something is awry.

There are, however, a couple of significant drawbacks to this test. First is that the test is only a measure of *average* blood sugars. Second, elevated blood sugars may take 24 hours to have any long-term effect on HgbA$_{1C}$, and if blood sugar is elevated for only part of each day and is normalized or too low the rest of the time, your HgbA$_{1C}$ results may appear deceptively low. Thus, if your blood sugars are only elevated for a few hours after meals, your HgbA$_{1C}$ may not be affected, but many tissues and organs throughout your body will be injured.

The other drawback is that the upper and lower ranges of "normal" values reported by most labs are usually erroneously high and low, respectively. In other words, the ranges are usually much too wide. Thus, it's up to your physician to decide, based upon his experience, what the proper normal range for his lab should be. Some doctors have their own formulas for estimating average four-month blood sugar levels from HgbA$_{1C}$. A normal value should correspond to blood sugars of about 75–86 mg/dl. The experience I've had with the lab I use (the largest in the United States) for my patients is that a truly normal HgbA$_{1C}$ ranges from 4.2 percent to 4.6 percent, which corresponds to blood sugars of about 72–86 mg/dl. A recent study of "nondiabetics" showed a 28 percent increase in mortality for every 1 percent increase in HgbA$_{1C}$ above 4.9 percent.

Because the blood contains more recently made red cells than older ones, recent blood sugars have more of an effect on HgbA$_{1C}$ than do earlier blood sugars. The test value therefore levels off after about three months. Any ailment that hastens red blood cell loss will cause a deceptive shortening of the time frame reflected by the HgbA$_{1C}$. Such ailments include liver and kidney disease, blood loss, hemoglobinopathies, et cetera. High doses of vitamins C and E can cause a deceptive lowering, and low serum levels of thyroid hormones can cause an increase without increasing blood sugars.

Serum C-peptide (Fasting)
C-peptide is a protein produced by the beta cells of the pancreas whenever insulin is made. The level of C-peptide in the blood is a crude index of the amount of insulin you're producing. The level is usually zero in type 1 diabetics, and within or above the "normal range" in mild type 2 obese (insulin-resistant) diabetics. If your serum C-peptide is elevated, this would suggest to your physician that your blood sugar may be controllable merely by diet, weight loss, and exercise. If, at the other extreme, your C-peptide is below the limits of measurability, you probably require injected insulin for blood sugar normalization. C-peptide measurements, to be most significant, should be checked after an 8-hour fast when blood sugars are normal. The test can be best interpreted if blood sugar is measured at the same time, because in nondiabetics high blood sugars cause more insulin (and C-peptide) production than do low blood sugars.

This test, while of interest, is not absolutely necessary.

Complete Blood Count (CBC)
Part of most medical workups, this is a routine diagnostic test that can disclose the presence of ailments other than diabetes. A CBC measures the number of various types of cells found in your blood—white cells,

red cells, and platelets. A high level of white blood cells, for example, can disclose the presence of infection, while too few red blood cells can indicate anemia. Many diabetics have inherited thyroid dysfunction, which can cause low-normal to low white cell counts. A white cell count less than 5.6 suggests that a full thyroid profile should be performed. This must include free and total T_3 and T_4.*

A CBC can also detect certain hematologic malignancies, which are usually more effectively treated the earlier they are discovered.

Standard Blood Chemistry Profile

This battery of twelve to twenty tests is part of most routine medical examinations. It includes gauges for such important chemical indicators of health as liver enzymes, blood urea nitrogen (BUN), creatinine, alkaline phosphatase, calcium, and others. If you have a history of hypertension, your doctor may want to add red blood cell magnesium to this profile.

Serum Ferritin

This is a measure of total body iron stores. Although usually used for diagnosing iron deficiency anemia, high ferritin levels can cause insulin resistance and type 2 diabetes. Sometimes this form of diabetes can be treated by diet, exercise, and regular blood donation.

Serum Albumin

Although serum albumin is usually included in the blood chemistry profile, it is not widely appreciated that low levels are associated with double the all-cause mortality of normal levels. It is thus very important that patients with low serum albumin receive further tests to determine the cause.

Serum Globulin

Globulins are antibodies produced by the immune system. They help the body to fight off infections and malignancy. If you experience frequent colds, sinusitis, diarrhea, cancer, or slow-healing infections of

---

* It's worth noting that one of the hallmarks of high blood sugars is fatigue. However, diminished thyroid function can cause profound fatigue, coldness, or muscle cramps. If you're still "always tired" or "always cold" after normalizing blood sugars, talk to your physician about a thyroid profile. This test can be costly.

any type, you may have an immunoglobulin deficiency. If your total serum globulins are low or even low normal, you should be tested for specific immunoglobulins, such as IgA, IgG, and IgM. We recently published evidence that at least 19 percent of diabetics have an inherited immune disorder (common variable immunodeficiency, or CVID) that may be treatable.

Cardiac Risk Factors

This is a battery of tests that measure substances in the blood that may predispose you to arterial and heart disease.

IMPORTANT NOTE: Sometimes, long before or even months to years after a patient has experienced normal or near-normal blood sugars and resultant improvements in the cardiac risk profile, we might see deterioration in the results of tests such as those for LDL, HDL, homocysteine, fibrinogen, and lipoprotein(a). All too often, the patient or his physician will blame our diet. Inevitably, however, we find upon further testing that his thyroid activity has declined. Hypothyroidism is an autoimmune disorder, like diabetes, and is frequently inherited by diabetics and their close relatives. It can appear years before or after the development of diabetes and is not caused by high blood sugars. In fact, hypothyroidism can cause a greater likelihood of abnormalities in the cardiac risk profile than can blood sugar elevation. The treatment of a low-thyroid condition is oral replacement of the deficient hormone(s) — usually 1–3 pills daily. The best screening test is free T_3 as measured by tracer dialysis. If this is low, then a full thyroid test profile should be performed. Correction of the thyroid deficiency inevitably corrects the abnormalities of cardiac risk factors that it caused. TSH, the inexpensive thyroid test performed by most physicians, does not correlate as well with symptoms of hypothyroidism as free T_3. My goal with these patients is to use supplemental T_3 and T_4 to get free T_3 and free T_4 to the middle of the normal range.

Lipid profile. This profile measures fatty substances (lipids) in your blood and includes total cholesterol, HDL (high-density lipoprotein), triglycerides, and "real" LDL (low-density lipoprotein). Other cardiac risk factors (discussed below) include C-reactive protein, fibrinogen, lipoprotein(a), and homocysteine, and may be more predictive. Abnormalities indicated by these tests are frequently treatable and tend to improve with normalization of blood sugars.

These tests should be performed after you have fasted for at least 8 hours. The easiest thing is to have them scheduled in the morning. If you haven't fasted before the test, the results will be difficult to interpret.

Maybe you've heard of "good" cholesterol and "bad" cholesterol?

Well, this is why a reading for total cholesterol by itself won't necessarily reflect cardiac risk. Most of the cholesterol in our bodies, both good and bad, is made in the liver; it does not come from eating so-called heart attack foods. If you've eaten a meal that's high in cholesterol, your liver will adjust to make less of the "bad" cholesterol, LDL. Serum triglyceride levels can vary dramatically after meals, with high-carbohydrate meals causing high triglyceride levels. Some people—because they're obese or have high blood sugars or are genetically predisposed—make more or dispose of less LDL than they should, which can put them at a higher risk for cardiac problems. High levels of LDL are thought to increase the risk of heart disease, which makes LDL the "bad" cholesterol. HDL, on the other hand, is a lipid that reduces the risk of heart disease and is the "good" cholesterol. So it is the ratio of total cholesterol to HDL (total cholesterol ÷ HDL) that is significant. You could have a high total cholesterol and yet, because of low LDL and high HDL, have a low cardiac risk. Conversely, a low total cholesterol with a low HDL would signify increased risk. Recently, as more has become known about cholesterol, research has shown that LDL occurs in at least two forms—small, dense LDL particles (or type B, the hazardous form) and large, buoyant LDL particles. LDL particle size is now being measured by commercial laboratories. Larger particles, classified as size A, are considered benign, while smaller particles carry cardiac risk. Associated with the test for particle size is apolipoprotein B. When the Apo B test result is lower than 120 mg/dl, or when LDL particle size is type A, even high LDL levels are considered benign and should not be treated with statin drugs.

The only truly accurate measure of LDL is the "real" LDL test. The customary, calculated measure of LDL is estimated mathematically, which can result in values that are sometimes grossly in error. The "real" test, however, may cost more than the rest of your lipid profile.

Recently a commercial lipid panel called "VAP cholesterol" has become available. It contains all of the lipid tests described above. It is costly but can be ordered from most commercial laboratories.

The role of serum lipids in heart disease has come into question by some studies showing that at least 50 percent of people who suffer heart attacks have normal lipid profiles. There is evidence that the new (difficult to obtain) tests for oxidized and glycated LDL may be even better predictors of cardiac risk.

Also important to remember is that—as we will discuss in Chapter 9, "The Basic Food Groups"—fats and cholesterol in the diet do not cause high-risk lipid profiles in most people. On the other hand, diabetics tend to have lipid profiles that suggest increased cardiac risk, if their blood sugars have been elevated for several weeks or months.

Thrombotic risk profile. This profile includes levels of fibrinogen, C-reactive protein, and lipoprotein(a). These are also "acute phase reactants," or substances that reflect ongoing infection or other inflammation. These three substances are associated with increased tendency of blood to clot or form infarcts (blockages of arteries) in people who have had sustained high blood sugars.

In the cases of elevated fibrinogen or lipoprotein(a), there is, additionally, often an increased risk of kidney impairment or retinal disease. Obesity, even without diabetes, can cause elevation of C-reactive protein. In my experience, all these tests are more potent indicators of impending heart attack than the lipid profile. Treatments are available for elevations of each of these. Blood sugar normalization will tend to reverse most of these elevations over the long term. Fibrinogen can be elevated by kidney disease, even in the absence of elevated blood sugars. It will tend to normalize if kidney disease reverses. Lipoprotein(a) will also tend to normalize somewhat with blood sugar normalization, although your genetic makeup (and low estrogen levels in women) can play a greater role than blood sugar. Abnormally low thyroid function is a common cause of low HDL and elevated LDL, homocysteine, and lipoprotein(a). Although serum homocysteine is also a cardiac risk factor, it was recently discovered that the usual treatment for elevated values (vitamin B-12 and folic acid supplements) actually increased mortality.

Serum transferrin saturation, ferritin, and total iron binding capacity (TIBC). These are all measures of total body iron stores. Iron is vital, but it is also potentially dangerous. Levels that are too high can indicate a cardiac risk, can cause insulin resistance, and are a risk factor for liver cancer. I will discuss insulin resistance at length in Chapter 6, "Strange Biology." Higher iron levels are more likely in men than in premenopausal women because of blood (iron) loss during menstruation. (This is why I recommend iron-enhanced vitamin supplements *only* for those with an established need.) Iron levels that are too low (iron deficiency anemia, which is more common in premenopausal women) can cause an uncontrollable urge to snack, which in turn can lead to uncontrollable blood sugars. Both high and low iron stores can be easily determined and readily treated.

Renal Risk Profile

Chronic blood sugar elevation for many years can cause slow deterioration of the kidneys. If caught early, it may be reversible by blood sugar normalization, as it was in my own case. Unless you think frequent hospital visits for dialysis might be a nice way to meet people, it's wise to have periodic tests that reflect early kidney changes. It is also wise to have all these periodically performed together, as the results of each can clarify the interpretation of all.

Several factors cause false positive results in some of these tests, so you should keep them in mind when your doctor schedules the tests. You should avoid strenuous or prolonged lower body exercise (which would include motorcycle or horseback riding) in the 48 hours preceding the tests. Additionally, if on the day the tests are to be performed you are menstruating or have a fever, a urinary tract infection, or active kidney stones, you should postpone the tests until these conditions have cleared.

A basic renal risk profile should include the following tests.

Urinary kappa light chains. If early diabetic kidney disease is present, this test reports "polyclonal kappa light chains present." This means that small amounts of tiny protein molecules may be entering the urine, due to leaky blood vessels in the kidneys. Because these molecules are so small, they are the first proteins to leak through tiny pores in the blood vessels of the kidneys that may have been affected by disease.

This test requires a small amount of fresh urine. If the test report states "monoclonal light chains present," there is a possibility of treatable malignancies of certain white blood cells.

Microalbuminuria. This less costly test can now be performed qualitatively (by dipstick) in your doctor's office, or quantitatively at an outside laboratory. It, like the urinary kappa light chain test, can also reflect leaky vessels in the kidneys, but at a later stage, since albumin is a slightly larger molecule.

A quantitative measurement requires a 24-hour urine specimen, which means you'll need to collect all the urine you produce in a 24-hour period in a big jug and deliver it to your physician or laboratory. Given the potential embarrassment of carrying a jug full of urine around at work, you might want to schedule your test on a Monday and collect the urine while at home on Sunday. Many of my women patients report that it's easier to collect urine initially in a clean paper cup, and then pour it into the jug. An easier screening test is the measurement of the albumin-to-creatinine ratio in a first morning urine sample.

24-hour urinary protein. This test detects kidney damage at a later stage than the preceding two tests; it also requires a 24-hour urine collection. As with the other tests, false positive results can occur following strenuous lower body exercise, as previously noted.

Creatinine clearance. Creatinine is a chemical by-product of muscle metabolism, and is present in your bloodstream all the time. Measuring the clearance of creatinine from the body is a way of estimating the filtering capacity of the kidneys. Test values are usually higher than normal when a person is spilling a lot of sugar in the urine, and eventually lower than normal when the kidneys have been damaged by years of elevated blood sugars. It is not surprising to see an appropriate drop in creatinine clearance when blood sugars are normalized and urine glucose vanishes.

The creatinine clearance test requires a 24-hour urine collection, and your lab will simultaneously draw a small amount of blood to measure serum creatinine. The most common cause of abnormally low values for this test is failure of the patient to collect all the urine produced in a 24-hour period. Therefore, if other kidney tests are normal, tests with low values for creatinine clearance should be repeated for verification.

A low creatinine clearance without excess urinary protein suggests a nondiabetic cause of kidney impairment.

When it is impractical to make a 24-hour urine collection, as for small children, a new test requiring a small amount of blood, **crystatin-C,** can be performed. Crystatin-C is believed to be a more accurate measure of kidney function than creatinine clearance, but unfortunately many insurers still consider this test to be "experimental" and won't pay for it.

25-OH vitamin D-3. This is the standard test for vitamin D. Normal values range from 50 to 80 mg/ml. People who are not regularly exposed to sunlight are usually deficient in this essential vitamin, which can be replaced by supplements. A deficiency can cause insulin resistance.

Serum beta$_2$ microglobulin. This is a very sensitive test for injury to the tubules of the kidneys, which pass urine filtered from the blood (see Figure A-1, page 469). As with fibrinogen levels, elevated values can also result from inflammation or infection anywhere in the body. Thus an isolated elevation of serum beta$_2$ microglobulin without the presence of urinary kappa light chains or microalbumin is probably due to some sort of infection or inflammation, not to diabetic kidney disease. Such elevation is commonplace in people with AIDS, lymphoma, and immunodeficiency disorders.

24-hour urinary glucose. This test too requires a 24-hour collection of urine, and is of value for proper interpretation of creatinine clearance.

NOTE: If, as you've been reading about these tests, you've imagined yourself lugging around multiple jugs of urine, most of us only need one 3-liter jug. This should give you an adequate specimen for your laboratory to perform creatinine clearance, microalbumin, 24-hour protein, and 24-hour glucose. Nevertheless, it's wise to bring home two empty jugs, just in case your urine output is very high.

As indicated under "Cardiac Risk Factors," significant kidney damage may also be accompanied by elevations of serum homocysteine and fibrinogen.

OTHER TESTS

Insulin-like Growth Factor 1 (IGF-1)
Rapid correction of very high blood sugars can, on occasion, cause exacerbation of a common complication of diabetes called proliferative retinopathy. This condition can cause hemorrhaging inside the eye and blindness. Such exacerbations are usually preceded by an

increase in serum levels of insulin-like growth factor 1. A baseline level of IGF-1 in the blood should be measured in people with proliferative retinopathy. Repeat determinations should be made every two to three months. If levels increase, blood sugars should then be reduced more slowly.

R-R Interval Study

The purpose of this study is to test the functioning of the vagus nerve, and it should be part of your initial diabetic physical examination. It is performed like an ordinary electrocardiogram, but it requires fewer electrical leads (i.e., only on the limbs, not the chest).

The vagus nerve is the largest nerve in the body, running from the brain to the lower body. It's the main neural component of the parasympathetic nervous system, or that part of the nervous system that takes care of vegetative, autonomic functions, the functions that run more or less on "automatic pilot" and that you don't actively have to think about to make happen. These include heart rate and digestion.

Like any other nerve in the body, the vagus nerve can be injured by long-term exposure to high blood sugars, but since it plays such a central role in bodily function, damage to it can cause many more disorders than damage to most other individual nerves.

The vagus plays a major role in a number of diabetic complications involving the autonomic nervous system, including rapid heart rate, erectile dysfunction in men, and digestive problems, particularly gastroparesis, or delayed stomach-emptying (which we will discuss in detail in Chapter 22). The good news is that when you've had your blood sugars normalized over an extended period, it can slowly recover proper function. (Many of my male patients who have been unable to achieve or maintain an erection report that after blood sugars have been normalized, that ability has returned.)

This nerve is unique in that its function can be investigated simply and cheaply. If the vagus nerve is working properly, there should be a considerable difference in heart rate between inhaling and exhaling. By measuring the variation of your heart rate with deep breathing, we can get a picture of just how much the function has been impaired. In nondiabetics, the heart rate increases when they inhale deeply and slows when they exhale fully. So a twenty-one-year-old nondiabetic's heart rate might typically slow as much as 85 percent from inhaling to exhaling. This may drop to about 30 percent for a seventy-year-old nondiabetic. A young type 1 diabetic with ten years of very high blood sugars may not have any heart rate variation at all. (The variation is measured by looking at the interval between "R-points," or peaks on the tracing of the electrocardiogram. As you're probably aware, each time your heart beats, the electrocardiograph traces a shape resembling a mountain. The tip of the mountain is the R-point, so the physician measures the intervals between R-points.)

I consider this test an important, reproducible, quantitative measure of an important diabetic complication and perform it on all of my new patients before blood sugars have been stabilized. I repeat it about every eighteen months, for several reasons. It's a very good index of how, with aggressive blood sugar control, neurologic complications can and do reverse, and it gives both patient and doctor good, concrete evidence of the success of treatment, and encouragement to keep it up. Additionally, the digestive disorder of gastroparesis, which I mentioned above, can be and frequently is one of the most difficult barriers to blood sugar normalization, and can even make blood sugar control virtually impossible in some people who require insulin. A low heart rate variability on the initial test can be a good indicator that the patient is likely to have a problem with delayed stomach-emptying. It can also give the doctor clues as to causes of other problems that a patient may be experiencing — sexual dysfunction, fainting upon standing when arising from bed, and so on.

If your physician would like to learn how to perform this study in his or her office, he or she should read my article "R-R Interval Studies: A Simple Office Protocol" (*Diabetes Care* 1984; 7:510–513). If he or she is unwilling to do an R-R study, there are several companies that offer it; just search the Internet for "tests for cardiac autonomic neuropathy."

Neurologic Examination

In addition to a standard physical examination, it is desirable (but not essential) that a routine neurologic exam be performed before blood sugars are corrected, and again every few years thereafter. These tests are not painful. They should include checking for sensation in the feet, reflexes of limbs and eyes, double vision, short-term memory, and muscle strength. In my experience, performance on a number of the neurologic tests improves after many months of essentially normal blood sugars. Performance tends to deteriorate if blood sugars remain high.

Eye Examination

One of the most valuable retinal studies, the Amsler grid test, can be performed by any physician or nurse in less than a minute without dilating your pupils. Since chronically high blood sugars frequently cause a number of disorders that can impair vision, your eyes, if normal, should be examined carefully by an ophthalmologist or retinologist every one to two years.

The ophthalmologist will evaluate the retina, lens, and anterior chamber in each eye, and you can expect to have your pupils dilated with special drops. A proper retinal exam requires the use of both direct and indirect ophthalmoscopes and a slit lamp. If an abnormality is found, certain examinations may have to be performed by a retinologist every few months.

Examination of the Feet

Because ulcers of the diabetic foot are avoidable, even when blood sugar is not well controlled, you should ask your physician to examine your feet at every routine office visit. Foot problems that aren't prevented or treated properly can lead to serious complications, even amputation. Your physician should train you in foot self-examination and preventive care. In Appendix D, I have reproduced the same instructions I give my own patients on how to care for their feet.

Oscillometric Study of Lower Extremities

This inexpensive test utilizes a simple blood pressure cuff connected to a small instrument that should be in every doctor's office. It gives an index of the adequacy of pulsatile circulation to the legs and feet. Since long-standing, poorly controlled diabetes can seriously impair peripheral circulation, this test is fairly important. All diabetics should take special care of their feet, but if you have an abnormal oscillometric study, you have to be extra careful. People who have diminished circulation in the legs usually also have significant deposits in the arteries that nourish the heart, brain, kidneys, and arteries necessary for penile erection. Therefore, if this study shows impaired circulation, your doctor may want you to undergo tests that would help diagnose coronary artery disease and, if you have certain symptoms, diagnose impaired circulation to the brain. Oscillometry can be performed by any trained physician in a few minutes. It is taught at many medical schools throughout the world but rarely in the United States, where hands-on care is diminishing. Your physician can search the Internet on "oscillometer" if he or she wishes to purchase one. Most insurers will compensate doctors for doing this test.

Musculoskeletal Examination

Prolonged high blood sugars can cause glycation of tendons. Glycation is the permanent fusing of glucose to proteins, and the simplest analogy is bread crust. Think of the soft inside of the bread as your tendons as they should be, and the crust as what happens when they're exposed to elevated blood sugars over a long period of time. Glycation of tendons occurs in such common diabetic complications as Dupuytren's contractures of the fingers, frozen shoulders, trigger fingers, carpal tunnel syndrome, and iliotibial band/tensor fascialata syndrome of the hips and upper legs. All of these conditions are easily treated if caught early and blood sugars are controlled. A musculoskeletal examination can identify these in their early, treatable stages.*

When to Perform These Tests

As valuable as they can be to you and your physician, none of these tests is crucial to our central goal of achieving blood sugar normalization. If you are without medical insurance, or if your insurance won't pay for these tests, and financial considerations are a top priority, all can be deferred. If, however, you are experiencing problems, such as impairment of vision, you should be tested immediately. Also, examination of your feet, and learning how to care for them properly, is vital and can prevent or forestall serious problems.

The most valuable of these tests for our purposes is the $HgbA_{1C}$, because it alerts your physician to the possibility that your self-monitored blood sugar data may not reflect the average blood sugar for the prior three months. This can occur if your blood sugar–measuring technique or supplies are defective. More commonly, some patients, with a scheduled visit to the doctor approaching, will improve their eating habits so that their blood sugar records improve. I have seen several teenagers whose falsified blood sugar data were

---

* For information on the proper treatment of these conditions, visit www .diabetes-book.com; select "Articles," then "Research," and then the article title that begins "Some Long-Term Sequelae of Poorly Controlled Diabetes."

discovered by this test. I therefore suggest that HgbA$_{1C}$ be measured at regular visits every two to three months. This test costs about $65 in the United States.

Ideally, the other blood and urine tests should be performed before attempting to normalize blood sugar and annually thereafter. If an abnormal value is found, your physician may wish to repeat that test and related tests more often. The exception is the fasting C-peptide test, as there is little value in repeating it except to see if pancreatic function is deteriorating or improving. I certainly like to repeat the thrombotic risk and lipid profiles about four months and then eight months after blood sugars or thyroid tests have been normalized. The improvement that I frequently see tends to encourage patients to continue their efforts at blood sugar normalization. The R-R interval test should be performed every eighteen months. *I consider it the second most important test I perform on my patients after the HgbA$_{1C}$.*

A FINAL NOTE: Dietary vitamin C is important to good health. In doses above 500 mg/day, however, vitamin C supplements can destroy the enzymes on blood sugar test strips and can also raise blood sugars. Finally, in levels higher than about 400 mg/day, vitamin C becomes an oxidant rather than an antioxidant and can cause neuropathies. If you are already taking supplemental vitamin C, I urge you to taper it off or lower your dose to no more than 250 mg daily. Use only the timed-release form.

I will personally answer questions from readers for one hour every month. This free service is available by visiting www.askdrbernstein.net.

3

Your Diabetic Tool Kit

SUPPLIES YOU WILL NEED AND
WHERE TO GET THEM

In order to monitor and control your blood sugar levels, you're going to need certain tools. This chapter lists and describes them; you'll learn more about them in later chapters. Also included are supplies for foot care and for treating dehydrating illnesses. For most items, approximate costs are listed. Some expenses will be onetime outlays, such as for your blood glucose meter outfit. Others will continue on an ongoing basis.

The tools that all diabetics will need are listed first. Tools that only insulin users will need are listed separately. Some are necessary, and some are optional. You can show your physician the list and he or she can decide which items are appropriate for your needs.

Following the tables of supplies is a brief description of each, what it's for, where you can purchase it, whether you'll need a prescription, and where in this book you'll find a complete description of its use.

If you can't locate some of these supplies in your area, all prescription items and most nonprescription items can be ordered via telephone and credit card, check, or money order from Rosedale Pharmacy, (888) 796-3348, or at www.rx4betterhealth.com.

SUPPLIES FOR ALL DIABETICS

For measuring and recording blood sugar	**Approximate cost**
Blood sugar meter outfit (including lancing device and lancets)	$30*
Blood sugar test strips (at least 1 box of 50)	$70/box less a likely discount of $50 during promotional periods
GLUCOGRAF III data sheets	$13/pad of 26 double-sided sheets (covers one year), at Rosedale Pharmacy

For removing blood from clothing	
Hydrogen peroxide	$1

For dehydration	
Morton Lite Salt, Featherweight Salt, Diamel Salt-It, Adolf's Salt, Nu-Salt, etc.	$4.50

For diarrhea	
Lomotil (diphenoxylate HCl with atropine sulfate)	$25/60 ml dropper bottle; $4/100 tablets (generics)

For severe vomiting	
Tigan injectable (trimethobenzamide HCl)	$25/20 ml vial (generic)

For low blood sugars (required if taking medication that lowers blood sugar)	
Dex4 tablets[†]	$7.50/50 scored tablets (4 gm glucose each)
Dex4 Bits	$2.99/60 bits (1 gm glucose)
Dextro Energy, Dextro Energen, SweeTARTS, or Winkies (kosher)	
MedicAlert identification bracelet[‡]	$10–$139

For urine testing during illness	
Ketostix (foil-wrapped), 1 package	$12

---

* See your pharmacist for current mail-in rebate or trade-in deals.
[†] Available at most pharmacies without a prescription under a variety of house label names.
[‡] This is an important product. The bracelet and accompanying contact information (see page 75) can provide paramedics or other medical professionals with considerable information in case of loss of consciousness.

For testing food for sugar

Diastix, 1 package $15

For foot care

Olive oil, vitamin E cream, coconut oil, $5–$15
  mink oil, emu oil, etc.
Bath thermometer $20

For menu planning

The Complete Book of Food Counts, 9th ed., $8.99 (paperback)
  Corinne T. Netzer (Dell, 2011)
Bowes & Church's Food Values of Portions $62.16 (plastic comb bound)
  Commonly Used, 19th ed., Jean A. T.
  Pennington and Judith Spungen
  (Lippincott Williams & Wilkins, 2009)
The NutriBase Complete Book of $5.98 (paperback)
  Food Counts (Avery, 2001)

Artificial sweeteners

Stevia extract $18.95/2 ounces liquid; $18/1
                                                  ounce powder
Saccharin tablets $6/1,000 tablets (1/2 grain)
Equal tablets $2.65/100 tablets

SUPPLIES FOR INSULIN-USING DIABETICS ONLY

Insulins and insulin supplies*

Humalog (Lilly) or Novolog (Novo), 2 vials $125/vial
regular insulin or Novolin R (Novo), 2 vials $55/vial
NPH insulin, 2 vials (to be diluted for small children only) $90/vial
Levemir (Novo), 2 vials $115/vial
Frio (to store insulin while traveling in hot climates) $29
30-unit short-needle insulin syringes with ½-unit markings, $25/box of 100
  such as BD Ultrafine II (get at least 200 to start)
30-unit standard-needle insulin syringes $25/box of 100
  such as BD Ultrafine, for correcting elevated blood sugars
  with *optional* intramuscular injections (get 100 to start)

---

* The particular insulins to be used will vary from one person to another, as indicated in Chapters 17–19.

For low blood sugar emergencies

Glutose 15 (Paddock Laboratories)	$15/3 tubes
Dex4 gel	$3.99/1 tube
Dex4 Liquid Blast	$2.99/2-ounce bottle
Dex4 bits	$2.99/60 bits
Dex4 tablets	$1.99/vial of 10
Dex4 tablets	$7.50/bottle of 50
Glucagon Emergency Kit	$125
Metoclopramide syrup	$20/4-ounce bottle

RECOMMENDED DIABETIC TOOLS — THE DETAILS

For All Diabetics

Blood sugar meter outfit. A blood sugar meter outfit should contain a blood sugar meter, a finger-stick device, and a small startup supply of disposable lancets and test strips. The meter does the same job as the one I bought decades ago, although my old one weighed 3 pounds and some of the new models have footprints smaller than a credit card. They work quite simply: with one drop of blood from a finger stick, the instrument gives you a reading of your blood sugar. (See Chapter 4, "How and When to Measure Blood Sugar.") The batteries for these meters usually die after about one year, so it is wise to store extra batteries in the freezer. It is also wise to own at least two meters, as they can permanently stop working when exposed to high or low temperatures or to high humidity.

Blood sugar meters are available at most pharmacies and chain drugstores. Some are more accurate and reliable than others. Because of the rapid advances in technology, it would be counterproductive to recommend a particular meter in this book.* If you want our current recommendation, call our Diabetes Center at (914) 698-7525, Monday through Thursday, 9:30 A.M. to 2:30 P.M. eastern standard time.

---

* The most accurate personal meter as of this writing is the HemoCue. It is much larger and more difficult to use than other meters and requires much more blood. It is great for calibrating more portable meters.

Disposable lancets. These are used with or without your finger-stick device to puncture your skin for glucose testing. I reuse mine until they become dull. The small supply packed with the various meter outfits may last a year.

Blood sugar test strips. When you stick your finger, you'll put the drop of blood on or into one of these. They work with your meter to give your blood sugar readings.

GLUCOGRAF III data sheets. See Chapter 5, "Recording Blood Sugar Data." These are essential to record your blood sugars and other important data properly. They are available from Rosedale Pharmacy and www.rx4betterhealth.com. These are the only data sheets that I recommend.

Hydrogen peroxide. Now and then, when you're sticking your fingers or injecting through your shirt, as I do, you may get a little blood on your clothing. Hydrogen peroxide is an effective way to eradicate it. You can get small bottles for home, office, car, or travel. Available at any drugstore and at many groceries. (See page 276 for tips on removing bloodstains.)

For dehydration. Dehydrating illnesses, such as vomiting, diarrhea, or fever, are potentially fatal for diabetics. If you become dehydrated, salt substitutes can help you replace lost electrolytes. Look for potassium chloride on the list of ingredients. These should be available at the supermarket or grocery store. Their use is covered in Chapter 21, "How to Cope with Dehydration, Dehydrating Illness, and Infection." They should be used as directed by a physician.

For diarrhea. Diarrhea can cause dehydration. The one product that appears always to work is Lomotil (diphenoxylate HCl with atropine sulfate). This is a prescription drug. Generic versions are available at lower cost. For small children, buy the liquid only. For adults, buy both the liquid and tablets. Alternatively, use 30 mg codeine tablets.

For vomiting. Vomiting can also cause dehydration, which, as noted above, can be life-threatening for diabetics. Injectable Tigan (trimethobenzamide HCl) frequently relieves vomiting and should be used for no more than 1–2 days at a time, unless directed otherwise by your physician. It is available in 20 ml vials, 110 mg/ml. Use as directed in Chapter 21. This product requires a prescription. Generic versions are available.

For low blood sugars. If you experience low blood sugars, glucose tablets are a good, controlled way of bringing them up by precise increments, while minimizing the risk of overshoot that you might experience with, say, a glass of fruit juice or a soft drink. Each Dex4 tablet will raise the blood sugar of a 140-pound person by about 20 mg/dl. Half a scored tablet has half the effect. Dex4 Bits each contain 1 gram of glucose and will raise blood sugar 5 mg/dl for a 140-pound person. If you run out of Dex4 tablets and need an emergency supply of glucose tablets, you can use one of the following: Dextro Energy will raise blood sugar approximately 15 mg/dl; Dextro Energen, 20 mg/dl; SweeTARTS, 10 mg/dl;* and Winkies, 2 mg/dl. (See Chapter 14, "Using Exercise to Enhance Insulin Sensitivity and Slow Aging," and Chapter 20, "How to Prevent and Correct Low Blood Sugars.") Most of these are available through most drugstores; Winkies are available only at kosher food stores. Glucose tablets will not work rapidly enough for people with severe gastroparesis (see page 78 and Chapter 22), so for these people we use Dex4 liquid.

MedicAlert identification bracelets. These bracelets should be worn at all times so that if you happen to become unconscious or confused (for example, after a motor vehicle accident or a cerebral concussion) when you're not with a trained companion, health care professionals will know you're a diabetic and take appropriate action. (Although necklaces are also available, they are less likely than bracelets to be noticed in an emergency. I therefore recommend only the bracelets.) Available by mail order, using forms that your physician should be able to provide, or by phone, (888) 633-4298. They're also available on the Web at www.medicalert.org. By registering with MedicAlert (the cost at this writing is $40 the first year and includes a stainless steel bracelet),† you can inform health care workers how you want to be treated, which is crucial for maintaining reasonable blood sugars. Furthermore, you can have your complete medical history

---

* The size of SweeTARTS varies with the packaging, so 10 mg/dl can likewise vary.
† MedicAlert also offers sterling silver and gold-plated bracelets and ID wristwatches at an additional cost.

available to EMS or emergency room personnel. This includes any directives for care you may have in place (such as not to use a glucose intravenous drip if your blood sugar is not too low). Phone or visit the MedicAlert website for more information.

Ketostix. These dipsticks are for testing your urine for ketones when you are in danger of dehydration. (See Chapter 21.)

Diastix. These are urine test strips for glucose similar to Ketostix, but we use them for testing food (even though they are marketed for testing urine). See Chapter 10, "Diet Guidelines Essential to the Treatment of All Diabetics," to learn how you can use them to determine whether packaged or restaurant foods contain sugar or flour. Available at most pharmacies.

Skin lubricants. In Appendix D you will find foot care guidelines, an important part of diabetic self-care. If your feet are dry, you should use an animal or vegetable oil lubricant. Don't use mineral oils or petroleum-based products, as your skin will not absorb them. Available at Rosedale Pharmacy, drugstores, and health food stores. Olive oil is available at most food markets.

Bath thermometer. Many diabetics have impaired sensation in their feet. Without knowing it, you can scald and seriously injure your feet if showers or baths are too hot. Don't take foot care lightly. Poor foot care for diabetics can lead to amputation, especially if you have poor circulation. Available at most pharmacies.

Books and publications. There are many books of food values that can be helpful in trying to figure out your meal plan (see Chapter 11, "Creating a Customized Meal Plan"). They are optional, but the table lists a few I think are valuable. They can be ordered at most bookstores and through Internet booksellers.

Artificial sweeteners. As we will discuss in Chapter 10, the little packets of artificial sweetener you see on restaurant tables in the United States are predominantly glucose, lactose, or other sugars. Stay away from powdered sweeteners (except pure stevia extract), and always scan the lists of ingredients for any word ending in *-ose* or *-ol*. Also avoid maltodextrin. In the United States, use only tablet sweeteners, stevia liquid, or stevia powder that doesn't have maltodextrin on the label. You can get saccharin or Equal (aspartame) tablets in many drugstores and groceries. Stevia is sold at health food stores. If you have a sweet tooth, there is no restriction on how much of these sweeteners you use. Cyclamates are available in Canada and elsewhere outside the United States. These won't affect your blood sugar.

For Insulin-Using Diabetics

Insulins. The types of insulins I recommend are Humalog (lispro insulin); Novolog (aspart insulin); Apidra (glulisine insulin); regular insulin or Novolin R; and Levemir (detemir insulin). For small children, I recommend NPH, the only longer-acting insulin currently available that can be diluted. These and other insulins are discussed at length in Chapter 17, "Important Information About Various Insulins."

You should keep at least two vials of the insulins selected by your doctor on hand at all times. You may need a prescription, and your physician will select the insulin(s) appropriate for you. A thorough discussion of their characteristics, use, storage, and administration appears in Chapters 16–19.

Frio. This very clever product, a reusable wallet-style cooler activated by immersion in water, will keep insulin cool when you are traveling in hot climates. Frio is available in the United States from Medicool, Inc., (800) 433-2469 or www.medicool.com/diabetes; Rosedale Pharmacy; and www.rx4betterhealth.com. It is available in the U.K. from www.friouk.com.

Insulin syringes. Any 25- or 30-unit short-needle insulin syringe with ½-unit markings should be satisfactory. The syringes come in boxes of 100, and you should get at least 200 to start. They are available with a prescription at most pharmacies. Their use is covered in Chapter 16, "Insulin: The Basics of Self-Injection." Syringes with longer needles for more rapid correction of elevated blood sugars should also be considered after reading Chapters 16–19. Insulin syringes may sometimes be needed by non–insulin users to lower elevated blood sugars caused by sickness (see Chapter 21).

Glutose 15 or Dex4 gel. You will want to show your friends and relatives how to administer this glucose gel if you experience confusion but not unconsciousness from dangerously low blood sugars. Your confusion should lift rapidly as your blood sugar increases toward the normal range. (See Chapter 20.)

Dex4 Liquid Blast. People with severe gastroparesis (see Chapter 22) may not be able to digest glucose tablets rapidly enough to bring blood sugars back to acceptable levels in a hypoglycemic event. This may also be true for athletes during a competition or for anyone anxious to get low blood sugars up as rapidly as possible. This glucose solution is the answer. For a 140-pound diabetic, 1 teaspoon should raise blood sugar by about 6 mg/dl (18 mg/dl per tablespoon). It comes in a 2-ounce bottle and contains 15 grams of glucose. If this product is not available in your country, purchase a 10-ounce bottle of oral glucose tolerance test drink (100 grams of glucose) from any surgical supply dealer. This is one-third stronger than Dex4.

Glucagon Emergency Kit. If you don't live alone, it's important that you have this for the remote possibility that you may become unconscious from dangerously low blood sugars. You will want to train your friends, colleagues, spouse, or other family members in its use. Available by prescription at most pharmacies. It's a good idea to attach a small bottle of metoclopramide syrup (below), by rubber band, to each of your Glucagon Emergency Kits. (See Chapter 20.)

Metoclopramide syrup. Glucagon can cause nausea, and a dose of this syrup when you regain consciousness should keep you from retching. A prescription is required.

I will personally answer questions from readers for one hour every month. This free service is available by visiting www.askdrbernstein.net.

4

How and When to Measure
Blood Sugar

T he nondiabetic body is constantly measuring its levels of blood sugar and compensating for values that are either too high or too low. A diabetic's body has lost much or all of this capability. With a little help from technology, you can take over where your body has left off and do what it once did automatically—normalize your blood sugars.

YOUR BLOOD GLUCOSE PROFILE

No matter how mild your diabetes or even "pre-diabetes" may be, it is very unlikely that any physician can tell you how to normalize your blood sugars throughout the day without knowing what your blood glucose values are around the clock. Don't believe anyone who tells you otherwise. The only way to know what your around-the-clock levels are is to monitor them yourself.

A table of blood sugar levels, with associated events (meals, exercise, and so on), measured at least 5 times daily over a number of days, is the key element in what is called a blood glucose profile. This profile, described in detail in the next chapter, gives you and your physician or diabetes educator a glimpse of how your medication, lifestyle, and diet converge, and how they affect your blood sugars. Without this information, it's impossible to come up with a treatment plan that will normalize blood sugars. Except in emergencies, I try not to treat someone's diabetes until I receive a blood glucose profile that covers at least one week.

Blood glucose data, together with information about meals, blood sugar medication, exercise, and any other pertinent data that affect blood sugar, is best recorded on the GLUCOGRAF III data sheet, illustrated on page 89.

How Frequently Are Glucose Profiles Necessary?

If your treatment includes insulin injections before each meal, your diabetes is probably severe enough to render it impossible for your body to automatically correct small deviations from a target blood glucose range. To achieve blood sugar normalization, it therefore may be necessary for you to record blood glucose profiles every day for the rest of your life, so that you can fine-tune any out-of-range values. If you are not treated with insulin, or if you have a very mild form of insulin-treated diabetes, it may be necessary to prepare blood glucose profiles only when needed for readjustment of your diet or medication. Typically, this might be for one to two weeks prior to every routine follow-up visit to your physician, and for a few weeks while your treatment plan is being fine-tuned for the first time. After all, your physician or diabetes educator cannot tell whether a new regimen is working properly without seeing your blood glucose profiles. It is wise, however, that you also do a blood glucose profile for 1 day at least every other week, so you will be assured that things are continuing as planned.

Selecting a Blood Glucose Measuring Outfit

The measuring system usually consists of a pocket-sized electronic meter with a liquid crystal display. The outfit will include a separate spring-driven finger-sticking device and a supply of lancets. The meter is designed for use with disposable plastic strips, into which a drop of blood is placed. These strips contain electrodes that conduct or generate more or less current depending upon the amount of glucose in the blood.

About seventy different blood glucose metering outfits are currently being marketed in the United States. A few of these have a degree of accuracy acceptable for our purposes. Some systems routinely report blood glucose values that are 20–100 percent in error. This can be very dangerous to the user. How these have secured approval from the Food and Drug Administration (FDA) is a matter of conjecture. Usually the problem involves poor quality control or poor design of the plastic strips, or inability to calibrate the meter accurately for different batches of strips.

Although your supplier should be in a position to advise you properly on the selection of systems for blood glucose monitoring, this is almost never the case. Even physicians and educators specializing in diabetes rarely conduct the studies necessary to evaluate these products. Reports in medical journals that purport to be evaluating different blood glucose self-measurement systems are frequently financed by one of the manufacturers and often present grossly deceptive conclusions. All this puts you, the consumer, in a difficult position.

Designs advance so rapidly that it's impossible to predict what will be available when you read this book. I frequently compare new meters for accuracy versus a major clinical lab, or versus my "gold standard" meter, the HemoCue. This meter is large and slow, making it inconvenient for everyday use. I also check the reproducibility of results. You can call our Diabetes Center at (914) 698-7525, Monday through Thursday between 9:30 A.M. and 2:30 P.M. eastern standard time, to find out what system we currently recommend for our patients.

There are two things to look for in a meter: accuracy and reproducibility (precision). Other "features" are nothing more than marketing gimmicks. You want a meter that would give you the same results if you were to take several readings, one immediately after the other. The meters that I recommend are selected with precision and accuracy in mind. Buy from a dealer who will refund your money if you find the system to be inconsistent or inaccurate. You can test the meter right in the store by taking four readings in succession. They should be within 5 percent of one another when blood sugars are within the 70–120 mg/dl range. I have not found any meters that are suitably precise or accurate above 200 mg/dl, but this upper range will not be important once your blood sugars are usually below 100 mg/dl (18.2 mmol/l). Ask your physician about the systems he has evaluated. He can secure virtually any system from its manufacturer for study at no cost.

A number of my patients have been tempted by advertising for blood sugar meters that contain a built-in device to puncture the skin at sites other than the fingertips (arms, buttocks, abdomen), where the puncture causes absolutely no pain. I have tested several of these products and found their blood sugar readings to be inaccurate. If blood sugar is changing rapidly, these alternative test site results may lag behind fingertip tests by as much as 20 minutes. In my experience, nearly all of the finger sticks that I perform on anyone are painless because I use the technique described in the following section.

MEASURING YOUR BLOOD SUGARS: IMPORTANT TECHNIQUES

Many instruction booklets give inadequate or erroneous directions for preparing and pricking the finger or putting the drop of blood into the test strip. If the instructions that follow conflict with what you've been told, believe mine. My techniques aren't based on something I read in medical school or in a medical journal. They're the ones I use on myself every day. I've been measuring my own blood sugars for more than forty years and have performed hundreds of thousands of finger sticks on myself and thousands of my patients.

1. If you've handled glucose tablets, skin lotion, or any food since last washing your hands, wash them again. Invisible material on your fingers can cause erroneously high readings. Certainly wash your hands if they are soiled. If you are sitting in a car or some other place where you cannot wash your hands, lick the appropriate finger enthusiastically and dry it on a handkerchief or clothing. Don't wipe your fingers with alcohol; this will dry out the skin and can eventually foster the formation of calluses. Neither I nor any of my patients have developed finger infections by not using alcohol, and I surely hold the world record for the number of self-inflicted finger sticks.

2. Unless your fingers are already warm, it may be necessary to rinse them under warm water. Blood will flow much more readily from a warm finger. If your blood sugar is below 60 mg/dl, your finger may not bleed until it is warmed. If you're outdoors in cold weather, store your meter in a pocket next to your body and put your finger under your tongue to warm it.

3. Lay out all the supplies you will need at your work area. These usually include a finger-stick device loaded with a lancet, your blood glucose meter, a blood glucose test strip, and a tissue for blotting your finger after the test. If you have no tissue, just suck off the blood (unless your religion forbids consuming human blood). Insert a disposable test strip into your blood sugar meter.

4. Many spring-activated finger-stick devices come with two rigid plastic covers for the end that touches your finger. Usually one cover is for thin or soft skin (as in small children), while the other is for thick or callused skin. To get a shallower puncture, use the thicker-tipped cover with the smaller hole at the tip. To get a deeper puncture, use the thinner-tipped cover, usually made of clear plastic. Most finger-stick devices have a rotary control that can be dialed to the depth of the puncture that you prefer. An even deeper puncture may be obtained by strongly pressing your finger against the lancet cover. A very shallow puncture may be obtained by barely touching the fingertip to the cover. The pressure of the finger on the cover determines how deep the puncture will go. It should be deep enough to provide an adequate drop of blood, but not be so deep as to cause bruising or pain. Contrary to common teaching, the best sites for pricking fingers are actually on the back (dorsum) of the finger. Prick your finger between the first joint and the nail, or between the first and second joints (not over the knuckles), as shown by the shaded areas in Figure 4-1. Pricking these sites should be less likely to cause pain and more likely to produce a drop of blood than will pricking your fingers on the palmar side of the hand. You will also be free from the calluses that occur after repeated punctures on the palmar surface of the fingers.* When using this technique, I press the tip of the lancing device *very gently* against the finger, as the skin is thinner there than on the palmar surface. If you find it repugnant to prick the dorsum (knuckle side) of your fingers, use the sites on the palmar surface illustrated in Figure 4-2. I actually use all of the sites shown in both diagrams. As you will not be sharing your finger-stick device, you need not discard the disposable

---

* My patients, myself, and many diabetic violinists are much indebted to Ron Raab, president of Insulin for Life, of Ballarat, Victoria, Australia (www.insulin forlife.org), for this not-so-obvious technique. Mr. Raab's attempts to publish this important finding were repeatedly scorned by medical journals and finally came to my attention via personal correspondence. He has had type 1 diabetes since 1956 and favors a low-carbohydrate diet. I use Mr. Raab's technique myself and find it far superior to the palmar technique, which I used for years. By the way, this technique was in common use by physicians eighty years ago. Like so many things in medicine, it had to be rediscovered.

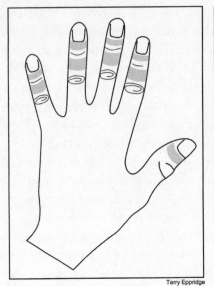

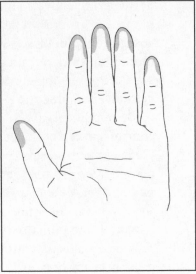

Terry Eppridge

Fig. 4-1. *Sites to prick on the dorsum*   Fig. 4-2. *Sites to prick on the palmar*
of your fingers.   *surface of your fingers.*

plastic lancets with the metal point after every finger stick. It is a good idea to discard them once a week, as they do eventually become dull.

5. Over a period of time, you should use all the fingers of both hands. There is no reason to prefer one finger over the others. Once you have pricked your finger, squeeze it (use a rhythmic action rather than steady pressure) with the opposite hand until the drop of blood is about ¹⁄₁₀ inch (2 mm) in diameter. As you squeeze, the index finger on your squeezing hand should be behind the distal (outermost) joint of the finger you are squeezing. If flow is inadequate (see items 7 and 8), perform a deeper finger stick.

6. Touch the drop of blood to the proper point on the test strip.*

7. Meters will start an automatic countdown as soon as the strip

---

* Most manufacturers provide strips that have an invisible hole at the tip. Blood is sucked into the strip by capillary action. The puncture site should point upward and the tip of the strip must be inserted into the drop of blood. With such strips, the blood should not be put on top of the strip as erroneously practiced by some users.

has absorbed enough blood. The countdown, in seconds, may appear on the display screen and concludes with the appearance of your blood glucose value.

8. Most meters have an automatic timer that begins a countdown preceded by an audible beep that repeats when the strip has been filled.

9. If you get a little blood on your clothing, rub on some hydrogen peroxide with a handkerchief. Wait for the foaming to stop. Then blot and repeat the process. Continue until the blood has disappeared. If you don't have any hydrogen peroxide, try milk or human saliva. This works best while the blood is still wet.

10. When your meter finishes its countdown (or countup, depending on the model), your blood sugar will be shown on the display screen. Write it down on your GLUCOGRAF III data sheet as instructed in Chapter 5.

11. If you are measuring someone else's blood sugars using your personal equipment (not a wise practice), install a fresh lancet each time, and wipe off the end cap of the finger-stick device with fresh bleach after each use. It is possible to transmit serious infectious diseases from one person to another via finger sticks.

The entire process, from pricking the finger to a final reading, takes as little as 3 seconds, and rarely more than 30 seconds.

NOTE: Do not expect accurate blood sugars (or $HgbA_{1C}$) if you have been taking more than 250 mg per day of a vitamin C supplement. Readings may be lower than the true values.

PREPARING FOR YOUR FIRST BLOOD SUGAR CONTROL VISIT TO YOUR PHYSICIAN OR DIABETES EDUCATOR

Make sure you have all the supplies you and your physician have checked off in Chapter 3. Put a string on your finger to remind you to ask someone at the doctor's office to watch you measure your blood sugar and to correct any errors you may make. (About 20 percent of my new patients are not measuring their blood sugars accurately when I first see them.) Bring along at least two weeks' worth of your blood glucose profiles. Ideally, these should be written on GLUCOGRAF III data sheets (see Chapter 5, "Recording Blood Sugar Data"), which have been designed for quick review by the physician or other health care professional. To compile your profiles, blood sugars should be measured:

- Upon rising in the morning
- Immediately before breakfast
- Five hours after every injection of rapid-acting insulin (if you use one of these before meals or to cover elevated blood sugars)
- Before each meal or snack
- Two hours after meals and snacks
- At bedtime
- Before and after exercising, shopping, or running errands
- Whenever you are hungry or suspect that your blood glucose may be higher or lower than usual
- Before driving a car or operating heavy machinery and hourly while engaging in these activities

Once your blood sugars have been fine-tuned, it may not be necessary for you to check them 2 hours after meals and immediately before breakfast. Appropriate times for testing will be specified in subsequent chapters.

I will personally answer questions from readers for
one hour every month. This free service is available by
visiting www.askdrbernstein.net.

5

Recording Blood Sugar Data

USING THE GLUCOGRAF III DATA SHEET

Your blood sugar levels are affected by a variety of things: what medications you are taking (such as insulin or oral hypoglycemic or insulin-sensitizing agents), what exercise you may have performed, whether you've got an infection or cold, what you ate, when you ate it, and others you will discover as you track your blood sugars. Many people find, for example, that such things as competitive exercise, public speaking, or arguments can raise blood sugars. All of these bits of information — not just your blood sugar levels — need to be recorded and taken into account. Without this detailed information — your own personal blood sugar profile — your physician or diabetes educator cannot assist you in developing an ongoing program for blood sugar normalization. To my knowledge, none of the many forms or computer programs currently available for this purpose show adequate information in a readily usable format. The GLUCOGRAF III data sheet,* like our program, was designed by a diabetic engineer (me) for diabetics.

GLUCOGRAF III data sheets are printed identically on both sides so

---

* GLUCOGRAF is a registered trademark owned by Richard K. Bernstein, MD. The data sheet form is protected by U.S. copyright, and may not be reproduced for sale without permission of the author. Readers of this book who wish to have some practice copies for immediate use may make photocopies of the form, which is reproduced at a reduced size on page 89 in order to make it fit into this book. Most photocopiers can enlarge the image in order to provide you with standard 8½ × 11 sheets. Pads containing enough pages to cover one year can be ordered by phone from Rosedale Pharmacy, (888) 796-3348, or from www.rx4betterhealth.com.

that each page provides space for two weeks' worth of data. If your physician wants detailed information about the content of each of your meals, use one side to list meal content and the reverse to list medication, blood sugars, exercise, the times of your meals, and so on. The data sheet is designed so that you can fold it up and carry it with you. I recommend carrying a fine-point pen (0.1 mm) with you as well. It will help when space is tight—which is likely, particularly in the MEDICATION, EXERCISE, FOOD, ETC. column, where much information must be written in a small space. If you will be faxing, scanning, or e-mailing your sheets to your physician, do not use pencil, as it doesn't always copy or transmit clearly.

The rest of this chapter is divided into sections corresponding to column and field headings on the GLUCOGRAF III form, and explains the sorts of things you ought to be recording and the most informative ways for doing so.

DATA FIELDS

Across the top of the data sheet, there are several fields with space for entering important information.

NAME. Entering your name will ensure that the form will end up in your chart at your doctor's office and not in someone else's.

DOCTOR'S PHONE. This field should contain the telephone number at which you can reach your physician when you are asked to discuss your blood sugar and other data.

DOCTOR'S FAX/E-MAIL. If you will be faxing your data sheets, enter your physician's fax number as well. Alternatively, if you would usually scan and e-mail your form, you might enter his e-mail address here—or just put it in your "address book."

TARGET BG. This is the blood sugar goal that your physician will assign and that you will try to maintain. Although normal is approximately 80–85 mg/dl, in certain instances your physician may opt for a higher value for a brief period. If you've endured very high blood sugar levels for an extended period of time, your physician will not instantly try to normalize your blood sugars, as you may at first feel uncomfortable

GlucograF III DATA SHEET

© 2006 Richard K. Bernstein, M.D., Mamaroneck, NY 10543

Name:

DOCTOR'S PHONE

DOCTOR'S FAX / E-MAIL

TARGET BG

USUAL DOSES OF INSULIN OR ORAL AGENT
Upon Arising
___ Min. pre / post bkfst.
___ Min. pre / post lunch
___ Min. pre / post dinner
___ Min. pre / post snacks
At Bedtime

1 Unit ___ Will ___
Lower Blood ___ mg/dl
Sugar

MISCELLANEOUS

BG EFFECTS OF SWEETS (mg/dl)
1 gm CHO →

EXERCISE ADJUSTMENTS

ABBREVIATIONS

DATE WEEK BEGINS / /

	SUNDAY		MONDAY		TUESDAY		WEDNESDAY		THURSDAY		FRIDAY		SATURDAY	
	TIME	BLOOD SUGAR	MEDICATION, EXERCISE, FOOD, etc.	TIME	BLOOD SUGAR	MEDICATION, EXERCISE, FOOD, etc.	TIME	BLOOD SUGAR	MEDICATION, EXERCISE, FOOD, etc.	TIME	BLOOD SUGAR	MEDICATION, EXERCISE, FOOD, etc.	TIME	BLOOD SUGAR	MEDICATION, EXERCISE, FOOD, etc.
1 AM THRU 6 AM															
6 AM THRU 9 AM															
9 AM THRU 12 NOON															
12 NOON THRU 3 PM															
3 PM THRU 6 PM															
6 PM THRU 9 PM															
9 PM THRU 1 AM															

(hypoglycemic) at a normal value. If you take insulin, he'll assign a series of intermediate target values, together with instructions for correcting blood sugars to reach these levels as you work toward blood sugar normalization. If your initial blood sugars show that you are in the 300–400 mg/dl range, he might set a target of, say, 175 mg/dl for a brief time. If you have gastroparesis (delayed stomach-emptying; see Chapter 22) and use insulin, you are at real risk for severe hypoglycemia. Your physician may therefore recommend a target well above normal for an indefinite period of time, to provide a safety factor that reduces the likelihood of very low blood sugars.

USUAL DOSES OF INSULIN OR ORAL AGENT. If you require insulin or an insulin-sensitizing or insulin-mimetic agent* to maintain your target range, you will have to follow a precise regimen. It will therefore be important to have your blood sugar medications spelled out so that even if you forget, you can always refer to the doses and times in this field. When you are to take a medication before a meal, cross out "post" (as shown below); when you are to take one after a meal, cross out "pre."

If your physician asks you to change the dose of one of your blood sugar–lowering medications, put a line through the prior dosage and enter the new dose to the right of the old one, as in the following example:

```
┌─────────────────────────────────────────────────────────────┐
│ USUAL DOSES OF INSULIN OR ORAL AGENT                          │
│ Upon  Arising    2 Lev  1½ Lev                                │
│ _____ Min. pre / post bkfst. _____│
│ _____ Min. pre / post lunch _____│
│  90   Min. pre / post dinner  3 X 500 Gluc 2 X 500 Gluc      │
│ _____ Min. pre / post snacks _____ │
│ At Bedtime                                                    │
└─────────────────────────────────────────────────────────────┘
```

In this fictitious example, the patient had been injecting 2 units of Levemir insulin on arising when this data sheet was started. In addition to insulin, he had been taking three 500 mg tablets of Glucophage (an insulin-sensitizing agent) 90 minutes before dinner. During the week the sheet covers, his dose of insulin on arising was reduced to 1½ units and his dose of Glucophage before dinner was reduced to two

---

* Insulin-sensitizing and insulin-mimetic agents are blood sugar–lowering pills that you may be using. They are discussed in detail in Chapter 15, "Oral Insulin-Sensitizing Agents, Insulin-Mimetic Agents, and Other Options."

500 mg tablets. Retaining the old doses in this field can give your physician an important at-a-glance history of the changes that were made.

1 UNIT ___ WILL LOWER BLOOD SUGAR [insert the abbreviation of your more-rapid-acting insulin]. This field is for use only by people who take insulin and use rapid-acting insulin to bring down elevated blood sugars. In Chapter 19, "Intensive Insulin Regimens," we'll discuss guidelines for calibrating the effect that 1 unit of rapid-acting insulin will have upon your blood sugar. Meanwhile, enter on the form the amount of blood sugar reduction (mg/dl) that your physician suggests will be achieved by injecting 1 unit.

MISCELLANEOUS. This field (box) is for any other pertinent guidelines or instructions that you may have difficulty recalling. Some people enter the times they should check their blood sugars. Thus, depending on your regimen, you might write:

✓ BG -on arising
     -before meals
     -2 hr post meals
     -bedtime
     -when hungry

If this field is too small for all you wish to enter, use the top margin of the form.

BG EFFECTS OF SWEETS. If you use insulin or oral agents, you will be taught how to use glucose tablets or liquid to raise your blood sugar rapidly. In Chapter 20, "How to Prevent and Correct Low Blood Sugars," we'll discuss how you will calibrate the effect that 1 tablet has on your blood sugar. Thus, if 1 Dex4 raises your blood sugar 18 mg/dl, you would write:

1 D4 → ↑18

Alternatively, if your brand of glucose tablet is Wacky Wafers (which might raise your blood sugar 10 mg/dl), you could write:

1 WW → ↑10

You will also learn to calibrate the effect 1 gram of carbohydrate has on your blood sugar. If 1 gram will raise your blood sugar 5 mg/dl, you would write:

1 gm CHO → ↑5

EXERCISE ADJUSTMENTS. This field is also used only if you use insulin or oral agents. It reminds you what to eat for various forms of exercise to prevent your blood sugar from dropping too low. Thus, if you were planning to spend the afternoon at a shopping mall (which can be treacherous, because this often requires considerably more walking than we realize), you may be advised to eat half a slice of bread at the start of every hour to keep your blood sugar from falling too low. Thus, you might write:

Mall — ½ brd/hr

ABBREVIATE NAMES OF ACTIVITIES AND MEDICATIONS. Space constraints make it necessary to use abbreviations. Use the first one to three letters of the name of each activity or medication. Using these abbreviations will help both you and your physician to know immediately the details of "events" that affect your blood sugar.

DAY-BY-DAY RECORD OF EVENTS

As you can see, each day is broken up horizontally into three columns — TIME; BLOOD SUGAR; and MEDICATION, EXERCISE, FOOD, ETC. Vertically, each column is broken up into 3-hour blocks, except the 9 PM THRU 1 AM and 1 AM THRU 6 AM blocks, which are 4-hour and 5-hour blocks, respectively. During each day, you will experience various "events" involving your blood sugar. An event may be a meal, a dose of medication, exercise, or even a blood sugar measurement itself. These should be recorded in the corresponding column and time block. You should not record a dose of medication that does not affect your blood sugar levels, such as blood pressure medication.

TIME. In this column, write the exact time of the event. If you measured your blood sugar at 1:30 P.M. on Tuesday, write 1:30 in the 12 NOON THRU 3 PM block of the time column for Tuesday.

BLOOD SUGAR. In this column, write all blood sugar readings. If for some reason you do not have your blood sugar meter with you (a minor crime) and you experience symptoms suggestive of low blood sugar, write "Low?" in this column in the appropriate time block and proceed with the instructions for correcting low blood sugar in Chapter 20.

MEDICATION, EXERCISE, FOOD, ETC. This column is a catchall where you should record all events other than blood sugar readings. Following are a few examples of events and how you would record them in abbreviated form in the proper blocks:

Injected 5 units of Levemir insulin	5 Lev
Ate breakfast	B
Consumed more food at dinner than prescribed	↑DIN
Took ½ Dex4 (glucose tablet)	½ D4
Took two 500 mg Glucophage (metformin) pills	2 × 500 GP
Walked 2 miles	Walk 2 mi
Went shopping for 3 hours	Shop 3 hr
Injected 1½ units Humalog insulin, intramuscularly (into a muscle)	1½ H — IM
Sore throat all day	Sore throat [enter at the top of the day's column]
Went to dentist	Dentist

UNUSUAL OR UNEXPECTED BLOOD SUGAR VALUES

Once your blood sugars have been fine-tuned on one of the regimens described in this book, we expect that they will remain within narrow limits of your target value most of the time. There will, in all likelihood, be instances when your blood sugars will deviate from your target range.

Show What Caused Blood Sugars to Deviate

Sometimes you may stick precisely to your diet and medication plan but then find yourself in a restaurant and simply incapable of letting the dessert cart go by without partaking of its wonders. Your blood sugars will naturally show a precipitous rise. Or you may get some exercise that makes your blood sugar go too low. To make it easy for both you and your physician to understand and evaluate such connections, circle the cause, then circle the resulting blood sugar value, and connect the two circles with a line. For example, a high morning blood sugar might be circled and connected to "snack" at bedtime the previous night.

Circle Puzzling Blood Sugar Values

Even though you stick to your regimen with an iron will, your data will sometimes show an unexpectedly high or low blood sugar value. Repeat the measurement after washing your hands (to remove any traces of food or glucose) and ensure that you haven't inadvertently slipped on your measurement technique. If the unexpected reading persists, circle this value, as it may require further investigation. There are several strange biologic phenomena that can affect your blood sugar, and these are detailed in the next chapter. Your physician or diabetes educator should help you figure out the cause of unexpected blood sugar readings so that you can prevent or anticipate them in the future.

Now that you have been exposed to blood sugar self-monitoring and the recording of data, you can begin using this knowledge to normalize your blood sugars.

I will personally answer questions from readers for
one hour every month. This free service is available by
visiting www.askdrbernstein.net.

6

Strange Biology

PHENOMENA PECULIAR TO DIABETES
THAT CAN AFFECT BLOOD SUGAR

S ometimes, even when you think you're doing everything right, your blood sugars may not respond as you expect. Often this will be due to one or more of the biologic curiosities that affect diabetics. The purpose of this chapter is to acquaint you with some real phenomena that can confound your plans, but which you can frequently circumvent if you are aware of them.

DIMINISHED PHASE I INSULIN RESPONSE

Figure 1-2 (page 47) illustrates the normal, nondiabetic blood insulin response to a meal containing carbohydrate and protein. When glucose from dietary carbohydrate enters the bloodstream, beta cells of the pancreas respond—or should respond—immediately by releasing stored insulin granules. These granules may have been stored for many hours in anticipation of what is known as a glucose challenge. This rapid release is called phase I insulin response.

The nondiabetic body will utilize this immediate release of insulin to prevent blood sugar from increasing significantly. As we discussed in Chapter 1, "Diabetes: The Basics," one of the hallmarks of type 2 diabetes is the diminished ability to do this. Therefore, blood sugars will shoot up after eating (carbohydrates in particular) and will be brought back into line only slowly by phase II insulin response (the release of newly manufactured insulin). This blood sugar rise can be minimized, primarily by dietary manipulation, but for some diabetics by diet and/or oral agents or injected insulin.

A possible but unproven explanation for diminished or absent phase I insulin response in diabetics is that the beta cells are still capable of making insulin but not capable of storing it. In this model, insulin would be released almost as soon as it is made. This inability to store insulin could also explain the inappropriate release of insulin that often occurs when blood sugar is already low in very early type 2 diabetes. Such individuals may experience blood sugars that are both too high and too low in the same day — even without medication. An alternative explanation is that the sensitivity of the beta cells to changes in blood sugar diminishes, so that they respond inadequately to such changes.

GLUCONEOGENESIS, THE DAWN PHENOMENON, AND DELAYED STOMACH-EMPTYING

You may begin to notice as you regularly monitor your blood sugars that your fasting blood glucose on waking in the morning is considerably higher than it was when you went to bed, even though you didn't get up for a midnight snack. There are three common causes for this: gluconeogenesis, the dawn phenomenon, and gastroparesis (delayed stomach-emptying).

Gluconeogenesis

Gluconeogenesis, which we discussed briefly in Chapter 1, is the mechanism by which the liver (and, to a lesser degree, the kidneys and intestines) converts amino acids into glucose. Dietary protein is not the only source of amino acids. The proteins of your muscles and other tissues continually receive amino acids from and return them to the bloodstream. This constant flux ensures that amino acids are always available in the blood for conversion to glucose (gluconeogenesis) by the liver or to protein by the muscles and vital organs. Some diabetics still make adequate insulin to prevent gluconeogenesis. However, once your insulin production drops below a certain level, your liver (and your kidneys and intestines) will inappropriately produce glucose and thus raise your blood sugar even while you're fasting.

In all likelihood, you won't be able to control this phenomenon by diet alone, particularly if you're a type 1 diabetic or a type 2 making far too little insulin to offset your insulin resistance. For type 2s, appropriate weight loss and vigorous exercise may be most helpful in improving the sensitivity of the liver and muscles to whatever insulin remains. The most reliable treatments will involve medication, either certain oral agents or insulin. If you're obese, however, large doses of insulin can make you more obese and more resistant to insulin. So a major goal should be to bring your weight into line.

The Dawn Phenomenon

As you know, I'm a type 1 diabetic. I may no longer make any insulin at all. If I decide to fast for 24 hours—eat absolutely nothing—I will need to inject 4 units of long-acting insulin in the morning to prevent gluconeogenesis for 18 hours. If I check my blood sugar every few hours, it will remain constant, confirming that the insulin is suppressing gluconeogenesis.

If, 18 hours after my first injection—and while still fasting—I inject another 4 units of insulin, common sense would maintain that this second dose should suppress gluconeogenesis overnight. In reality it doesn't. I must set an alarm for 4 hours later and then insert another 4 units.

So I go to sleep and awaken 9–10 hours later. On arising, I check my blood sugar. Instead of being constant, as it was during my waking hours, it's now 20–100 mg/dl higher than it was at bedtime.

If I were to try the same experiment a week later, I'd experience about the same overnight rise in blood sugar. Why?

Although the mechanics of the dawn phenomenon aren't yet entirely clear, research suggests that the liver deactivates more circulating insulin during the early morning hours than at other times of the day. It doesn't matter whether you made the insulin yourself or injected it; the liver has no preference. With inadequate circulating insulin to prevent gluconeogenesis, your blood sugars may be higher in the morning than they were at bedtime.* This isn't a problem for a nondiabetic, because a body with fully functional pancreatic beta cells will just make more insulin.

Investigators have actually measured blood sugar every hour throughout the night. They have found that the entire blood sugar increase occurs about 8–10 hours after bedtime for most people who

---

* Consuming alcohol at bedtime can inhibit gluconeogenesis overnight, but not in a predictable fashion.

are so affected. That doesn't mean, however, that you should sleep only 7 hours a night to try to avoid it. Both the time it takes for blood sugar to increase and the amount of the increase vary from one person to another. An increase may be negligible in some and profound in others. This is one of many reasons why any truly workable program for blood sugar normalization must be tailored to the individual.

Though it is more apparent in type 1 diabetics, many type 2 diabetics also show signs of the dawn phenomenon. As you will see, the treatments described in this book enable us to circumvent this blood sugar rise.

Gastroparesis

This condition has a chapter all its own (Chapter 22, "Delayed Stomach-Emptying"), and we will discuss it there in detail. However, it's important to mention it in any list of factors that can lead to puzzling blood sugar readings.

Most people who've had long-standing diabetes develop some degree of damage to the nerves that govern the muscles of the stomach and intestines. Gastroparesis diabeticorum (the weak or paralyzed stomach of diabetics) is caused by many years of elevated blood sugars. If you're a type 1, or a type 2 who isn't making significant amounts of insulin, it can have unpredictable effects on blood sugar.

Like diabetes itself, gastroparesis can be mild to severe. In extreme cases, people may walk around for days with constipation, belching or vomiting, midchest burning, and bulging stomachs. Much more common, however, is mild gastroparesis in which physical symptoms are not apparent but blood sugars are erratic.

The big problems with gastroparesis arise if you're taking insulin. If you take your insulin before a meal to prevent a subsequent rise in blood sugar but the meal remains in your stomach and glucose doesn't enter the bloodstream as predicted, the insulin can take your blood sugar dangerously low. I know three individuals who experienced daily episodes of unconsciousness and seizures from time to time after meals for several years before I met them and diagnosed this condition.

There are, however, ways of greatly improving blood sugars in spite of the unpredictability of this condition, and these are discussed in Chapter 22.

STRESS AND BLOOD SUGAR

Sustained Emotional Stress

For years, many physicians have been blaming emotional stress for the frequent unexplained blood sugar variations that many patients experience. This is an evasive and possibly self-serving diagnosis. It puts the responsibility for unexplained variations in blood sugar on the patient's shoulders and leaves the physician with no obligation to examine the treatment regimen. Certainly there is no question that stress can have adverse effects upon your health. I have reviewed more than a million blood sugar entries from many patients, including myself. One common feature of all this data is that most prolonged emotional stress rarely has a direct effect upon blood sugar. This kind of stress can, however, have a secondary effect by precipitating over-eating, binge eating, or indulgence in kinds of eating that will increase blood sugar.

I know many diabetics who've been involved in stressful marriages, divorces, loss of a business, slow death of a close relative, and the countless other sustained stresses of life we all must endure. These stresses have one thing in common: they aren't sudden but usually last days, or even years. I have yet to see such a situation directly cause blood sugar to increase — or, for that matter, decrease. An important thing to remember during sustained periods of life when everything seems out of control is that at least you can control one thing: your blood sugar.

Adrenaline Surges

Many patients have reported sudden blood sugar spurts after brief episodes of severe stress. Examples have included an automobile accident without physical injury; speaking in front of a large audience; taking very important exams in school; and having arguments that nearly become violent. I am occasionally interviewed on television, and I always check — and, if necessary, adjust — my blood sugar immediately before and after such appearances. Until I eventually became accustomed to this, my blood sugar would inevitably increase 75–100 mg/dl, even though on the surface I might have appeared relaxed. As a rule of thumb, from personal experience and from observing my patients, I would say that if an acute event is stressful enough to start your epinephrine (adrenaline) flowing, as indicated by rapid heart rate and tremors, it is likely to raise your blood sugar. Epinephrine is one of the counterregulatory hormones that cause the liver to convert stored glycogen to glucose. This is part of what is often called the "fight or flight" response, your body's attempt to provide you with enough extra energy either to overcome an enemy or run like heck to get away. Type 2 diabetics who make a lot of insulin are less likely to have their blood sugar reflect acute stress than are those who make little or none.

An occasional blood sugar increase after a very stressful event may well have been brought on by the event. On the other hand, unexplained blood sugar increases extending for days or weeks can rarely be properly attributed to stress. I know of no instances where prolonged emotional stress caused abnormal blood sugars in diabetic or nondiabetic individuals. Therefore, if you experience a prolonged unexplained change in your blood sugar levels after extended periods of normal blood sugars, it is wise to seek out a cause other than emotional stress.

General Anesthesia
If not treated with special dosing of insulin, type 1 and most type 2 diabetics with previously level, normal blood sugars may experience a blood sugar increase during surgery that is accompanied by general anesthesia.

Insulin Resistance Caused by Elevated Blood Sugars
There are at least five causes of insulin resistance — inheritance, dehydration, infection, obesity, and high blood sugars. Insulin's ability to facilitate the transport of glucose from the blood into liver, muscle, fat, and other cells is impaired as blood sugar rises. This reduced effectiveness of insulin, known as insulin resistance, has been attributed to a phenomenon called postreceptor defects in glucose utilization. If, for example, 1 unit of injected or self-made insulin will usually lower blood sugar from 130 to 90 mg/dl, someone with insulin resistance caused by elevated blood sugars may require 3 units to lower it from 430 to 390 mg/dl.

Consider what might happen if I, a type 1 diabetic, am fasting and inject just enough long-acting insulin to keep my blood sugar at 90 mg/dl for 18 hours. If I eat 8 grams of glucose — enough to raise my blood sugar to 130 mg/dl — the chances are that, because of the elevated blood sugar, my blood sugar won't just rise to 130 mg/dl and remain there. It will continue to rise slowly throughout the day, so that 12 hours after I consumed the glucose, my blood sugar might actually be 165 mg/dl. Insulin resistance, at least for type 1 diabetics, occurs as blood sugar increases, and so elevated blood sugar should be corrected as soon as it's feasible. Delay will only permit it to rise higher. Because type 2s still produce some insulin, their bodies are more likely to eventually correct the blood sugar rise automatically.

We will discuss dehydration as a cause of insulin resistance in Chapter 21. Infections are discussed at the end of this chapter and also in Chapter 21.

THE CHINESE RESTAURANT EFFECT

Many years ago a patient asked me why her blood sugar went from 90 mg/dl up to 300 mg/dl every afternoon after she went swimming. I asked what she ate before the swim. "Nothing, just a freebie," she replied. As it turned out, the "freebie" was lettuce. When I asked her just how much lettuce she was eating before her swims, she replied, "A head."

A head of lettuce contains about 10 grams of carbohydrate, which can raise a type 1 adult's blood sugar about 50 mg/dl at most. So what accounts for the other 160 mg/dl rise in her blood sugar?

The explanation lies in what I call the Chinese restaurant effect. Often Chinese restaurant meals contain large amounts of protein or slow-acting, low-carbohydrate foods, such as bean sprouts, bok choy, mushrooms, bamboo shoots, and water chestnuts, which can make you feel full.

How can these low-carbohydrate foods affect blood sugar so dramatically?

The upper part of the small intestine contains cells that release hormones into the bloodstream when they are stretched, as after a meal. These hormones signal the pancreas to produce some insulin to prevent the blood sugar rise that might otherwise follow the digestion of a meal. Large meals will cause greater stretching of the intestinal cells, which in turn will secrete proportionately larger amounts of these "incretin" hormones. Since a very small amount of insulin released by the pancreas can cause a large drop in blood sugar, the pancreas simultaneously produces the less potent hormone glucagon to offset the potential excess effect of the insulin. If you're diabetic and deficient in producing insulin, you might not be able to release insulin, but you will still release glucagon, which will cause gluconeogenesis and glyco-genolysis and thereby raise your blood sugar. Thus, if you eat enough to feel stuffed, your blood sugar can go up by a large amount, even if you eat something indigestible, such as sawdust. Even a small amount of an indigestible substance will cause a blood sugar increase in type 1 diabetics if not covered by an insulin injection.

Complicating matters further, pancreatic beta cells also make a hormone called amylin. Amylin inhibits the effectiveness of glucagon and works on the brain to cause satiety. It also slows stomach-emptying to discourage overeating. With few or no beta cells, diabetics don't make enough amylin, and consequently they tend to remain hungry after eating and show an exaggerated Chinese restaurant effect. Since the first edition of this book, amylin substitutes have become available and have found an important use in the prevention of overeating (see page 214).

The first lesson here is: *Don't stuff yourself.* The second lesson is: *There's no such thing as a freebie.** Any solid food that you eat can raise your blood sugar.[†] If you can't control your overeating, see page 260.

THE EFFECTS OF EXERCISE UPON BLOOD SUGAR

Exercise can have varying effects upon blood sugar, depending upon a number of variables, including the type of exercise, how vigorously it's performed, when it is performed, and what type of medication you are using, if any. These effects are too varied and numerous to discuss in this brief space. Please see Chapter 14, "Using Exercise to Enhance Insulin Sensitivity and Slow Aging," if you are embarking on an exercise program or find your blood sugars unpredictably affected by your existing exercise program.

---

* Except for noncaloric fluids that flow through the intestines without causing distention.
† Several readers from China have e-mailed me that their restaurants don't use sweet sauces, so this effect shouldn't apply to them. This is a misunderstanding of the effect—the Chinese restaurant effect is caused by any solid foods. It is also caused by nutrient-loaded foods containing carbohydrate, protein, or fat.

THE HONEYMOON PERIOD

At the time they are diagnosed, type 1 diabetics usually have experienced very high blood sugars that cause a host of unpleasant symptoms, such as weight loss, frequent urination, and severe thirst. These symptoms subside soon after treatment with injected insulin begins. After a few weeks of insulin therapy, many patients experience a dramatic reduction of insulin requirements, almost as if the diabetes were reversing. Blood sugars may become nearly normal, even with discontinuation of insulin injections. This benign "honeymoon period" may last weeks, months, or even as long as a year. If the medical treatment is conventional, the honeymoon period eventually terminates and the well-known roller coaster of blood sugar swings ensues.

Why doesn't the honeymoon period last forever? My experience with patients indicates that it can, *with proper treatment*. But there are several likely reasons why it does not with conventional treatment. At this writing, however, they still remain speculative.

- The normal human pancreas contains many more insulin-producing beta cells than are necessary for maintaining normal blood sugars. For blood sugar to increase abnormally, at least 80 percent of the beta cells must have been destroyed. In early type 1 diabetes, many of the remaining 20 percent have been weakened by glucose toxicity from constant high blood sugars and by beta cell overwork. These beta cells can recover if they are given a rest with the help of injected insulin. Even if they recover, however, they still must work at least five times as hard to match the job of a normal pancreas working at 100 percent capacity. Eventually, with conventional treatment, this overwork helps cause them to burn out.
- It is now believed that high blood glucose levels are toxic to beta cells. Even a brief blood sugar increase after a high-carbohydrate meal may take a small toll. Over time, the cumulative effect may wipe them out completely.
- The autoimmune attack upon beta cells, the presumed cause of type 1 diabetes, is focused upon several proteins. One is insulin, and another is GADA, present on the special vesicles—or bubbles—that are formed at the outer membrane of the beta

cell. These vesicles contain insulin granules. Normally, they burst at the surface of the cell, releasing insulin granules into the bloodstream. The more vesicles created when more insulin is manufactured, the greater the autoimmune attack upon the beta cell. If less insulin is released, less GADA is exposed to attack.

Based upon my experience with the fair number of type 1 diabetics I've treated from the time of diagnosis, I'm convinced that the honeymoon period can be prolonged indefinitely. The trick is to assist the pancreas and keep it as quiescent as possible. With the meticulous use of small doses of injected insulin and with the essential use of a very low carbohydrate diet, the remaining capacity of the pancreas, I believe, can be preserved.

TESTOSTERONE AND INSULIN RESISTANCE

Low serum free testosterone levels can cause insulin resistance in men, and elevated levels can cause insulin resistance in women. Since the situation for women is discussed in Appendix E, "Polycystic Ovarian Syndrome," here we will cover only low testosterone in men.

The clues that remind me to test men for low free serum testosterone are:

- Excessive breast tissue
- Abdominal obesity without overeating
- A need to inject large doses of insulin (typically more than 65 units per day) in order to normalize blood sugar

These three clues need not all appear — any one of them is good reason to perform a blood test.

When serum free testosterone is below the lower fifth of the normal range, I prescribe self-injection of testosterone cipionate (200 mg/ml) once or twice per week. We then periodically retest on a day midway between two injections and repeat testing until the level is in the middle of the normal range. I usually start with injections of 0.2 ml in a "tuberculin" syringe or 20 units in a long-needle insulin syringe.

I don't prescribe testosterone gel or skin patches because most men find them to be irritating or difficult to remember to use. They would rather inject once or twice weekly.

With testosterone use, I usually see about a one-third drop in insulin requirement and more rapid weight loss.

INFECTION AND ITS EFFECT ON BLOOD SUGARS

Another kind of stress to which your body can become subject—and which can muddy and in some instances wreak havoc on your best efforts to control blood sugars—is infection. I have saved this category of stress for last not because it is the least important, but because, when present, it can be the most important.

A kidney infection, for example, can triple insulin requirements overnight. When blood sugar rises unexpectedly after weeks of normal values, it is wise to suspect infection. I have noted that my own blood sugars rise 24 hours before the onset of a sore throat or cold. Everyone in my family takes Sambucus lozenges (made from an extract of the black elderberry tree) at the first sign of a cold, and I highly recommend it. You can purchase them by mail order from Rosedale Pharmacy, (888) 796-3348; from www.rx4betterhealth.com; or at most health food stores.

Dental Infections

Quite often, dental infections won't be obvious, but high blood sugars cause dental infections, and in the typical vicious circle of diabetes, these infections can cause very high blood sugars. You cannot easily control blood sugars under these circumstances. I have seldom met a long-standing diabetic over age forty (with a history of uncontrolled blood sugars) who had all his teeth.

Frequent dental infections can be a sign of diabetes for those who have not already been diagnosed. I have had many patients who have undergone multiple root canals or gum treatments prior to the diagnosis of diabetes.

If your insulin* "isn't working"—that is, your normal dose isn't acting as you think it should be—and you have determined that your insulin isn't contaminated (for example, by reusing syringes) or expired, the first place to look is in your mouth.

---

* Or oral agents for controlling blood sugar.

First, look at your gums to see if there's any sign of infection—e.g., redness, swelling, tenderness to pressure. Put some water with crushed ice in your mouth for 30 seconds. If a tooth hurts, you should suspect an infection.

Get an emergency appointment with your dentist immediately. He can determine if you have a superficial infection, and can X-ray where your teeth are sensitive, but he should refer you to an endodontist (a dentist who deals with root canals and the jawbone) or a periodontist (who treats infected gums). This kind of infection is extremely common in diabetics and should be addressed as rapidly as possible in order to allow you to bring your blood sugars under control. We will discuss this subject further in Chapter 21.

INFLAMMATION — POSSIBLY THE UNDERLYING CAUSE OF INSULIN RESISTANCE

As you know by now, type 2 diabetes involves two metabolic defects—insulin resistance and inadequate insulin production to overcome this resistance. Although insulin resistance can occur at many sites along the pathways involved in glucose metabolism, there appears to be a common factor causing defects at a variety of sites—inflammation. Inflammation results from the response of the immune system to intrusions such as infection. When a wound becomes infected, the pain, swelling, redness, warmth, and production of pus or fluids are all part of the immune response that aims to destroy the intruding organisms. Other causes of inflammation that can generate insulin resistance include mesenteric fat that covers the intestines (abdominal obesity), autoimmune disorders such as systemic lupus erythematosus, juvenile rheumatoid arthritis, and celiac disease. It is likely that even unlucky genetic inheritance can cause other, unknown inflammatory disorders.

I've had several diabetic patients who also had lupus. Their lupus often became more severe in warm weather and at night. These were the times when their blood sugars would also dramatically increase.

Sometimes, but certainly not always, markers of inflammation will show up when testing the blood. Such tests include serum beta$_2$ microglobulin, C-reactive protein, ferritin, complement C3, erythrocyte sedimentation rate, tumor necrosis factor alpha, and serum fibrinogen activity. When one or more of these tests are positive, further workup by an immunologist may be warranted.

I have seen reports of many studies where anti-inflammatory antioxidants have supposedly been successfully used to reduce insulin resistance, but I have never observed this firsthand. I do not object to experimentation, but I also do not expect dramatic results. Some of the treatments discussed include green tea and green tea extract, R-alpha lipoic acid (R-ALA), and sources of omega-3 fatty acids such as fish oil, flaxseed, and perilla oil.

> I will personally answer questions from readers for one hour every month. This free service is available by visiting www.askdrbernstein.net.

7

The Laws of Small Numbers

Big inputs make big mistakes; small inputs make small mistakes." That is the first thing my friend Kanji Ishikawa would say to himself each morning on arising. It was his mantra, the single most important thing he knew about diabetes.

Kanji was, until 2009, the oldest surviving type 1 diabetic in Japan. Though younger than I, he was afflicted with numerous long-term diabetic complications, because of many years of uncontrolled blood sugar, prior to reading my first book.

Many biological and mechanical systems respond in a predictable way to small inputs but in a chaotic and considerably less predictable way to large inputs. Consider for a moment traffic. Put a small number of automobiles on a given stretch of highway and traffic acts in a predictable fashion: cars can maintain speed, enter and merge into open spaces, and exit with a minimum of danger. There's room for error. Double the number of cars and the risks don't just double, they increase geometrically. Triple or quadruple the number of cars and the unpredictability of a safe trip increases exponentially.

The name of the game for the diabetic in achieving blood sugar normalization is *predictability*. It's very difficult to use medications safely unless you can predict the effects they'll have. Nor can you normalize blood sugar unless you can predict the effects of what you're eating.

If you can't accurately predict your blood sugar levels, then you can't accurately predict your needs for insulin or oral blood sugar–lowering agents. If the kinds of foods you're eating give you consistently unpredictable blood sugar levels, then it will be impossible to normalize blood sugars.

One of the prime purposes of this book is to give you the information you need to learn to predict your blood sugar levels and how to ensure that your predictions will be accurate. Here the Laws of Small Numbers are exceedingly important.

Predictability. How do you achieve it?

THE LAW OF CARBOHYDRATE ESTIMATION

The 2010 American Diabetes Association (ADA) Internet food pyramid recommendations advocate at least 84 grams of carbohydrate per meal if you are eating three meals per day. This, as you may know by now, is grossly excessive for people trying to control their blood sugars. Here is one reason why.

Typically, 84 grams of carbohydrate would be a good-sized bowl of cooked pasta. You may think that by reading the ingredients label on the package you can precisely compute how much of the dry pasta you must weigh out to dispense exactly 84 grams of carbohydrate. Now, if you're a nonobese type 1 diabetic who weighs 140 pounds (63 kg) and makes no insulin, 1 gram of carbohydrate will raise your blood sugar by about 5 mg/dl. By using methods that we'll later describe, you can calculate exactly how much insulin you must inject to keep your blood sugar at the same point after the meal as it was before the meal. This may sound elegant, but it will rarely work for a high-carbohydrate meal. What neither the ADA nor the package tells you is that food producers are permitted a margin of error of plus or minus 20 percent in their labeling of ingredients. Furthermore, many packaged products—for example, vegetable soup—cannot even match this error range, in spite of federal labeling requirements. So even if you perform the necessary calculations, your blood sugar after the meal can be off by a carbohydrate error of 5 mg/dl multiplied by ±17 grams (±20 percent of 84 gm), or by a whopping ±85 mg/dl for just this one meal. If your blood sugar level before the meal was approximately 85 mg/dl, you've now got a blood glucose level anywhere between 170 mg/dl and 0 mg/dl. Either situation is clearly unacceptable.

Let's try another example. Say you're a type 2 diabetic, obese, and make some insulin of your own but also inject insulin. You've found that 1 gram of carbohydrate raises your blood sugar by only 3 mg/dl. Your blood sugar would be off by ±51 mg/dl. If your target blood sugar value is, say, 90 mg/dl, you're looking at a postmeal blood sugar level of anywhere from 141 mg/dl to 49 mg/dl.

That's one of the many problems with the ADA guidelines. Big inputs cause big uncertainty.

But if you eat an amount of carbohydrate that will affect your blood sugar by a much smaller margin of error, then you're going to have a much simpler time of normalizing blood sugar levels. My diet plan, which we will get into in Chapters 9–11, aims to keep these margins in the realm of ±10–20 mg/dl for type 1 diabetics and less for most of those who produce insulin. How do we accomplish this? Small inputs.

Eating only half a teacup of pasta is not the answer. Even small amounts of some carbohydrates can cause rapid swings in blood sugar. And anyway, who would feel satisfied after such a small serving of pasta? The key is to eat foods that will affect your blood sugar in a very small, slow way.

Small inputs, small mistakes. Sounds so simple and straightforward that it may make you want to ask why no one has told you about it before.

Say that instead of eating pasta as the carbohydrate portion of your meal, you eat salad. If you estimate 2 cups of salad to total 12 grams of carbohydrate and are off not by 20 percent but by 30 percent, that's still an uncertainty of only 4 grams of carbohydrate—a maximum potential 20 mg/dl rise or fall in blood sugar. A big bowl of pasta for a couple of cups of salad? Not much of a trade, you may say. Well, we don't intend that you starve. As you decrease the amount of fast-acting carbohydrate you eat, you can often simultaneously increase the amount of protein you eat. Protein can, as you may recall, also cause a blood sugar rise, but this takes place much more slowly, to a much smaller degree, and is therefore more easily covered with medication. In addition, unlike the pasta, which can leave you feeling hungry after a meal—I will explain this further in later chapters—protein leaves you feeling satisfied longer.

In theory, you could weigh everything you eat right down to the last gram and make your calculations based on information provided by the manufacturer or derived from some of the books we use. This information, as noted above, is only an estimate, with considerable margin for error. You will have only a vague idea of what you're actually consuming, and of the effect it will have on blood sugar.

The idea here is to stick with low levels of slow-acting, nutritious carbohydrates. In addition, stick with foods that will make you feel satisfied without causing huge swings in blood sugar. Simple.

THE LAW OF INSULIN DOSE ABSORPTION

If you do not take insulin, you can skip this section.

Think again of traffic. You're driving down the road and your car drifts slightly toward the median. To bring it back into line, you make a slight adjustment of the steering wheel. No problem. But yank the steering wheel and it could carry you into another lane, or could send you careening off the road.

When you inject insulin, not all of it reaches your bloodstream. Research has shown that there's a level of uncertainty as to just how much absorption of insulin actually takes place, and even as to how sensitive the body is to insulin from one day to the next. The more insulin you use, the greater the level of uncertainty.

When you inject insulin, you're putting beneath your skin a substance that isn't, according to your immune system's way of seeing things, supposed to be there. So a portion of it will be destroyed as a foreign substance before it can reach the bloodstream. The amount that the body can destroy depends on several factors. First is how big a dose you inject. The bigger the dose, the more inflammation and irritation you cause, and the more of a "red flag" you send up to your immune system. Other factors include the depth, speed, and location of your injection.

Your injections will naturally vary from one time to the next. Even the most fastidious person will unconsciously alter minor things in the injection process from day to day. So the amount of insulin that gets into your bloodstream is always going to have some variability. The bigger the dose, the bigger the variation.

A number of years ago, researchers at the University of Minnesota demonstrated that if you inject about 20 units of insulin into your arm, you'll get on average a 39 percent variation in the amount that makes it into the bloodstream from one day to the next. They found that abdominal injections had only a 29 percent average variation, and so recommended that we use only abdominal injections. On paper that seems fine, but in practice the effects on blood sugar are still intolerable.

Say you do inject 20 units of human insulin at one time. Each unit lowers the blood sugar of a typical 140-pound adult by 40 mg/dl. A 29 percent variability will create about a 6-unit discrepancy in your 20-unit injection, which means a 240 mg/dl blood sugar uncertainty (40 mg/dl × 6 units). The result is totally haphazard blood sugars and complete unpredictability, just by virtue of the varying amounts of insulin absorbed from such a large dose.

Research and my own experience demonstrate that the smaller your dose of insulin, the less variability you get. For type 1 adult diabetics who are not obese, we'd ideally like to see doses anywhere from ¼ unit to 6 units or at the most 7. Typically, you might take 3–5 units in a shot. At these lower doses, the uncertainty of absorption approaches zero, so that there is no need to worry about whether you should inject in your arm or abdomen or buttock.

I have a very obese patient who requires 27 units of long-acting insulin at bedtime. He's so insulin-resistant that there's no way to keep his blood sugar under control without this massive dose. In order to ameliorate the unpredictability of large doses, he splits his bedtime insulin into four small shots given into four separate sites using the same disposable syringe. *As a rule, I recommend that a single insulin injection not exceed 7 units for adults and proportionally less for children, depending on their weight.*

THE LAW OF INSULIN TIMING

Again, it's very difficult to use any medication safely unless you can predict the effect it will have. With insulin, this is as true of *when* you inject as it is of how much you take. If you're a recent-onset type 1 diabetic, fast-acting (regular) insulin can be injected 40–45 minutes prior to a meal tailored to your diet plan to prevent the ensuing rise in blood sugar. Regular, "fast-acting" insulin, despite its designation, doesn't act very fast, and cannot come close to approximating the phase I insulin response of a nondiabetic. To a lesser degree this is also true of the new, faster-acting lispro (Humalog), glulisine (Apidra), or aspart (Novolog) insulins. Still, these are the fastest we have. Small doses of regular insulin start to work in about 45 minutes and do not finish for at least 8 hours; lispro starts to work in about 20 minutes and takes well over 5 hours to finish. This is considerably slower than the speed at which fast-acting carbohydrate raises blood sugar.

Many years ago, John Galloway, then medical director and senior scientist of Eli Lilly and Company, performed an eye-opening experiment. He gave one injection of 70 units of regular insulin (a very large dose) to a nondiabetic volunteer who was connected to an intravenous glucose infusion. Dr. Galloway then measured blood sugars every few minutes and adjusted the glucose drip to keep the patient's blood sugars clamped at 90 mg/dl. How long would you guess the glucose infusion had to be continued to prevent dangerously low blood sugars, or hypoglycemia?

It took a week, even though the package insert says that regular insulin lasts only 4–12 hours. So the conclusion is that even the timing of injected insulin is very much dependent upon how much is injected. In practice, larger insulin injections start working sooner, last longer, and have less predictable timing of action.

If you eat a meal not specifically tailored to our restricted-carbohydrate diet and try to cover it with insulin, you'll get a postprandial (after-eating) increase in blood sugar, eventually followed by a decrease as the fast-acting insulin catches up. This means that you'll have high blood sugars after every meal, and you could still fall prey to the long-term complications of diabetes. If you try to prevent the inevitable postprandial blood sugar spike by waiting to eat until after the start time of your insulin, you may easily make yourself hypoglycemic, which could in turn cause you to overcompensate by overeating — that is, presuming you don't lose consciousness first.

Type 2 diabetics have a diminished or absent phase I insulin response, and so they face a problem similar to that of type 1s. They have to wait hours for the phase II insulin to catch up if they eat fast-acting carbohydrate or large amounts of slow-acting carbohydrate.

The key to timing insulin injections is to know how carbohydrates and insulin affect your blood sugar and to use that knowledge to minimize the swings. Since you can't approximate phase I insulin response, you have to eat foods that allow you to work within the limits of the insulin you make or inject. If you think you'll miss out on the ADA's great high-carb, low-fat diet — which, statistically, has only succeeded in raising levels of obesity, elevating triglycerides and LDL, and causing an epidemic of diabetes and early death — there is considerable evidence that restricting carbohydrate is healthier not only for diabetics but for everyone. This is supported by a twenty-year study of 82,802 nondiabetic nurses published in the November 9, 2006, issue of the *New England Journal of Medicine*. (For more details on this point, see *Protein Power*, by Drs. Michael and Mary Dan Eades, Bantam Books, 1996.)

If you consume only *small amounts* of slow-acting carbohydrate, you can actually prevent postprandial blood sugar elevation with injected preprandial rapid-acting insulin. In fact, by restricting carbohydrate intake, many type 2 diabetics will be able to prevent this rise with their phase II insulin response and will not need injected insulin before meals.

OBEYING THE LAWS OF SMALL NUMBERS

Essential to obeying the Laws of Small Numbers is to eat only small amounts of slow-acting carbohydrate when you eat carbohydrate, and no fast-acting carbohydrate. Even the slowest-acting carbohydrate can outpace injected or phase II insulin if consumed in greater amounts than recommended later in this book (Chapters 9–11).

If you eat a small amount of slow-acting carbohydrate, you might get by with a very small or no postprandial blood sugar increase. If you double the amount of slow-acting carbohydrate, you'll more than double the potential increase in blood sugar (and remember that high blood sugar leads to even higher blood sugar). If you *fill up* on slow-acting carbohydrate, it will work as fast as a lesser amount of fast-acting carbohydrate, and if you feel stuffed, you'll compound it with the Chinese restaurant effect (see pages 101–102).

All of this not only points toward eating less carbohydrate, it also implies eating smaller meals 4 or 5 times a day rather than three large meals. If you're a type 2 diabetic and require no medication, eating like this may work well for you. The difficulty with this sort of plan is its inconvenience, but some people don't mind and actually prefer to eat this way.

For the type 2 diabetic who doesn't need insulin injections, smaller meals throughout the day can be a very effective way of maintaining a constant level of blood sugar. Since this kind of diet would be tailored to work with a phase II insulin response, blood sugars should never go too high. It would, however, involve a certain amount of daily preparation and routinization that could be thrown off by changes in schedule— illness, travel, houseguests, and so forth. People who cover their meals with injected insulin and also correct small blood sugar elevations with very rapid-acting insulin, however, cannot get away with more than three daily meals (see Chapter 19, "Intensive Insulin Regimens").

I will personally answer questions from readers for one hour every month. This free service is available by visiting www.askdrbernstein.net.

8

Establishing a Treatment Plan

THE BASIC TREATMENT PLANS AND
HOW WE STRUCTURE THEM

Now that you know the different factors that can affect blood sugar, we can begin to discuss treatment plans. Blood sugar normalization for most diabetics can be achieved through one of four basic plans. Although there are only two major types of diabetes—type 1 and type 2—there are so many variations, particularly in type 2, that a treatment plan that works for one diabetic won't necessarily work for another. Each plan has to be tailored to the individual.

The basic treatment plans increase in complexity with the severity of the disease.

For type 2 diabetes

Level 1: Diet (and appropriate weight loss)*
Level 2: Diet (and appropriate weight loss) *plus* exercise
Level 3: Diet (and appropriate weight loss) *plus* exercise *plus* an
     oral insulin-sensitizing or insulin-mimetic agent
Level 4: Diet (and appropriate weight loss) *plus* exercise *plus*
     insulin injections, with or without an oral agent

For type 1 diabetes

Same as level 4 above, with the addition of multiple daily insulin injections, with questionable benefit from exercise in controlling blood sugars, and with benefit from oral insulin-sensitizing

---

* Since 80 percent or more of type 2 diabetics are overweight, weight loss should be an important part of treatment for the majority.

agents only when insulin requirements are excessive, as with those who are obese or who have polycystic ovarian syndrome (PCOS; see Appendix E).

STRUCTURING A TREATMENT PLAN

What are normal blood sugar levels? What range do we find in non-diabetics? The answers depend upon whom you ask. I've seen figures in the scientific literature over the years ranging anywhere from 60 to 140 mg/dl. My experience checking random blood sugar readings on nonobese nondiabetics, as well as figures from large population studies, tells me that for most nondiabetics, blood sugar levels cover a pretty narrow range of about 75–90 mg/dl (by finger stick), except after meals containing large amounts of fast-acting carbohydrates.

After initial fine-tuning of blood sugar, I usually select a target of 83 mg/dl for most of my patients. This target is not an average, but one we try to maintain 24 hours a day. Even if you *average* 83 mg/dl but your blood sugars are bouncing back and forth between 60 and 140 mg/dl, you're still on the roller coaster. Our object is to find a treatment plan that will get you off the roller coaster and keep you off.

Type 1 diabetics with severe gastroparesis (unpredictable stomach-emptying) are at such great risk for severe hypoglycemia after meals that I frequently set their target blood sugar higher, to play it safe. (See Chapter 22.)

One of the most important considerations in setting up an initial target is that people who have had high blood sugar levels for many months or years usually experience unpleasant symptoms of hypoglycemia as blood sugars approach normal. Someone who has grown accustomed to blood sugars consistently over 300 mg/dl may feel "shaky" at 120 mg/dl. In such a case, we might start with 160 mg/dl as the initial target. We'd then lower the target to its ultimate value over a period of weeks or months as treatment proceeds.

It's unusual when an initial meal plan and dosage of medication instantly result in the desired blood sugar profiles. Some people, a few days into their regimen, may find something objectionable, such as not enough to eat for a certain meal. Because of this, it's often necessary to experiment with a plan, making small changes based upon personal preferences and blood sugar profiles.

People tend to become discouraged if they cannot see rapid

improvement, and so, where warranted, I try to make adjustments to the regimen every few days in order to demonstrate that our efforts are accomplishing positive results. To this end, I ask patients to bring, e-mail, or fax to my office their blood sugar profiles about one week after their final training visit, if initial treatment is by diet alone. If I've prescribed insulin, I like to see profiles within a few days. I certainly try to make sure that no blood sugars are below 70 mg/dl during this trial period. I ask all new patients to phone me at any time of the day or night if they experience a blood sugar under 70 or become confused about their instructions. Additional repeat visits or phone calls may be necessary every few days or weeks, depending upon how rapidly blood sugar profiles reach our ultimate target.

Many new patients come to my office from out of town, some traveling distances of thousands of miles. Clearly, frequent office visits would be impractical in such cases. For these patients, I often schedule follow-up "telephone visits" instead of office visits. Patients fax or e-mail their blood sugars to me on GLUCOGRAF III data sheets.

These subsequent office or telephone interactions enable me to fine-tune the original plan, and also to reinforce the training program by catching any mistakes that a patient may inadvertently make. This interactive training is much more effective for patients than just reading a book or hearing a few lectures.*

BEGINNING TREATMENT WITH YOUR DOCTOR OR DIABETES EDUCATOR

Although the protocol will likely differ at every doctor's office, in the next several pages, I'll try to give you an idea of how things work at our Diabetes Center. This way, you'll get a general notion of how a comprehensive diabetes treatment program should work.

In my experience, most patients will cooperate with a treatment plan that shows them concrete results. Greatly improved blood sugars, weight normalization, halting or reversing diabetic complications,

---

* Nevertheless, I record my 4–6 hour training sessions for my patients and give them the tapes. Readers of this book can purchase CD recordings of actual training sessions at www.rx4betterhealth.com.

and a sense of improved overall health can go a long way toward convincing an individual to stick with a treatment program.

Much is written in the diabetes literature about the key role of patient "compliance." Treatment failures are often blamed upon "lack of compliance." I think it's unreasonable to expect anyone to comply with a treatment plan that explains little and, as in the case of the standard ADA approach, isn't really effective and offers little incentive to continue. What we must do is set up a sensible, workable plan that you understand and agree with. When I work with my patients in the office, I don't just have my staff hand them a photocopied diet and expect automatic acceptance. This is something that has to be negotiated, worked out. Do you like turnips? Great, we can probably fit them into your diet, even though I don't think I've ever eaten one in my life. Call it "physician compliance," but the point is that it's unreasonable to try to force my personal preferences on my patients. Only when one understands and agrees with the plan can we expect cooperation. For cooperation to continue, however, patients have to see positive, rapid results.

Not all people are able to follow a given treatment plan. For example, someone who's been overeating carbohydrate for a lifetime may find it next to impossible to begin to follow a restricted diet immediately, but we have ways around this (see Chapter 13, "How to Curb Carbohydrate Craving or Overeating"). Some absolutely resist exercise. But for most people we are still able to develop a treatment plan that works. If, for example, someone whose blood sugar should be controllable with diet and exercise refuses to exercise, I might instead prescribe medication that lowers insulin resistance.

YOUR FIRST FEW VISITS

When seeing new patients, for those who live nearby, my preference is an introductory visit followed later by a series of treatment/training visits lasting 2–3 hours each. The continuity of time is invaluable to showing rapid results. However, most insurance companies don't like to pay for lengthy office visits—especially for diabetes training—and so it may be necessary to break down the initial workup and training into multiple brief visits. Although I don't like to, I may do this with local patients; but with patients who live a great distance from my office, it's simply not workable to have successive short visits.

At the first visit I always get a drop of fingertip blood to measure the patient's baseline (initial) HgbA$_{1C}$. As time goes on and the patient sticks with the program, the inevitable progression of reduced blood sugar over the next few months can provide tremendous encouragement.

My preferred procedure for the first few days of treatment is to break down visits into three sessions. Before seeing a new patient, however, I send him or her a lab order form for the blood and urine tests listed in Chapter 2.

Introductory Visit

In addition to taking a brief history of the patient's diabetes experience, I review with him or her the laboratory test results that I have received. We then negotiate plans for dealing with any abnormal results.

Since blood glucose profiles are so essential to formulating a treatment plan, prior to the introductory visit I usually ask a new patient to procure blood glucose testing supplies—GLUCOGRAF III data sheets and the other supplies listed in Chapter 3. I provide guidelines for blood glucose self-monitoring (like those you have seen in Chapter 4), and ask the patient to learn how to use the equipment so that later, on the first treatment/training visit, I can look over one or two weeks' worth of blood glucose profiles. I also may give the patient a couple of large bottles so that a 24-hour urine specimen can be collected for a subsequent visit.

First Treatment/Training Visit

If I haven't done so in the introductory visit, I take a medical history and begin a physical exam geared toward uncovering long-term complications of diabetes. For patients who have had diabetes more than about five years, I inevitably find a good number of these long-term sequelae (consequences), some of which may be reversed by blood sugar normalization. The exam will include some or all of the tests described in Chapter 2. We check to ensure that the patient has purchased the right supplies. If we haven't done so already, we provide a supply list (Chapter 3) with the appropriate items checked off.

We discuss plans for treatment of medical problems other than blood glucose control. These may include conditions the patient already knows about, but also anything uncovered by blood testing or by the history and physical exam.* If the patient has already acquired supplies and begun measuring blood sugars, I review his or her technique and correct it if necessary.

Second Treatment/Training Visit

Many of my patients come from out of town, and so the second visit may take place the day after the first. For local patients, however, it may be approximately a week later. At this visit we finish the physical examination. We also recheck the patient's blood glucose measurement technique and proper use of the GLUCOGRAF form.

If I feel that the patient should be taking insulin, I give instructions for insulin doses to be taken the night before and the morning of the third visit. I also provide training in self-injection (see Chapter 16) to patients who have never injected before. For those who are veteran insulin users, I evaluate their self-injection techniques and correct them if necessary. It's my experience that most insulin-using patients have previously been taught improper techniques for filling syringes and injecting insulin. Because anyone can get an infection (see Chapter 21) or may undergo treatment with steroids, both of which can dramatically raise blood sugars, I teach every diabetic how to inject.

To this visit the patient is expected to bring the blood sugar data he or she has collected over the prior week(s), together with a separate list of what he or she eats on a typical day. This information enables me to estimate if the patient will need medication for blood glucose control and tells me about foods the patient likes that might be included in our meal plans. The blood glucose profile also provides a snapshot of the patient's status before beginning the new treatment regimen. We can review this at a later date to evaluate progress. As with each of the other initial visits, the bulk of our time will be devoted to training.†

Most important, this is the visit where we negotiate the meal plan (see Chapter 11).

---

* Your physician, if interested, may order a copy of my eight-page examination for diabetic complications by contacting me as instructed on page 73.
† My training program consists essentially of the material covered in this book. It's my hope that physicians who have little time to educate patients will use this book to assist in that task.

Third Treatment/Training Visit

This visit may take place anytime after the second. I continue training and enter all the "data to remember" at the top of a Glucograf data sheet (see Chapter 5). I use this visit to give verbal instructions and a printed handout regarding foot care (see Appendix D).

On this day, if the patient arises with a blood glucose above our target value, she'd have instructions to take a trial dose of fast-acting insulin to bring blood sugar down to the target value. If blood sugar on awakening is below the target, she'd use glucose tablets to bring blood glucose up to the target. By this means, we confirm or correct my estimation of how much a given amount of insulin or glucose will lower or raise the individual's blood sugar.

SETTING A BLOOD SUGAR TARGET

Whenever I talk about blood sugars in this book, I'm referring to finger-stick, plasma blood glucose measurements. When I discuss "normal" blood sugar values, I am referring to those found in non-obese nondiabetics—and to those *not* taken within 5 hours of a high-carbohydrate meal.

In my experience, given the right blood sugar meter, these values will be almost exactly the same as you would get from plasma measurements of venous blood that your doctor would send to a clinical laboratory. I've seen finger-stick blood sugars measured on many nondiabetic, nonobese adults (for example, salespeople who come into the office trying to sell me meters—I insist on demonstrations;* or the nondiabetic spouses, parents, or siblings of patients). It usually is about 83 mg/dl. I therefore tell my patients that a normal to shoot

---

* I used to have some fun with nondiabetic sales reps when they came into the office selling blood sugar meters. They'd be demonstrating a meter, which I would compare to my own meter. I always used their blood because I've had enough finger sticks. I'd "guess" their blood sugar. I'd make a show of examining their skin, then give them a number. It was always the same, but they didn't know that. The number was 83 mg/dl. Inevitably I'd be within ±3 mg/dl. You know, of course, that I didn't have any special powers—it was just that I'd seen so many random finger-stick readings from nondiabetics that I knew what number the nondiabetic was likely to show.

for is 83 mg/dl, no matter what age. I haven't had the opportunity to test a great number of nondiabetic children, but the literature shows that normal blood sugars in children will be lower.*

With respect to hemoglobin A_{1C}, I have a sophisticated machine in my office that I've found correlates almost exactly with measures from a major clinical laboratory. I therefore check $HgbA_{1C}$ values on every patient at every routine visit, and frequently on nondiabetic relatives. Essentially what I see is that nondiabetics who are not obese have $HgbA_{1C}$ levels in the range of 4.2–4.6 percent. I have a number of diabetic patients who, under treatment, now have $HgbA_{1C}$ readings as low as 4.1 percent. This is a considerable deviation from the ADA's recommendation of under 6 percent—with no intervention unless levels exceed 7 percent. In my opinion, this is yet another example of "the rape of the diabetic."

The ADA recommendation for "tight control" of blood sugars, from its website, is as follows:

> Ideally, this means levels between 90 and 130 mg/dl before meals and less than 180 two hours after starting a meal, with a glycated hemoglobin level less than 7 percent.

The recommendations go on to state that tight control (what I advocate) "isn't for everyone," which I believe is nonsense. But the ADA's tight control as defined above isn't very tight at all. I would call it "out of control."

---

* A study published in the *New England Journal of Medicine* found that nondiabetic men with fasting blood sugars of 87 mg/dl or more had greater risk of developing diabetes than those with values less than 81 mg/dl. Another study of about two thousand healthy men, published in *Diabetes Care* in January 1999, showed that over a period of twenty-two years the risk of cardiac death was 40 percent greater for those with fasting blood sugars greater than 85 mg/dl.

To my amazement, a medical director of a major insulin manufacturer recently told me that it found most nondiabetic men to have blood sugars in the 70s. Dr. Stan De Loach, a diabetes specialist in Mexico, tested three hundred nondiabetic children and found them all to have blood sugars in the 70s.

CONVERTING HgbA₁c TO BLOOD SUGAR VALUES

Many years ago, I reviewed dozens of HgbA$_{1C}$ values and thousands of blood sugars from data sheets submitted by my patients and came up with a formula for converting HgbA$_{1C}$ to mean (average) blood sugar.

My formula does not jibe with some other formulas, perhaps because others haven't collected blood sugars throughout the day running into the hundreds or even thousands of patients covering four-month periods. The formula is very simple. An HgbA$_{1C}$ of 5 percent is equivalent to an average blood sugar reading of 100 mg/dl, and every 1 percent above 5 corresponds to an additional 40 mg/dl increase in blood sugars. So an HgbA$_{1C}$ of 7 percent would correspond to an average blood sugar of 180 mg/dl.

The formula is, in my experience, useless for HgbA$_{1C}$ values of less than 5 percent, and it may not work for average blood sugars greater than 200 mg/dl, for the simple reason that for a new patient running blood sugars greater than 200 mg/dl, we rapidly get them down into the 100s or less. Such new patients don't come in bringing me hundreds of data points above 200 for me to compute an accurate formula at these values — nor would I ask them to.

In February 2002 a study published in *Diabetes Care* reported a formula that is valid for average blood sugars over a much wider range than mine, including values well above and below 100 mg/dl. It gives results close to mine in the 100–200 mg/dl range. The formula is:
mean plasma glucose = $(35.6 \times HgbA_{1C}) - 77.3$ mg/dl.

So how do we go about setting a target normal value given all these numbers? Let's take a look at a type 2 diabetic whose disease can be controlled by diet and exercise. Here, we'll certainly shoot for blood sugars of about 83 mg/dl before, during, and after meals. It will then be up to both me and the patient jointly — if his blood sugars are, say, in the 90s — to decide whether we want to introduce medications to further lower blood sugar. Many patients these days are hesitant to take any medication that's been approved by the FDA, despite many such medications being quite benign. If we have a type 2 diabetic who requires the insulin-sensitizing drugs like metformin, we certainly can shoot for a target blood sugar of 83 mg/dl before, during, and after meals, and indeed, I will work with the patient to juggle the medications, using long- or short-acting versions in order to achieve that target.

Type 2 diabetics who require very small amounts of insulin (say, 1–2 units per dose) are at very low risk for hypoglycemia and will usually automatically "turn off" the insulin they make themselves if blood sugars are too low. Such people are also good candidates for a target of 83 mg/dl.

When it comes to type 1 diabetics, where virtually all of the needed insulin is going to be injected, I temporarily increase the target to 90 mg/dl or higher, even though we know that the mortality rate— even in the general, nondiabetic population—is slightly greater for those with fasting or postprandial blood sugars of 90 mg/dl than it is for those with blood sugars of 83. If at all feasible without frequent hypoglycemic episodes, I will eventually lower the target to 83 mg/dl. I've been using 83 as a target for myself.

A target may imply corrections to get you to your target. As a rule, if you're a type 2, your blood sugar goes down eventually—maybe quickly, maybe over many hours. If you're a type 1 and injecting significant doses of insulin, if you make a mistake in your diet and your blood sugar goes up, you have to inject additional, calibrated doses of fast-acting insulin deliberately to bring down your blood sugar and, if it's too low, take glucose tablets to raise it.

For a new patient in the very early stages of type 2 diabetes, I may see both hypo- and hyperglycemia. This is probably because one of the early "lesions" of type 2 is difficulty in storing the insulin granules your body makes. So such a person would make insulin for a meal, then make more after the meal. A nondiabetic would store that additional insulin as it's being made, but the early type 2 might release some or all of it into the bloodstream as it's generated, thereby bringing blood sugar too low. This explanation also accounts for attenuated (diminished) phase I insulin response—just not having enough insulin stored to cover a meal adequately (another reason to follow a low-carbohydrate diet). Such an individual could experience blood sugars in the 70s or even mid-60s from time to time, and these individuals must carry glucose tablets with them to bring blood sugars up to their target, usually 83. They don't take injected insulin to bring blood sugar down if it goes too high when they make a mistake, because their bodies will do that for them, probably faster than injected insulin would.

SETTING GOALS OF TREATMENT

On the third visit, it's generally appropriate to prepare a list of treatment goals. Exactly what are we going to accomplish, how, and over what time frame? The patient and I discuss a list of goals to make sure that he or she understands and agrees. The following list is typical of the things I want to see any given patient accomplish. (Remember, the training I provide to my patients is the substance of this book, so if you don't entirely understand all of these goals right now, don't be discouraged. Mark this chapter and come back to it when you've finished the book. By then you should understand the whole philosophy of my approach and the goals will make sense. You may also by that time have developed—if you haven't already—conscious goals of your own.)

- Normalization of blood glucose profiles.
- Improvement or normalization of the following laboratory tests that respond to blood glucose control (see Chapter 2):
    hemoglobin A_{1C}
    red blood cell magnesium
    lipid profile
    thrombotic risk profile
    renal profile
- Attainment of ideal weight (where appropriate).
- Full or partial reversal of diabetic complications, including pain or numbness in feet, diabetes-related retinal or kidney problems, gastroparesis, cardiac autonomic neuropathy, neuropathic erectile dysfunction, postural hypotension, and so on. If blood sugars are kept normal, some of these improvements will appear within weeks to years, depending upon the particular problem and its severity.
- Reduction in frequency and severity of hypoglycemic episodes (where appropriate).
- Relief of chronic fatigue and short-term memory impairment associated with high blood sugars.
- Improvement or normalization of hypertension.
- Reduction of demand upon beta cells. If C-peptide is present before starting our program (that is, if the pancreas is producing

measurable amounts of insulin), glucose tolerance should improve if a regimen is pursued that minimizes the demand upon the beta cells. This is a very important goal. Remember that for type 2 patients, small sacrifices now can prevent the need for 5 or more daily insulin doses down the road. Beta cell burnout (see page 103) can frequently be prevented or partially reversed.

- Increased strength, endurance, and feeling of well-being.
- About 40 percent of my new patients show low thyroid function on initial testing. We therefore try to normalize blood levels of T_3 and T_4 by prescribing T_3 and/or T_4 replacement. When blood levels are normalized we expect correction of prior tiredness, coldness, hair loss, poor memory, dyslipidemia, and so on.

The patient may wish to add some personal goals. The doctor should respect these if at all possible. For example, I have several patients who are willing to do whatever I ask, provided I do not put them on insulin. I consider this a reasonable preliminary goal for some, even though it may increase the risk of beta cell burnout. After all, if we cannot enlist a patient's cooperation, we achieve nothing.

I will personally answer questions from readers for one hour every month. This free service is available by visiting www.askdrbernstein.net.

PART TWO

Treatment

9

The Basic Food Groups

OR MUCH OF WHAT YOU'VE BEEN TAUGHT
ABOUT DIET IS PROBABLY WRONG

In Chapter 1 we discussed how diabetics and nondiabetics might react to a particular meal. Here we'll talk about how specific kinds of foods can affect your blood sugar.

A curious fact about diet, nutrition, and medication is that while we can make accurate generalizations about how most of us will react to a particular diet or medical regimen, *we cannot predict exactly* how each individual will react to a given food or medication—but we can find out by trial and error.

The foods we consume, once you take away the water and indigestible contents, can be grouped into three major categories that provide calories or energy: protein, fat, and carbohydrate. (Alcohol also provides calories, and will be discussed later in this chapter.) Seldom will food from one of these groups contain solely one type of nutrient. Protein foods often contain fat; carbohydrate foods frequently contain some protein and some fat. The common foods that are virtually 100 percent fat are oils, butter, some types of margarine, and lard.

Since our principal concern here is blood sugar control, we'll concentrate on how these three major sources of calories affect blood sugar. If you're a long-standing diabetic and have followed standard ADA teachings for years, you'll find that much of what you're about to read is radically at odds with the ADA's dietary guidelines—and with good reason, as you'll soon learn.

When we eat, the digestive process breaks down the three major food groups into their building blocks. These building blocks are then absorbed into the bloodstream and reassembled into the various products our bodies need in order to function.

PROTEIN

Proteins are constructed of building blocks called amino acids.
Through digestion, dietary proteins are broken down by enzymes in
the digestive tract into their amino acid components. These amino
acids can then be reassembled not only into muscle, nerves, and vital
organs, but also into hormones, enzymes, and neurochemicals. They
can also be converted to glucose, but very slowly and inefficiently.

We acquire dietary protein from a number of sources, but the foods
that are richest in it—egg whites, cheese, and meat (including fish
and fowl)—contain virtually no carbohydrate. Protein is available in
smaller amounts from vegetable sources such as legumes (beans),
seeds, and nuts, which also contain fat and carbohydrate.*

Protein and carbohydrate are our two dietary sources of blood
sugar. Protein foods from animal sources are only about 20 percent
protein by weight (about 6 grams per ounce), the rest being fat, water,
and/or indigestible "gristle." Our liver (and to a lesser degree, our
kidneys and intestines), instructed by the hormone glucagon,† can
very slowly transform as much as 36 percent of these 6 grams per
ounce into glucose‡—if blood sugar descends too low, if serum insulin levels are inadequate, or if the body's other amino acid needs have
been met. Neither carbohydrate nor fat can be transformed into
protein.

In many respects—and going against the grain of a number of
the medical establishment's accepted notions about diabetics and
protein—protein will become the most important part of your diet

---

* Phosphate, a by-product of protein digestion, requires calcium in order to be
eliminated from the body—about 1 gram of calcium for every 10 ounces of
protein foods. If you don't eat much cheese, cream, milk (too high in carbohydrate), yogurt, or bones, all good sources of calcium, it would be wise to take a
calcium supplement. This will prevent the slow loss of calcium from your
bones. I recommend calcium citrate in formulations supplemented with magnesium and vitamin D.
† And other so-called counterregulatory hormones, such as cortisol and growth
hormone.
‡ This amounts to about 7.5 percent of the total weight of a protein food. Say you
eat a 3-ounce (85-gram) hamburger, no bun, for lunch—the protein in it can
slowly be transformed by the liver into no more than 6½ grams of glucose.

if you are going to control blood sugars, just as it was for our hunter-gatherer ancestors.

If you are a long-standing diabetic and are frustrated with the care you've received over the years, you have probably been conditioned to think that protein is more of a poison than sugar and is the cause of kidney disease. I was conditioned the same way—many years ago, as I mentioned, I had laboratory evidence of advanced proteinuria, signifying potentially fatal kidney disease—but in this case, the conventional wisdom is just a myth.

Nondiabetics who eat a lot of protein don't get diabetic kidney disease. Diabetics with normal blood sugars don't get diabetic kidney disease. High levels of dietary protein do not cause kidney disease in diabetics or anyone else. There is no higher incidence of kidney disease in the cattle-growing states of the United States, where many people eat beef at virtually every meal, than there is in the states where beef is more expensive and consumed to a much lesser degree. Similarly, the incidence of kidney disease in vegetarians is the same as the incidence of kidney disease in nonvegetarians. *It is the high blood sugar levels that are unique to diabetes, and to a much lesser degree the high levels of insulin required to cover high carbohydrate consumption (causing hypertension), that cause the complications associated with diabetes.**

FAT

The Big Fat Lie

Call it the Big Fat Lie. Fat has, through no real fault of its own, become the great demon of the American dietary scene. It is no myth that more than half of Americans are overweight, and the number of obese Americans is growing.

Current dietary recommendations from the government, and nearly every "reputable" organization with an opinion, are to eat no more than 35 percent of calories as fat—which very few people can maintain—and there are some recommendations for even lower percentages than that. The low-fat mania in our culture has spawned an increase in carbohydrate intake. All a candy or cookie has needed is the label "fat-free" to send its sales through the roof. The fallacy that

---

* This is discussed further in Appendix A.

eating fat will make you fat is about as scientifically logical as saying that eating tomatoes will turn you red.

This is the kind of fallacious thinking behind the prevailing "wisdom," which maintains that there is an unavoidable link between dietary fat and high serum cholesterol. And that if you want to lose weight and reduce cholesterol, all you need to do is eat lots of carbohydrate, limit consumption of meat, and cut out fat as much as possible. But many contemporary researchers exploring this phenomenon have begun to arrive at the conclusion that a high-carbohydrate diet, especially rich in fruit and grain products, is not so benign. In fact, it has been shown—and it is my own observation in myself and in my patients—that such a diet can increase body weight, increase blood insulin levels, and raise most cardiac risk factors.

In an unbiased, clearheaded, and award-winning article published in the respected journal *Science* on March 30, 2001, the science writer Gary Taubes explores what he calls "The Soft Science of Dietary Fat." (The full text of this article is available at www.diabetes-book.com/articles/ssdf.shtml.) Taubes cites the failure of the antifat crusade to improve the health of Americans:

> Since the early 1970s, for instance, Americans' average fat intake has dropped from over 40% of total calories to 34%; average serum cholesterol levels have dropped as well....
>
> Meanwhile, obesity in America, which remained constant from the early 1960s through 1980, has surged upward since then—from 14% of the population to over 22%. Diabetes has increased apace. Both obesity and diabetes increase heart disease risk, which could explain why heart disease incidence is not decreasing. That this obesity epidemic occurred just as the government began bombarding Americans with the low-fat message suggests the possibility... that low-fat diets might have unintended consequences—among them, weight gain. "Most of us would have predicted that if we can get the population to change its fat intake, with its dense calories,* we would see a reduction in weight," admits [Bill] Harlan [of the NIH]. "Instead, we see the exact opposite."

---

* Contrary to traditional thinking, a study published in the *Journal of the American College of Nutrition* demonstrated that the metabolizable calories in fats are about the same as in carbohydrates.

I urge you to have a look at Taubes's article, which will give you a notion of the kinds of competing personal, economic, and political interests that go into the formulation of "scientific" guidelines. You might also give your physician a copy of Taubes's book *Why We Get Fat* (Knopf, 2010), which is available at Amazon.com.

According to the NIH, the National Health and Nutrition Examination Survey (NHANES) for 2003–2006 and 2007–2008 showed that more than two-thirds (68 percent) of Americans are overweight and more than a third (33.8 percent) are obese. NHANES also showed that 12.5 percent of children ages two to five and 17 percent of those ages six to eleven are overweight, and nearly 18 percent of adolescents ages twelve to nineteen are overweight.

The advent of our agricultural society is comparatively recent in evolutionary terms—that is, it began only about ten thousand years ago. For the millions of years that preceded the constant availability of grain and the more recent year-round availability of a variety of fruits and vegetables, our ancestors were hunters and ate what was available to them in the immediate environment, primarily meat, fish, some fowl, reptiles, and insects—food that was present year-round, and predominantly protein and fat. In warm weather, some may have eaten fruits, nuts, and berries that were available locally in some regions and not deliberately bred for sweetness (agriculture didn't exist). If they stored fat in their bodies during warm periods, much of that fat was burned up during the winter. Although for the past two centuries, fruit, grain, and vegetables have, in one

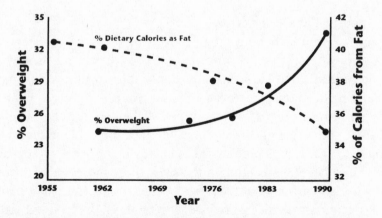

Fig. 9-1. *From 1955 to 1990, even as the percentage of calories consumed as fat declined, the percentage of overweight Americans increased by nearly half.*

form or another, been available to us in this country year-round, our collective food supply has historically been interrupted often by famine—in some cultures more than others. The history of the planet as best as we can determine is one of feast (rarely) and famine, and suggests that famine will strike again and again as it has in the past few decades in a variety of places.

Curiously, what today seems in our society to be a genetic predisposition toward obesity functioned during the famines of prehistory as an effective method of survival. Ironically, the ancestors of those who today are most at risk for type 2 diabetes were, during prehistory, not the sick and dying, but the survivors. If famine struck today in the United States, guess who would survive most easily? The same people who are most at risk for type 2 diabetes. For those living in a harsh environment where the availability of food is uncertain, bodies that store fat most efficiently when food is available (for example, by being insulin-resistant and craving carbohydrate, like most type 2 diabetics) survive to reproduce.

If you give it some thought, it makes perfect sense: If a farmer wants to fatten up his pigs or cows, he doesn't feed them meat or butter and eggs, he feeds them grain. If you want to fatten yourself up, just start loading up on bread, pasta, potatoes, cake, cereal, and cookies—all high-carbohydrate foods. If you want to hasten the fattening process, consume dietary fat with your carbohydrate. Indeed, two studies showed that dietary fat, when consumed as part of a high-carbohydrate diet, was converted to body fat. Fat consumed as part of a low-carbohydrate diet was metabolized, or burned off.

The Insulin-Fat Connection

The primary source of body fat for most Americans is not dietary fat but carbohydrate, which is converted to blood sugar and then, with the aid of insulin, to fat by fat cells. Remember, insulin is our main fat-building hormone. Eat a plate of pasta. Your blood sugar will rise and your insulin level (if you have type 2 diabetes or are not diabetic) will also rise in order to cover, or prevent, the jump in blood sugar. All the blood sugar that is not burned as energy or stored as glycogen is turned into fat. So you could, in theory, acquire more body fat from eating a high-carbohydrate "fat-free" dessert than you would from eating a tender steak nicely marbled with fat. Even the fat in the steak is more likely to be stored if it is accompanied by bread, potatoes, corn, and so on.

The fatty-acid building blocks of fats can be metabolized (burned), stored, or converted by your body into other compounds, depending on what it requires. Consequently, fat is always in flux in the body, being stored, appearing in the blood, and being converted to energy. The amount of triglycerides (the storage form of fat) in your bloodstream at any given time will be determined by your heredity, your level of exercise, your blood sugar levels, your diet, your ratio of visceral (abdominal) fat to lean body mass (muscle), and *especially your recent consumption of carbohydrate.* The slim and fit tend to be very sensitive (i.e., responsive) to insulin and have low serum levels not only of triglycerides but insulin as well. But even their triglyceride levels will increase after a high-carbohydrate meal, as excess blood sugar is converted to fat. The higher the ratio of abdominal fat (and, to a lesser degree, total body fat) to lean body mass, the less sensitive to insulin you'll tend to be. In the obese, triglycerides tend to be present at high levels in the bloodstream all the time. (This is sometimes exaggerated during weight loss because fat is appearing in the bloodstream as it comes out of storage to be converted into energy.) Not only are high triglyceride levels a direct cause of insulin resistance, but they also contribute to fatty deposits on the walls of your blood vessels (atherosclerosis). Research demonstrates that if high concentrations of triglycerides or fatty acids are injected into the blood supply of the liver of a well-conditioned athlete, someone very sensitive to insulin, she will become temporarily insulin-resistant. (The most important thing to note here is that insulin resistance, as well as other risk factors for diabetic complications, can be reversed by eating less carbohydrate, normalizing blood sugars, and slimming down, which we'll discuss in greater detail later on.)

If you become overweight, you'll produce more insulin, become insulin-resistant (which will require you to produce yet more insulin), and become even more overweight because you'll create more fat and store more fat. You'll enter the vicious circle depicted in Figure 1-1 (page 43).

Consider that steak I mentioned earlier. As you know, the body can convert protein to blood sugar, but it does so at a very slow rate, and inefficiently. Serum insulin levels derived from the phase II insulin response or even from insulin injected before a meal may thus be sufficient to prevent a blood sugar rise from protein consumption by itself. Dietary fat cannot be converted to blood sugar, and therefore it doesn't cause serum insulin levels or requirements for injected insulin to increase.* Say you eat a 6-ounce steak with no carbohydrate side dish—this won't require much insulin to keep your blood sugar steady, and the lower insulin level will cause only a small amount of the fat to be stored.

Now consider what would happen if you instead ate a "fat-free," high-carbohydrate dessert with exactly the same number of calories as that steak. Your insulin level will jump dramatically in order to cover the sugar and starches in the dessert. Remember, insulin is the fat-building and fat-storage hormone. Since it's dessert, you probably won't be going out to run a marathon after eating, so the largest portion of your newly created blood sugar won't get burned. Instead much of it will be turned into fat and stored.

Interestingly enough, eating fat with carbohydrate can actually slow the digestion of carbohydrate, so the jump in your blood sugar level might thereby be slowed. This would probably be relatively effective if you're talking about eating a green salad with vinegar-and-oil dressing. But if you're eating a regular dessert, or a baked potato with your steak, the slowdown in digestion would not prevent blood sugar elevation in a diabetic.

Despite what the popular media would have us believe, fat is not evil. In fact, many researchers are becoming quite concerned about the dangerous potential of "fat substitutes." Fat is absolutely necessary for survival. Much of the brain is constructed from fatty acids. Without essential fatty acids—which, like essential amino acids, cannot be manufactured by the body and must be eaten—you would die.

Diabetics are affected disproportionately by diseases such as atherosclerosis. This has led to the long-standing myth that diabetics have abnormal lipid profiles because they eat more fat than nondiabetics.[†] It was likewise once thought that dietary fat *caused* all the long-term complications of diabetes. For many years, this was taken as gospel by most in the medical community. In truth, however, the high lipid profiles in many diabetics with uncontrolled blood sugar have nothing to do with the fat they consume. Most diabetics consume

---

* Except for the Chinese restaurant effect (see pages 101–102).
† A lipid profile is the measurement of cholesterol, HDL (good cholesterol), LDL (bad cholesterol), and triglyceride levels in the blood. Some physicians now consider lipoprotein(a) to be an essential component of the lipid profile. (See Chapter 2, "Tests: Baseline Measures of Your Disease and Risk Profile.")

very little fat—they've been conditioned to fear it. High lipid profiles are a symptom not of excess dietary fat, but of high blood sugars. Indeed, even in most nondiabetics, the consumption of fat has little if anything to do with their lipid profiles.

On the other hand, high consumption of carbohydrate, as we will discuss shortly, can cause "nondiabetics" to develop some of the complications usually associated with diabetes.

When I was on a very low fat, high-carbohydrate diet about forty-five years ago, I had high fasting triglycerides (usually over 250 mg/dl) and high serum cholesterol (usually over 300 mg/dl), and I developed a number of vascular complications. When I went on a very low carbohydrate diet and did not restrict my fat, my lipids plummeted. Now, in my late seventies, I have the lipid profile of an Olympic athlete, apparently from eating a low-carbohydrate diet in order to normalize my blood sugars. That I exercise regularly probably doesn't hurt my lipid profile, either—but I was also exercising when my lipid profile was abnormal.

Dare your physician. Ask her if her lipid profile on a low-fat diet can remotely compare to mine, on a high-fat, low-carbohydrate diet:

- LDL—the "bad" cholesterol—53 (below 100 is considered normal)
- HDL—the "good" cholesterol—123 (above 39 is considered normal)
- Triglycerides—45 (below 150 is considered normal)
- Lipoprotein(a)—undetectable (below 10 is considered normal)

Contrary to popular myth, fat is not a demon. It's the body's way of storing energy and maintaining essential organs such as the brain. Without essential fatty acids, your body would cease to function.

CARBOHYDRATE

I've saved carbohydrate for last because it's the food group that adversely affects blood sugar most profoundly. If you're like most diabetics—or virtually everyone who lives in an industrialized society—you probably eat a diet that's mostly carbohydrate. Grains. Fruit. Bread. Cake. Beans. Snack foods. Rice. Potatoes. Pasta. Breakfast cereal. Bagels. Muffins. They look different, but dietarily speaking, they're essentially the same.

If you are already obese, you know and I know that you crave — and consume — these foods and probably avoid fats. As studies show, you would be better off eating the fat than the carbohydrate. Fat alone will be burned off. A combination of high-carbohydrate foods and fat will foster fat storage.

It is, therefore, a myth that Americans are overweight due to excessive fat consumption. Americans are fat largely because of sugar, starches, and other high-carbohydrate foods.

In a study that looked at the relationship between dietary sugar intake and cardiovascular health, the American Heart Association (AHA) found that Americans on average consume more than 70 pounds of added sugars each year.* This represents an increase during the period 1970–2004 of almost 20 percent. The key word here is "added." This doesn't account for starches and sugars naturally present in food. According to a report from the Oregon Health Sciences University, a 12-ounce Starbucks Grande Caramel Mocha drink contains 45 teaspoons of added sugar.

This increase in sugar consumption not coincidentally corresponds with the timing of recommendations to eat less fat. It was 1984 when the National Institutes of Health (NIH) began advising everyone within shouting distance to cut fat intake. It also corresponds quite neatly with the creation of a whole new, multibillion-dollar industry in low-fat and nonfat foods, many of which are extremely high in sugar. For more than fifteen years, the government had planned to issue a report once and for all damning fat as the demon some scientists were sure it was. The problem was, researchers couldn't "reverse engineer" the actual data to make the science fit the assumption. Unfortunately, the program to indict fat was left to die a quiet death, and not so much as a press release was issued to say, "We were wrong." And so many of us *still* don't know the truth. *They guessed wrong.*

No doubt the popular media have made you aware of the endless procession of books and diets and advertisements for foods all touting the value of high "complex carbohydrate" in the diet. Athletes "carbo-load" before big games or marathons. TV and radio commercials extol the virtues of Brand X sports drink over Brand Y because it contains more "carbs." That AHA study showed a strong enough link

---

* You can read about this study, described in the journal *Circulation* in 2009, at http://circ.ahajournals.org/cgi/content/full/120/11/1011.

between elevated triglycerides and "bad cholesterol," not to mention increased likelihood of overweight and obesity, that it recommended drastic reductions in added sugar intake. I'd say the AHA didn't go far enough, even if it was the strongest such statement the organization had ever made.

As stunning as it sounds—and unbelievable, given the popular media's recent love affair with a high "complex carbohydrate," low-fat diet—you can quite easily survive on a diet in which you eat no carbohydrate. There are essential amino acids and essential fatty acids, but there is no such thing as an essential carbohydrate. Furthermore, by sticking to a diet that contains no carbohydrate but has high levels of fat and protein, you can reduce your cardiac risk profile—serum cholesterol, triglycerides, LDL, et cetera—although you'd deprive yourself of all the supposed "fun foods" that we crave most.* We've all been trained to think that carbohydrates are our best, most benign source of food, so how can this be?

What if I, a physician, told you, a diabetic, to eat a diet that consisted of 60 percent sugar equivalents, 20 percent protein, and 20 percent fat? More than likely, you'd think I was insane. *I'd* think I was insane, and I would never make this suggestion to a diabetic (nor would I even make it to a nondiabetic). But this is just the diet the ADA recommended to diabetics for decades. On the surface, these recommendations seemed to make sense because of kidney disease, heart disease, and our abnormal lipid profiles. But this is what is known as single-avenue thinking. It seemed logical to insist that dietary intake of protein and fat be reduced, because no one had looked at elevated blood sugars and the high levels of insulin necessary to bring them down as the possible culprits.

So if you eat very little fat and protein, what's left to eat? Carbohydrate.

As I discovered in my years of experimentation on myself, and then in my medical training and practice, the real dietary problem for diabetics is not only fast-acting carbohydrate but also large amounts of any carbohydrate. In either case, the result is high blood sugars requiring large amounts of insulin to try to contain them.

So what are carbohydrates?

---

* You'd also be missing the vitamins and other nutrients contained in low-carbohydrate vegetables, so a zero-carbohydrate diet is not in my game plan.

The technical answer is that carbohydrates are chains of sugar molecules. The carbohydrates we eat are mostly chains of glucose molecules. The shorter the chain, the sweeter the taste. Some chains are longer and more complicated (hence, "simple" and "complex" carbohydrates), having many links and even branches. But simple or complex, carbohydrates are composed entirely of sugar.

"Sugar?" you might ask, holding up a slice of coarse-ground, seven-grain bread. "This is sugar?"

In a word, yes, at least after you digest it.

With a number of important exceptions, carbohydrates, or foods derived primarily from plant sources that are starches, grains, and fruits, have the same ultimate effect on blood glucose levels that table sugar does. (The ADA has recognized officially that, for example, bread is as fast-acting a carbohydrate as table sugar. But instead of issuing a recommendation against eating bread, its response has been to say that table sugar is therefore okay, and can be "exchanged" for other carbohydrates. To me, this is nonsense.) Whether you eat a piece of the nuttiest whole grain bread, drink a Coke, or have mashed potatoes, the effect on blood glucose levels is essentially the same — blood sugar rises, rapidly, and in proportion to carbohydrate content.

As noted in the introduction to this chapter, the digestion process breaks each of the major food groups down into its basic elements, and these elements are then utilized by the body as needed. The basic element of most carbohydrate foods is glucose. We usually think of simple carbohydrates as sugars and complex carbohydrates as fruits and grains and vegetables. In reality, most fruit and grain products, and some vegetables, are what I prefer to talk about as "fast-acting" carbohydrates. Our saliva and digestive tract contain enzymes that can rapidly chop the chains down into free glucose. We haven't the enzymes to break down some carbohydrates, such as cellulose, or "indigestible fiber." Still, our saliva can break starches into the shorter chains on contact and then convert those into pure glucose.

Pasta, which is often made from durum wheat flour and water (but can also be made from plain white flour and egg yolks, or other variants), has been touted as a dream food — particularly for runners carbo-loading before marathons — but it quickly becomes glucose, and can raise blood sugar very rapidly for diabetics.

In the type 2 diabetic with impaired phase I insulin response, it takes hours for the phase II insulin to catch up with the postprandial levels of glucose in the blood, and day after day, during that time, the high blood sugars can wreak havoc. In the diabetic who injects insulin, there is a tremendous amount of (rarely successful) guesswork involved in finding the proper dosage and timing of insulin to cover a carbohydrate-heavy meal, and the injected insulin not only doesn't work fast enough, it is also highly unpredictable when taken in large doses in attempts to cover large amounts of carbohydrate (see Chapter 7, "The Laws of Small Numbers").

Some carbohydrate foods, like fruit, contain high levels of simple, fast-acting carbohydrates. Maltose and fructose—malt sugar and fruit sugar—for example, are slower-acting than sucrose—table or cane sugar—but they will cause the same increase in blood sugar levels. It may be the difference between nearly instant elevation and elevation in 2 hours, but the elevation is still high, and a lot of insulin is still required to bring it into line. And, if the insulin is injected, there's the further problem of guesswork in timing and dosage. Despite the old admonition that an apple a day keeps the doctor away, I haven't had fruit since 1970, and I am considerably healthier for it. Some whole-plant vegetables—that is, those that come mostly from the stalks and leaves—are of value to the diabetic and nondiabetic alike because they contain considerable amounts of vitamins, minerals, and other nutrients. (The recipe section of this book shows you a number of tasty and satisfying ways to work these vegetables into your diet.)

As noted previously, most Americans who are obese are overweight not because of dietary fat, but because of excessive dietary carbohydrate. Much of this obesity is due to "pigging out" on carbohydrate-rich snack foods or junk foods, or even on supposed healthy foods like whole grain bread and pasta. It's my belief that this pigging out has little to do with hunger and nothing at all to do with being a pig.

I'm convinced that people who crave carbohydrate have inherited this problem. To some extent, we all have a natural craving for carbohydrate—it makes us feel good. The more people overeat carbohydrates, the more they will become obese, even if they exercise a lot. But certain people have a natural, overwhelming desire for carbohydrate that doesn't correlate to hunger. These people in all likelihood have a genetic predisposition toward carbohydrate craving, as well as a genetic predisposition toward insulin resistance and diabetes. (See "The Thrifty Genotype," page 194.) This craving can be reduced for many by eliminating such foods from the diet and embarking upon a low-carbohydrate diet.

In light of the above, you might guess that I advocate a no-carbohydrate diet. In fact, in the next chapter you'll discover that I include small amounts of slow-acting carbohydrate in my meal plan. Back in 1970, as I was still experimenting with blood sugar normalization, I remembered that during the twentieth century a new vitamin had been discovered every fifteen years or so. While there may be no such thing as an essential carbohydrate, it seemed reasonable to conclude that, since our prehistoric ancestors consumed some plants, plant foods might well contain essential nutrients that were not yet present in vitamin supplements and had not even been discovered. I therefore added small amounts of low-carbohydrate vegetables (not starchy or sweet) to my personal meal plan. All of a sudden I was eating salads and cooked vegetables instead of the bread, fruit, cereal, skim milk, and pasta that I had been eating on my prior ADA diet. It took a while to get used to salads, but now I relish them. Only recently, in my lifetime, have phytochemicals (essential nutrients found in plant foods) been discovered. Phytochemicals are now incorporated into some vitamin pills, but research on the use of isolated phytochemicals is still in its early stages. You may have heard of such phytochemical supplements as lutein, lycopene, and so on. It would appear that many chemicals — large numbers of which are likely not even known about yet — work together to provide beneficial effects. So at this point, it certainly makes sense to eat low-carbohydrate salads and vegetables. (Although fruits contain the same phytochemicals as vegetables, they are too high in fast-acting carbohydrate to be part of a restricted-carbohydrate diet, as the next chapter will explain.)

Physicians and anyone interested in reading scientific studies that compare low-carb and low-fat diets should visit the archives of the Nutrition and Metabolism Society at http://locarbvslofat.org.

SOME WORDS ABOUT ALCOHOL

Alcohol can provide calories, or energy, without directly raising blood sugar, but if you're an insulin-dependent diabetic, you need to be cautious about drinking. Ethyl alcohol, which is the active ingredient in hard liquor, beer, and wine, has no direct effect on blood sugar because the body does not convert it into glucose. In the case of distilled spirits and very dry wine, the alcohol generally isn't accompanied by enough carbohydrate to affect your blood sugar very much.

For example, 100-proof gin has 83 calories per ounce. These extra calories can increase your weight slightly if accompanied by carbohydrate, but not your blood sugar. Different beers—ales, stouts, and lagers—can have varying amounts of carbohydrate, which is slow enough in its action that if you figure it into your meal plan, it may not raise your blood sugar. Mixed drinks and dessert wines can be loaded with sugar, so they're best avoided. Exceptions would be a dry martini or mixed drinks that can be made with a sugar-free mixer, such as sugar-free tonic water.

Ethyl alcohol, however, can indirectly lower the blood sugars of some diabetics if consumed at the time of a meal. It does this by partially paralyzing the liver and thereby inhibiting gluconeogenesis so that it can't convert enough protein from the meal into glucose. For the average adult, this appears to be a significant effect with doses greater than 1½ ounces of distilled spirits, or one standard shot glass. If you have two 1½-ounce servings of gin with a meal, your liver's ability to convert protein into glucose may be impaired. If you're insulin-dependent and your calculation of how much insulin you'll require to cover your meal is based on, say, two hot dogs, and those hot dogs don't get 7.5 percent converted to glucose, the insulin you've injected will take your blood sugar too low. You'll have hypoglycemia, or low blood sugar.

The problem of hypoglycemia itself is a relatively simple matter to correct—you just eat some glucose and your blood sugar will rise. But this gets you into the kind of messy jerking up and down of your blood sugar that can cause problems. It's best if you can avoid hypo- and hyperglycemia (high blood sugar) entirely.

Another problem with alcohol and hypoglycemia is that if you consume much alcohol, you'll have symptoms typical of both alcohol intoxication and hypoglycemia—light-headedness, confusion, and slurring of speech. The only way you'll know the cause of your symptoms is if you've been monitoring your blood sugar throughout your meal. This is unlikely. So you could find yourself thinking you've consumed too much alcohol when in fact your problem is dangerously low blood sugar. In such a situation, it wouldn't even occur to you to check your blood sugar. Remember, that early blood sugar–measuring device I got was developed in order to help emergency room staffs tell the difference between unconscious alcoholics and unconscious diabetics. Don't make yourself an unconscious diabetic. A simple oversight could turn fatal.

Many of the symptoms of alcohol intoxication mimic those of ketoacidosis, or the extreme high blood sugar and ketone buildup in the body that can result in diabetic coma. The great buildup of ketones causes a diabetic's breath to have an aroma rather like that of someone who's been drinking. If you don't die of severe hypoglycemia, then you might easily die of embarrassment when you come to and your friends are aghast and terrified that the emergency squad had to be called to bring you around.

In small amounts, alcohol is relatively harmless — one glass of dry wine or "lite" beer with dinner — but if you're the type who can't limit drinking, it's best to avoid it entirely. For the reasons already discussed, and contrary to the guidelines of the ADA, alcohol can be more benign between meals than it is at meals. One benevolent effect of alcohol is that it can enable some diabetics to consume one "lite" beer or one small Bloody Mary (tomato juice mixed with an ounce and a half of vodka) without raising blood sugar.

I will personally answer questions from readers for
one hour every month. This free service is available by
visiting www.askdrbernstein.net.

10

Diet Guidelines Essential to the Treatment of All Diabetics

Research into creating replacement cells for burned-out insulin-producing pancreatic beta cells is so promising that it's tempting to think of a "cure" not in terms of if but when. The reality is, however, less rosy. There may one day be a cure, but to put off normalizing your blood sugars until then is simply to ignore the reality of your situation. If you're going to control your diabetes and get on with a normal life, you will have to change your diet, and the *when* is now. No matter how mild or severe your diabetes, the key aspect of all our treatment plans for normalizing blood sugars and preventing or reversing complications of diabetes is diet. In the terms of the Laws of Small Numbers, the single largest "input" you can control is what you eat.

THE FUNDAMENTAL IMPORTANCE OF A RESTRICTED-CARBOHYDRATE DIET

The next several pages may well be the most difficult pages of this book for you to accept—as well as some of the most important. They're full of the foods you're going to have to restrict or eliminate from your diet if you're going to normalize your blood sugars. You may see some of your favorite foods on our No-No list, but before you stop reading, keep in mind a few important things. First, toward the end of this chapter we discuss the foods you can safely eat. Second, while you will have to eliminate certain foods, there are some genuinely sugar-free and low-carbohydrate alternatives.

One purpose of blood glucose self-monitoring is to learn through your blood sugar profiles how particular foods affect you. Blood sugar self-monitoring is the ultimate measure of the effect foods have on your blood sugar. If you don't believe what you're reading here, check your blood sugars every 2 hours after consuming food you are certain must be benign. Over years of examining profiles like the ones you will create, I've observed that some people are more tolerant of certain foods than other people. For example, bread makes my own blood sugar rise very rapidly. Yet one or two of my patients with mild type 2 diabetes eat a sandwich of thin bread every day with only minor problems. Inevitably I find this is related to delayed stomach-emptying (see Chapter 22). In any case, you should feel free to experiment with food and then perform blood sugar readings. It's likely that for many diabetics most or all of our restrictions will be necessary.

Patients often ask, "Can't I just take my medication and eat whatever I want?" It almost seems logical, and would be fine if it worked. But just taking your medication and eating whatever you want doesn't work—because of the Laws of Small Numbers—so we have to find something that does.

Many diabetics can be treated with diet alone, and if your disease is relatively mild, you could easily fall into this category. Some patients who have been using insulin or oral agents find that once on our diet they no longer need blood sugar–lowering medication. But even if you require insulin or other agents, diet will still constitute the most essential part of your treatment.

Think small inputs. You may recall from prior chapters that—for even the mildest diabetic—the impairment or loss of phase I insulin response makes normalizing blood sugars impossible for at least a few hours after a high-carbohydrate meal. Eating even small amounts of fast-acting carbohydrate raises blood sugar so rapidly that any remaining phase II insulin response cannot promptly compensate. This is true if you're injecting insulin or if you're still making your own insulin.

Any sensible meal plan for normalizing blood sugar takes this into account and follows these basic rules:

- First, eliminate all foods that contain simple sugars. As you should know by now—but it bears repeating—"simple sugar" does not mean just table sugar; that's why I prefer to call them fast-acting carbohydrates. Breads and other starchy foods, such as potatoes and grains, become glucose so rapidly that they can cause serious postprandial increases in blood sugar.

- Second, limit your total carbohydrate intake to an amount that will work with your injected insulin or your body's remaining phase II insulin response, if any. In this way, you avoid a postprandial blood sugar increase, and avoid overworking any remaining insulin-producing beta cells of your pancreas (research has demonstrated that beta cell burnout can be slowed or halted by normalizing blood sugars).
- Third, stop eating when you no longer feel hungry, not when you're stuffed. There's no reason for you to leave the table hungry, but there's also no reason to be gluttonous. Remember the Chinese restaurant effect (see page 101).
- Keep the protein and carbohydrate content for each meal consistent from one day to the next. If you are taking blood sugar–lowering agents, undereating can result in severe hypoglycemia.
- Finally, for best results, follow a predetermined meal plan (see Chapter 11).

TESTING FOR STARCH OR SUCROSE IN FOODS

Sometimes you'll find yourself at a restaurant, hotel, or reception where you cannot predict if foods have sugar or flour in them. Your waiter probably has little idea of what's in a given recipe, so don't even ask him; his response will likely be incorrect. I've found that the easiest way to make certain is to use the Diastix that should have been checked off on your supply list (Chapter 3). These are manufactured to test urine for glucose. We use them to test food. If, for example, you want to determine if a soup or salad dressing contains table sugar (sucrose) or a sauce contains flour, just put a small amount in your mouth and mix it with your saliva. Then spit a tiny bit onto a test strip. Any color change indicates the presence of sugar or starch. Saliva is essential to this reaction because it contains an enzyme that releases glucose from sucrose (table sugar) or from flour in the food, permitting it to react with the chemicals in the test strip. This is how I found that one restaurant in my neighborhood uses large amounts of sugar in its bouillon while another restaurant uses none.*

Solid foods can also be tested this way, but you must chew them first. The lightest color on the color chart label of the test strip container indicates a very low concentration of glucose. Any color paler than this may be acceptable for foods consumed in small amounts. The Diastix method works on nearly all the foods on our No-No list except milk products, which contain lactose. It will also not react with fructose (fruit sugar; also present in some vegetables, in all fruits, and in honey). If in doubt, assume the worst.

NO-NO FOODS: ELIMINATING SIMPLE SUGARS

Named below are some of the common foods that contain simple sugars, which rapidly raise blood sugar or otherwise hinder blood sugar control and should be eliminated from your diet. All grain products, for example — from the flour in "sugar-free" cookies to pasta to wheat or non-wheat grain products except pure bran — are converted so rapidly into glucose by the enzymes in saliva and farther down in the digestive tract that they are, as far as blood sugar is concerned, essentially no different than table sugar or even pure glucose. There are plenty of food products, however, that contain such tiny amounts of simple sugars that they will have a negligible effect on your blood sugar. One gram of carbohydrate will not raise blood sugar more than 5 mg/dl for most diabetic adults (but considerably more for small children). A single stick of chewing gum or a single tablespoon of salad dressing made with only 1 gram of sugar certainly poses no problems. In these areas, you have to use your judgment and your blood sugar profiles. If you're the type who, once you start chewing gum, has to have a new stick every 30 minutes, then you should probably avoid chewing gum. If you have delayed stomach-emptying (see Chapter 22), small amounts of "sugar-free" chewing gum may help facilitate your digestion.

---

* I use this test on television to show that even "whole grain" breads, contrary to claims of the ADA, become instant glucose when exposed to saliva.

Powdered Artificial Sweeteners

At this writing, several artificial sweeteners are available. They are available from different manufacturers under different names, and some, such as Equal and Sweet'n Low, can have brand names under which more than one form of sweetener is sold. Here, to simplify your shopping, are *acceptable* products currently available:

saccharin tablets or liquid (Sweet'n Low)
aspartame tablets (Equal, NutraSweet)*
acesulfame-K (Sunett, The Sweet One)
stevia (Most stevia powder is now made with the sugar maltodextrin. A few brands are available as pure stevia.)
sucralose tablets and liquid Splenda — now available in some parts
   of the United States, overseas, and on the Internet.† (These
   forms are benign in spite of containing minute amounts of
   lactose.)
neotame tablets
cyclamate tablets and liquid (not yet available in the United States)

These are all noncarbohydrate sweeteners that vary in their availability and can be used to satisfy a sweet tooth without significantly affecting blood sugars. *But when sold in powdered form, under such brand names as Sweet'n Low, Equal, The Sweet One, Sunett, Sugar Twin, Splenda, SweetLeaf, and others, these products usually contain a sugar to increase bulk, and will rapidly raise blood sugar.* They are all orders of magnitude sweeter-tasting than sugar. When you buy them in packets and powdered form, with the exception of a few stevia formulations, they usually contain about 96 percent glucose or maltodextrin and about 4 percent artificial sweetener. In powdered form, Splenda (like other powdered sweeteners with the exception of stevia) is principally a mixture of sugars to provide bulk and should be avoided. If you read the Nutrition Facts label on granulated Splenda, for example, it lists, as such labels must, ingredients in order from most to least: dextrose

---

* Many websites falsely perpetuate the myth that aspartame is toxic because its metabolism produces the poison methanol. In reality, one 12-ounce can of an aspartame-sweetened soft drink generates only 1/25 as much methanol as does a glass of milk.
† You can find the liquid at www.leansupplements.com.

(glucose), maltodextrin (a mixture of sugars), and finally sucralose. Most powdered sweeteners are sold as low-calorie and/or sugar-free sweeteners because they contain only 1 gram of a sugar as compared to 3 grams of sucrose in a similar paper packet labeled "sugar." More suitable for diabetics are tablet sweeteners such as saccharin, cyclamate, and aspartame. As noted above, the same brand name can denote multiple products: Equal is a powder containing 96 percent glucose and also a tablet containing a minuscule (acceptable) amount of lactose. Sweet'n Low powder is saccharin with 96 percent glucose. Stevia liquid (sold in health food stores) contains no sugar of any kind and only minute amounts of carbohydrate.

A new "natural artificial" sweetener called tagatose (no brand name as of this writing) has been approved for sale in the United States. Derived from milk, it's claimed to be 92 percent as sweet as sugar, with no aftertaste and no effect on blood sugars. This last claim — that it has no effect on blood sugars — remains to be seen. In many cases, what's termed "no effect" or "negligible effect" usually has a significant enough effect to make blood sugar control difficult.

Another new artificial sweetener, neotame, is being sold as an additive by the makers of NutraSweet. It is supposedly eight thousand times as sweet as table sugar. Its use as a food additive should pose no problems, but if it becomes available to consumers as a powder, it will probably be mixed with a sugar as in the instances cited above.

Yet another powdered sweetener, erythritol (Zsweet), is promoted as being 70 percent as sweet as table sugar, but to my taste it is much less sweet, so that a considerable amount must be used. Since erythritol is a sugar alcohol, it will raise diabetic blood sugars significantly when consumed by the tablespoon, as I found.

So-Called Diet Foods and Sugar-Free Foods
Because U.S. food-labeling laws in the recent past have permitted and thus encouraged products to be called "sugar-free" if they do not contain common table sugar (sucrose), the mere substitution of another sugar for sucrose has permitted the packager to deceive the consumer legally. Most so-called sugar-free products have been, for many years, full of sugars that may not promote tooth decay but most certainly will raise your blood sugar. If you've been deceived, you're not alone. I've been in doctors' offices that have candy dishes full of "sugar-free" hard candies for their diabetic patients! Sometimes the label will disclose the name of the substitute sugar.

Here is a partial list of some of the many sugars you can find in "sugar-free" foods. All of these will raise your blood sugar.

carob	honey	saccharose
corn syrup	lactose	sorbitol
dextrin	levulose	sorghum
dextrose	maltodextrin	treacle
dulcitol	maltose	turbinado
fructose	mannitol	xylitol
glucose	mannose	xylose
	molasses	

Some, such as sorbitol and fructose, raise blood sugar more slowly than glucose but still too much and too rapidly to prevent a postprandial blood sugar rise in people with diabetes.

Other "diet" foods contain either sugars that are alternates to sucrose, large amounts of rapid-acting carbohydrate, or both. Many of these foods (e.g., sugar-free cookies) are virtually 100 percent rapid-acting carbohydrate, usually flour, so that even if they were to contain none of the above added sugars, consumption of a small quantity would easily cause rapid blood sugar elevation.

There are exceptions:

- Most diet sodas—with some glaring exceptions, so always check the Nutrition Facts label and look for 0 under carbohydrate.*
- Sugar-free Jell-O brand gelatin desserts—the ready-to-eat variety, not the powdered mix (see page 169).†
- DaVinci brand sugar-free syrups (see page 169).

All of these are made without sugar of any kind. These you need not restrict. See "So What's Left to Eat?" later in this chapter.

---

* Looking for 0 under carbohydrate may not tell you everything you want to know. Also look in the list of ingredients to see if the product contains any of the sugars listed. If it does, check your blood sugars after drinking, if you choose to drink them, and see what effect they have on you.

† Unfortunately, the manufacturers of sugar-free Jell-O brand gelatin add maltodextrin to the powdered version. I expect that they will soon add it also to the ready-to-eat version. A suitable substitute would be Knox unflavored gelatin with added liquid stevia and your choice of DaVinci sugar-free syrup or Crystal Light powder for flavoring.

Candies, Including "Sugar-Free" Brands

A tiny "sugar-free" hard candy containing only 2.5 grams of sorbitol can raise blood sugar almost 13 mg/dl. Ten of these can raise blood sugar 125 mg/dl. Since sorbitol, for example, has only one-third the sweetening power of sucrose, the manufacturer uses three times as much to get the same effect. This will raise blood sugars almost three times as much as, although more slowly than, table sugar.

Honey and Fructose

In recent years a number of "authorities" have claimed that honey and fructose (a sugar occurring in fruits, some vegetables, and honey) are useful to diabetics because they are "natural sugars." Well, glucose is *the* most natural of the sugars, since it is present in all plants and all but one known species of animal, and we already know what glucose can do to blood sugars. Fructose, which is sold as a powdered sweetener, is often derived from corn (a grain) and is a significant ingredient in many food products (as in high-fructose corn syrup). Honey and fructose, "natural" or not, will raise blood sugar far more rapidly than phase II insulin release, injected insulin, or oral hypoglycemic agents can bring it down. Just eat a few grams of honey or fructose and check your blood sugar every 15 minutes. You will readily prove that "authorities" can be wrong.

Desserts and Pastries

With the possible exception of products marked "carbohydrate—0" on the Nutrition Facts label, virtually every food commonly used for desserts will raise blood sugar too much and too fast. This is not only because of added sugar but also because flour, milk, and other components of desserts are very high in rapid-acting carbohydrate.

Bread and Crackers

One average slice of white, rye, or whole grain bread contains 12 or more grams of carbohydrate. The "thin" or "light" breads are usually cut at half the thickness of standard bread slices and therefore contain half the carbohydrate. So-called high-protein breads contain only a small percentage of their calories as protein and are not significantly reduced in carbohydrate unless they are thinly cut. Brown bread, raisin bread, and corn bread all contain as much (or more) fast-acting carbohydrate as rye, white, or whole wheat. Some diabetics with severe gastroparesis (see Chapter 22) can tolerate the inclusion of 1 slice of thin bread or a few small crackers as part of their low-carbohydrate meal limits. Unfortunately, nearly all of us experience very rapid increases of blood sugar after eating even small amounts of such products (bread, crackers, cereals, pastry shells, et cetera) made from any grain. This includes those made from less common grains, such as barley, kasha, oats, sorghum, and quinoa.

Rice and Pasta

Both pasta and wild rice (which is actually not a true variety of rice but another grain entirely) are claimed by some nutrition authorities to raise blood sugar quite slowly. Just check your blood sugar levels after eating them and you'll again prove the "authorities" wrong. Alternatively, you might try the Diastix test described on page 147. Like wild rice and pasta, white rice and brown rice also raise blood sugar quite rapidly for most of us and should be avoided. (According to the glycemic index, a measure of how rapidly foods are metabolized into glucose, brown rice actually raises blood sugar faster than white rice.) The same is true of rice cakes. Some Internet sites offer low-carb pasta for diabetics. In my experience these products raise blood sugar less and much more slowly than regular pasta but are not "free foods."

Breakfast Cereals

Most cold cereals, like snack foods, are virtually 100 percent carbohydrate, even those claiming to be "high-protein." Additionally, many contain large amounts of added sugars. Since they are made from grain, small amounts, even of whole grain cereals, will cause a rapid rise in blood sugar. Even bran flakes are mostly flour. If you have been eating bran flakes to improve bowel function, you can substitute very small amounts (1 tablespoon) of psyllium husks powder, which is entirely indigestible fiber. Alternatively, use the sugar-free variety of Metamucil or other such products. (You can get the husks powder at a health food store and mix it with water. If you don't care for the texture or taste, you can drink it mixed in diet soda.) You can also make your own "cereal" from GG Scandinavian FiberSprinkle, which is available at www.brancrispbread.com.

Cooked cereals generally contain about 10–25 grams of fast-acting carbohydrate per half-cup serving. I find that even small servings make blood sugar control impossible.

Snack Foods

These are the products in cellophane bags that you find in vending machines and supermarkets. They include not just candy, cookies, and cakes, but pretzels, potato chips, taco chips, tiny crackers, and popcorn. These foods are virtually 100 percent carbohydrate and frequently have added sucrose, glucose (the label may say dextrose), corn syrup, et cetera. Although some nuts (e.g., macadamias) are relatively low in carbohydrate, who can sit down and eat only six macadamia nuts (about 1 gram of carbohydrate)? It's simpler just to avoid them, but see page 168 for possible exceptions.

So-Called Protein Bars

Although drugstore and grocery shelves are full of bars that claim to be "protein bars," most are really nothing more than candy bars with "healthy" packaging. The FDA analyzed twenty different brands and found that all but two contained much more carbohydrate than stated on the labels. These were removed from the marketplace, but many more remain. This is another case of when it sounds too good to be true, it probably is.

Milk and Cottage Cheese

Milk contains a considerable amount of the simple sugar lactose and will rapidly raise blood sugar. Skim milk actually contains more lactose per ounce than does whole milk. One or 2 teaspoons of milk in a cup of coffee will not significantly affect blood sugar, but ¼ cup of milk will make a considerable difference to most of us. Cream, which you have probably been instructed to avoid, is okay. One tablespoon has only 0.5 gram of carbohydrate. Furthermore, it tastes much better than substitutes and has considerably more "lightening power." The powdered lighteners for coffee contain relatively rapid-acting sugars and should be avoided if you use more than a teaspoonful at a time or drink more than 1 cup of coffee at a meal. A coffee lightener that some people use is WestSoy brand soymilk, which is sold in health food stores throughout the United States. Although several WestSoy flavors are marketed, only the ones marked "Organic Unsweetened" are unsweetened. It comes in plain, vanilla, chocolate, and almond and usually contains 5 grams of carbohydrate in 8 ounces. Other unsweetened brands, such as Vitasoy and Yü, are available in various parts of the country. One catch — soymilk curdles in very hot coffee or tea.

Cottage cheese also contains a considerable amount of lactose because, unlike most other cheeses (hard cheese, cream cheese), which are okay, it is only partly fermented. I was unaware of this until several patients showed me records of substantial blood sugar increases after consuming a container of cottage cheese. It should be avoided except in very small amounts, say about 2 tablespoons.

Fruits and Fruit Juices

These contain varying mixtures of simple sugars and more complex carbohydrates, all of which will act dramatically on blood sugar levels, which you can prove by doing a few experiments with blood sugar measurements. Bitter-tasting fruits such as grapefruit and lemon contain considerable amounts of simple sugars. They taste bitter because of the presence of bitter chemicals, not because sugar is absent. Orange juice, which may be high in vitamin C, also contains about as much sugar as a nondiet soft drink. Although eliminating fruit and fruit juices from the diet can initially be a big sacrifice for many of my patients, they usually get used to this rapidly, and they appreciate the effect upon blood sugar control. I haven't eaten fruit in over forty years, and I haven't suffered in any respect. Some people fear that they will lose important nutrients by eliminating fruit, but that shouldn't be a worry. Nutrients found in fruits are also present in the vegetables you can safely eat.

In our society, we generally reserve the name "fruit" for sweet fruits, such as apples, oranges, and bananas, all of which you should avoid. There are, however, a number of biological fruits (the part of certain plants that contains pulp and seeds) that are benign for the diabetic, such as summer squash, cucumbers (including many types of pickles), eggplant, bell and chili peppers, and avocados. These tend to have large amounts of cellulose, an indigestible fiber, rather than fast-acting carbohydrate. (It's worth noting that cellulose, found in vegetables and fruits, is essentially the same fiber that makes up much of the shady elm on the corner. It has indigestible calories our bodies won't metabolize because we don't have the enzymes to break down the special cellulose chains of sugars into digestible form.)

Vegetables

Beets. Like most other sweet-tasting vegetables, beets are loaded with sugar. Sugar beets are a source of table sugar.

Carrots. After cooking, carrots taste sweeter and appear to raise blood sugar much more rapidly than when raw. This probably relates to the breakdown of complex carbohydrates into simpler sugars by heat. Even raw carrots should be avoided. If, however, you are served a salad with a few carrot shavings on top for decoration, don't bother to remove them. The amount is insignificant, just like a teaspoon of milk.

Corn. Not a vegetable at all but a grain, as noted above. Nearly all of the corn grown in the United States is used for two main purposes. One is the production of sugars. Most of the sugar in Pepsi-Cola, for example, comes from corn. The other major purpose is animal feed (i.e., fattening up hogs, cattle, and chickens). Corn for consumption by people, as a "vegetable" or as snack foods, comes in third. Diabetics should avoid eating corn, whether popped, cooked, or in chips. Even 1 gram of corn (a couple of kernels of popcorn) will rapidly raise my blood sugar by about 5 mg/dl.

Potatoes. For most diabetics, cooked potatoes raise blood sugar almost as fast as pure glucose, even though they may not taste sweet. Giving up potatoes is a big sacrifice for many people, but it will also make a big difference in your postprandial blood sugars.

Tomatoes, tomato paste, and tomato sauce. Tomatoes, as you know, are actually a fruit, not a vegetable, and as with citrus fruits, their tang can conceal just how sweet they are. The prolonged cooking necessary for the preparation of tomato sauces releases a lot of glucose, and you would do well to avoid them. If you're at someone's home for dinner and are served meat or fish covered with tomato sauce, just scrape it off. The small amount that might remain should not significantly affect your blood sugar. If you are having them uncooked in a salad, limit yourself to one slice or a single cherry tomato per cup of salad. (See page 414 for a recipe for a low-carbohydrate, tomato-free, Italian-style red sauce that can be good over, say, a broiled, sautéed, or grilled chicken breast or veal scallopini.) Onions fall into this same category—despite some sharp flavor, they're quite sweet, some varieties sweeter than others. There are other vegetables in the allium family that can be easily substituted, although in smaller quantities, such as shallots and elephant garlic.

Commercially prepared soups. Believe it or not, most commercial soups marketed in this country can be as loaded with added sugar as a soft drink. The taste of the sugar is frequently masked by other flavors—spices, herbs, and particularly salt. Even if there were no added sugar, the prolonged cooking of vegetables can break the special glucose bonds in the cellulose of slow-acting carbohydrates, turning them into glucose. As you know from above, the amount of carbohydrate claimed on the Nutrition Facts label can vary considerably from what's actually in the can. Add to that the common inclusion of potatoes, barley, corn, rice, and other unacceptable foods, and you have a product that you should avoid. There are still some commercial soup possibilities that fit into our scheme. See the corresponding heading on page 162.

Health foods. Of the hundreds of packaged food products that you see on the shelves of the average health food store, perhaps 1 percent are low in carbohydrate. Many are sweetened, usually with honey or other so-called natural sugars. Indeed, many so-called natural foods can be very high in carbohydrate. Since the health food industry shuns artificial (nonsugar) sweeteners like saccharin and aspartame, if a food tastes sweet, it probably contains a sugar. There are a few foods carried by these stores that are unsweetened and low in carbohydrate. You'll find some of these listed later in this chapter.

SO WHAT'S LEFT TO EAT?

It's a good question, and the same one I asked myself over forty years ago as I discovered that more and more of the things that the American Diabetes Association had been telling me were perfectly fine to eat made blood sugar control impossible. In the following pages, I'll give you a broad overview of the kinds of food my patients and I usually eat. Please remember that with the exception of the no-calorie beverages (including seltzer water and mineral water with no added carbohydrate) and moderate portions of sugar-free Jell-O without maltodextrin, there are no "freebies." Virtually everything we eat will have some effect upon blood sugar if enough is consumed. You may discover things I've never heard of that have almost no effect on your blood sugar. If so, feel free to include them in your meal plan, but check your blood sugar every half hour for a few hours before assuming that they are benign.

Vegetables

Most vegetables, other than those listed in the No-No section, are acceptable. Acceptable vegetables include <u>asparagus, avocados, broccoli, brussels sprouts, cabbage and sauerkraut, cauliflower, eggplant, onions (in small amounts), peppers (any color except yellow), mushrooms, spinach, string beans, summer squash, and zucchini.</u> As a rule of thumb, ⅔ cup of whole cooked vegetables, ½ cup of diced or sliced cooked vegetables, ¼ cup of mashed cooked vegetables, or 1 cup of mixed salad acts upon blood sugar as if it contains about 6 grams of carbohydrate. Remember that <u>cooked vegetables tend to raise blood sugar more rapidly than raw vegetables</u> because the heat makes them more digestible and converts some of the cellulose to sugar. Generally, more cooked vegetables by weight will occupy less volume in a measuring cup, so a cup of cooked spinach will weigh considerably more than a cup of uncooked. On your self-measurements, note how your favorite vegetables affect your blood sugar. Raw or unmashed vegetables can present digestive problems to people with gastroparesis (see Chapter 22).

Of the following cooked vegetables, each acts upon blood sugar as if it contains about 6 grams of carbohydrate in ⅔ cup (all cooked except as noted):

artichoke hearts

asparagus

bamboo shoots

beet greens

bell peppers (green and red
   only, no yellow; cooked
   or raw)

bok choy (Chinese cabbage)

broccoli

brussels sprouts

cabbage

celery

celery root (celeriac)

collard greens

daikon radish

dandelion greens

eggplant

endive

escarole

hearts of palm

kohlrabi

mushrooms

mustard greens

okra

patty pan squash

pumpkin (¼ cup)

radicchio

rhubarb

sauerkraut

scallions

snow peas	turnips
spinach	water chestnuts
string beans	watercress
summer squash	zucchini
turnip greens	zucchini flowers

In addition to the above, you should keep the following in mind:

- Onions are high in carbohydrate and should only be used in small amounts for flavoring—small amounts of chives or shallots can pack a lot of flavor.
- One-half small avocado contains about 6 grams of carbohydrate.
- One cup mixed green salad without carrots and with a single slice of tomato or onion has about the same impact on blood sugars as 6 grams of carbohydrate.
- One-quarter cup mashed pumpkin contains about 6 grams of carbohydrate. My own opinion is that without some flavoring, pumpkin tastes about as appetizing as Kleenex. Therefore I flavor it with much stevia and spice (cinnamon) and warm it to make it a bit like pumpkin pie filling. (For other vegetables from this list, such as turnips, assume that ¼ cup of the mashed product acts like it contains 6 grams of carbohydrate.)

Meat, Fish, Fowl, Seafood, and Eggs

These are usually the major sources of calories in the meal plans of my patients. The popular press is currently down on meat and eggs, but my personal observations and recent research implicate carbohydrates rather than dietary fat in the heart disease and abnormal blood lipid profiles of diabetics and even of nondiabetics. If you are frightened of these foods, you can restrict them, but depriving yourself will be unlikely to buy you better health. Appendix A details the current controversy and the shaky science behind the present, faddish high-carbohydrate dietary recommendations, and lays out my concerns and opinions. Egg yolks, by the way, are a major source of the nutrient lutein, which is beneficial to the retina of the eye. Organic eggs contain large amounts of omega-3 fatty acids, which are good for your arteries.

No-No's in a Nutshell
Here is a concise list of foods to avoid that are discussed in this chapter. You may want to memorize it or copy it, as it is worth learning.

Sweets and Sweeteners
- Powdered sweeteners (other than pure stevia)
- Candies, especially so-called sugar-free types
- Honey and fructose
- Most "diet" and "sugar-free" foods (except sugar-free Jell-O brand gelatin when the label doesn't mention maltodextrin, and diet sodas that do not contain fruit juices or list carbohydrate on the label)
- Desserts (except Jell-O brand gelatin without malto-dextrin—no more than ½ cup per serving) and pastries: cakes, cookies, pies, tarts, et cetera
- Foods containing, as a significant ingredient, products whose names end in *-ol* or *-ose* (dextrose, glucose, lactose, mannitol, mannose, sorbitol, sucrose, xylitol, xylose, et cetera), except cellulose; also, corn syrup, molasses, maltodextrin, et cetera

Sweet or Starchy Vegetables
- Beans: chili beans, chickpeas, lima beans, lentils, sweet peas, et cetera (string beans, snow peas, and bell and chili peppers, which are mostly cellulose, are okay, as are very limited amounts of many soybean products)
- Beets
- Carrots
- Corn
- Onions, except in small amounts
- Packaged creamed spinach containing flour
- Parsnips
- Potatoes

- Cooked tomatoes, tomato paste, tomato sauce, and raw tomatoes except in small amounts
- Winter squash

Fruits and Juices
- All fruits (except avocados)
- All juices (including tomato and vegetable juices—except for some people, in a small Bloody Mary)

Certain Dairy Products
- Milk
- Sweetened, flavored, and low-fat yogurts
- Cottage cheese (except in very small amounts)
- Powdered milk substitutes and coffee lighteners
- Canned milk concentrate

Grains and Grain Products
- Wheat, rye, barley, corn, oats, and lesser-known "alternative" grains, such as kasha, quinoa, and sorghum
- White rice, brown rice, wild rice, or rice cakes
- Pasta
- Breakfast cereal
- Pancakes and waffles
- Bread, crackers, and other flour products, including "whole grain" breads

Prepared Foods
- Most commercially prepared soups
- Most packaged "health foods"
- Snack foods (virtually anything that comes wrapped in cellophane, including nuts)
- Balsamic vinegar (compared to wine vinegar, white vinegar, or cider vinegar, balsamic contains considerable sugar)

Tofu, and Soybean Substitutes for Bacon, Sausage, Hamburger, Fish, Chicken, and Steak

About half the calories in these products come from vegetable fats, and the balance from varying amounts of protein and slow-acting carbohydrate. They are easy to cook in a skillet or microwave. Protein and carbohydrate content should be read from the labels and counted in your meal plan. Their principal value is for people who are vegetarian or want to avoid red meat. Health food stores stock many of these products. For the purpose of our meal plans, as described in the next chapter, remember to divide the *grams* of protein listed on the package by 6 in order to get "*ounces*" of protein (see page 180).

Certain Commercially Prepared and Homemade Soups

Although most commercial and homemade soups contain large amounts of simple sugars, you can learn how to buy or prepare low- or zero-carbohydrate soups (see suggestions below). Many but not all packaged bouillon preparations have no added sugar and only small amounts of carbohydrate. Check the labels or use the Diastix test, observing the special technique described on page 147. Plain consommé or broth in some restaurants may occasionally be prepared without sugar. Again, check with Diastix.

Homemade soups, cooked without vegetables, can be made very tasty if they are concentrated. You can achieve this by barely covering the meat or chicken with water while cooking, rather than filling the entire pot with water, as is the customary procedure. Alternatively, let the stock cook down (reduce) so you get a more concentrated, flavorful soup. You can also use herbs and spices, all of which have negligible amounts of carbohydrates, to enhance flavor. (See "Mustard, Pepper, Salt, Spices, and Herbs" later in this chapter.) Clam broth (not chowder) is usually very low in carbohydrate. In the United States you can also buy clam juices (not Clamato), which contain only about 2 grams of carbohydrate in 3 fluid ounces. Campbell's canned beef bouillon and consommé contain only 1 gram carbohydrate per serving. College Inn brand canned chicken broth contains no carbohydrate. Most bouillon cubes are also low in carbohydrate; read the labels.

Cheese, Butter, Margarine, and Cream

Most cheeses (other than cottage cheese) contain approximately equal amounts of protein and fat and small amounts of carbohydrate. The carbohydrate and the protein must be figured into the meal plan, as I will explain in Chapter 11. For people who want (unwisely) to avoid animal fats, there are some special soybean cheeses (not very tasty). There's also hemp cheese, which I know nothing about. Cheese is an excellent source of calcium. Every ounce of whole-milk cheese contains approximately 1 gram carbohydrate, except cottage cheese, which contains more. Generally speaking, where dairy products are concerned, the lower the fat, the higher the sugar lactose, with skim milk and "no-fat" cheeses containing the most lactose and the least fat, and butter containing no lactose and the most fat.

Neither butter nor margarine in my experience will affect your blood sugar significantly, and they shouldn't be a problem as far as weight is concerned if you're not consuming a lot of carbohydrate along with them. Margarine and most vegetable oils contain trans fatty acids, which are now considered unhealthy for the heart. Butter is now a "healthy" fat. Organic coconut oil is perhaps the healthiest oil for cooking and salads. Since it is solid at room temperature, it should be warmed slightly for salads. It can be found on the Internet and in health food stores.

One tablespoon of cream has only 0.5 gram carbohydrate—it would take 8 tablespoons to raise my blood sugar 20 mg/dl.

The cheese puffs I describe on page 188 are low in carbohydrate and can be used instead of bread to make sandwiches.

Yogurt

Although I personally don't enjoy yogurt, many of my patients feel they cannot survive without it. For our purposes plain whole-milk yogurt—unflavored, unsweetened, and without fruit—is a reasonable food. A full 7-ounce container of plain, unflavored Fage brand whole-milk Greek yogurt contains only 6 grams of carbohydrate and 2⅓ ounces of protein. You can even throw in some chopped vegetables and not exceed the 12 grams of carbohydrate limit we suggest for lunch. Do not use nonfat yogurt. The carbohydrate goes up to 17 grams per 8-ounce container. Yogurt can be flavored with cinnamon, with DaVinci brand sugar-free syrups, with flavor extracts, with Crystal Light powder, or with the powder from sugar-free Jell-O brand gelatin (if the package doesn't list maltodextrin as an ingredient) without affecting the carbohydrate content. It can be sweetened with stevia or sucralose liquid or with Equal or Splenda tablets that have been dissolved in a small amount of hot water. Fage brand yogurt is available at supermarkets throughout the United States. If you read the labels, you may find other brands low in carbohydrate, including Erivan, Stonyfield Farm, and Brown Cow Farm. Always be sure to use only the whole-milk and not the low-fat products.

Soymilk

There are many soy products that can be used in our diet plan, and soymilk is no exception. It's a satisfactory lightener for coffee and tea, and one of my patients adds a small amount to diet sodas. Others drink it as a beverage, either straight or with added flavoring such as those mentioned for yogurt. Personally, I find the taste too bland to drink without flavoring, and I much prefer cream diluted with water. When used in small amounts (up to 2 tablespoons/1 ounce), soymilk need not be figured into the meal plan. It will curdle if you put it into very hot drinks.

As noted in the No-No foods section, of the many brands of soymilk on the market, WestSoy offers the only unsweetened ones I've been able to find, although other unsweetened brands are available in various parts of the United States.

Soybean Flour

If you or someone in your home is willing to try baking with soybean flour, you will find a neat solution to the pastry restriction. One ounce (by weight) of full-fat soybean flour (about ¼ cup) contains about 7.5 grams of slow-acting carbohydrate. You could make chicken pies, tuna pies, and even sugar-free Jell-O pies or pumpkin pies. Just remember to include the carbohydrate and protein contents in your meal plan.

Soybean flour usually must be blended with egg to form a batter suitable for breads, cakes, and the like. Each egg is equivalent to 1 ounce of protein. Creating a blend that works requires either experience or experimentation. Some recipes using soy flour appear in Part Three, "Your Diabetic Cookbook."

Bran Crackers

Of the dozens of different crackers that I have seen in health food stores and supermarkets, I have found only two brands that are truly low in carbohydrate.

- GG Scandinavian Bran Crispbread, produced by G. Gundersen Larvik A/S, Larvik, Norway (distributed in the United States by

Cel-Ent, Inc., Box 1173, Beaufort, SC 29901, [800] 437-5334, opt. 5, www.brancrispbread.com). Each 9-gram slice contains about 3 grams of digestible carbohydrate. If this product is not available locally, you can order it directly from the importer. One case contains thirty 4-ounce packages. It is also available from Rosedale Pharmacy, (888) 796-3348, and at www.rx4better health.com.

- Wasa Crisp'n Light 7 Grain crackerbread. This product is available in most supermarkets in the United States and in some other countries and on the Internet. One cracker contains about 5 grams of digestible carbohydrate. Many of my patients feel that this is the tastier of these two products. Do not use other Wasa products, as they contain more carbohydrate.

Although some people eat these without a spread, to me they taste like cardboard. My preference is to enjoy them with chive-flavored cream cheese or butter. Crumbling two GG crispbreads into a bowl and covering them with cream or cream diluted with water can create bran cracker cereal. Add some Equal or Splenda tablets (dissolved in a bit of hot water) or some stevia or sucralose liquid and, if desired, flavor extracts (banana flavor, butter flavor, et cetera), DaVinci sugar-free syrups, or Crystal Light powder. Bran Crispbread is now available fully crumbled in a 10.6-ounce plastic container; it's called FiberSprinkle.

If eaten in excessive amounts, bran crackers can cause diarrhea. They should be eaten with liquid. They are not recommended for people with gastroparesis (delayed stomach-emptying), since the bran fibers can form a plug that blocks the outlet of the stomach. The carbohydrate in these crackers is very slow to raise blood sugar. They are great for people who need a substitute for toast at breakfast.

NOTE: In the United States, labeling regulations require that fiber be listed as carbohydrate. There are many different kinds of fiber, soluble and insoluble, digestible and indigestible, and so, because there is no requirement to distinguish in labeling between them, these listings can complicate computation of carbohydrate content. Use the carbohydrate amounts that I have listed above instead of those listed on the package labels.

If you use thyroid pills, do not take them within 2 hours of eating bran products or more than 1 ounce of soy products. Bran and soy can bind thyroid hormones and thereby prevent their absorption.

Toasted Nori

When my friend Kanji Ishikawa sent me a beautifully decorated canister from Japan, I was most impressed and intrigued. You can imagine my dismay when I removed the cover and found seaweed. My dismay was only temporary, however. I reluctantly opened one of the cellophane envelopes and pulled out a tissue-thin slice. My first nibble was quite a surprise — it was delicious. When consumed in small amounts, I found, it had virtually no effect upon blood sugar. Once addicted, I combed the health food stores searching for more. Most of the seaweed I tried tasted like salty paper. Eventually, a patient explained to me that Kanji's seaweed is a special kind called toasted nori. It contains small amounts of additional ingredients that include soybeans, rice, barley, and red pepper. It is available at most health food stores, and can be a very tasty snack if you can find a good brand. Five or six pieces at a time have had no effect upon my blood sugar. The Diastix test showed no glucose after chewing. A standard slice usually measures 1¼ × 3½ inches and weighs about 0.3 gram. Since the product contains about 40 percent carbohydrate, each strip will have only 0.12 gram carbohydrate. Larger sheets of toasted nori should be weighed in order to estimate their carbohydrate content.

Sweeteners: Saccharin, Aspartame, Stevia, Splenda, Sucralose, and Cyclamate

I carry a package of Equal (aspartame) tablets with me, particularly when I go out to eat. Aspartame is destroyed by cooking, but it works for sweetening hot coffee or tea. It is much more costly than saccharin, which has a slightly bitter aftertaste, but I find that using one ½-grain saccharin tablet for every Equal tablet, rather than two saccharin tablets or two Equal tablets, eliminates saccharin's aftertaste and keeps costs down. Equal tablets are available in most pharmacies and many supermarkets. Although Equal tablets contain lactose, the amount is too small to affect blood sugar.

Acesulfame-K is a new artificial sweetener being marketed in tablet form outside the United States by Hoechst, AG, of Germany. It is not degraded by cooking. It is added to some "sugar-free" foods in the United States under the brand name Sunett, and is combined with glucose in the packaged powder called The Sweet One, which you obviously should avoid. There are, however, some questions about its causing cancer, so there may be better choices.

Other noncaloric tablet sweeteners will be appearing on grocery shelves in the United States in the future. Stevia is an herbal sweetener that has been available in health food stores for many years. It is not degraded by cooking and is packaged in tablet, powder, and liquid forms. The liquid must be refrigerated to prevent spoiling. Stevia has not yet been approved in the European Union because of fears that it may cause cancer. Studies of this "possibility" are under way. Most providers of stevia powder in the United States mix it with maltodextrin to reduce cost and provide bulk. Read the label very carefully before buying powdered stevia.

Splenda (sucralose) tablets and liquid are available now in some parts of the United States, overseas, and on the Internet.* They are benign in spite of containing minute amounts of lactose. In powdered form, Splenda, like the others except stevia, is principally a mixture of sugars to provide bulk and should be avoided.

Cyclamate is not currently available in the United States, but may be returning.

DaVinci Gourmet Sugar-Free Syrups

These syrups are available from several Internet distributors, including www.davincigourmet.com, and from Rosedale Pharmacy. DaVinci currently produces more than forty flavors. Internet prices range from $7.49 to $8.95 for a 750 ml bottle. Flavors include banana, blueberry, caramel, cherry, chocolate, coconut, cookie dough, pancake, peanut butter, and watermelon, among others. Sometimes I like to mix the toasted marshmallow syrup into my morning omelet. For a list of distributors, phone DaVinci Gourmet, Ltd., at (800) 640-6779. The product is certified kosher. DaVinci also sells syrups that are not sugar-free, so be sure to specify sugar-free when ordering.

Fox's U-bet Sugar Free Chocolate Flavor Syrup

This is probably the best-tasting of all the sugar-free chocolate syrups I have encountered. It is also a true syrup and not watery. It is sweetened with sucralose and manufactured by H. Fox & Co., Inc., in Brooklyn, New York. It is kosher and sold in some supermarkets.

---

* You can find Splenda liquid online at www.leansupplements.com.

Flavor Extracts

There are numerous flavor extracts often used in baking that you can use to make your food more exciting. They usually can be found in small brown bottles in the baking supply aisles of supermarkets. Read carbohydrate content from the label. Usually it's zero and therefore won't affect your blood sugar.

Mustard, Pepper, Salt, Spices, and Herbs

Most commercial mustards are made without sugar and contain essentially no carbohydrate. This can readily be determined for a given brand by reading the label or by using the Diastix test. Pepper and salt have no effect upon blood sugar. Hypertensive individuals with proven salt sensitivity should, of course, avoid added salt and highly salted foods (see page 472).

Most herbs and spices have very low carbohydrate content and are used in such small amounts that the amount of ingested carbohydrate will be insignificant. Watch out, however, for certain combinations, such as ground cinnamon with sugar. Just read the labels. By the way, I mix ground cinnamon with powdered stevia and cream cheese and eat it off the plate with bites of smoked salmon for lunch.

Low-Carbohydrate Salad Dressings

Most salad dressings are loaded with sugars and other carbohydrates. The ideal dressing for someone who desires normal blood sugars would therefore be oil and vinegar, perhaps with added spices or mustard, and followed by grated cheese or even real or soy bacon bits. Some commercial salad dressings with only 1 gram carbohydrate per 2-tablespoon serving are now available. This is low enough that such a product can be worked into our meal plans. Be careful with mayonnaise. Most brands are labeled "carbohydrate—0 grams," but may contain up to 0.4 grams per tablespoon. This is not a lot, but it adds up if you eat large amounts. Some imitation mayonnaise products have 5 grams of carbohydrate per 2-tablespoon serving. I personally use olive oil and vinegar on my salads, but I like to mix the vinegar with DaVinci sugar-free raspberry syrup.

Nuts

Although all nuts contain carbohydrate (as well as protein and fat), some usually raise blood sugar slowly and can be worked into meal plans in small amounts. As with most other foods, you will want to look up your favorite nuts in one of the books listed on page 72 in order to obtain their carbohydrate content. By way of example, 10 pistachio nuts (small, not jumbo) contain only 1 gram of carbohydrate, while 10 cashew nuts contain 5 grams of carbohydrate. Although a few nuts may contain little carbohydrate, the catch is in the word "few." Very few of us can eat only a few nuts. In fact, I have only one patient who can count out a preplanned number of nuts, eat them, and then stop. So unless you have unusual willpower, beware. Just avoid them altogether. Also beware of peanut butter, another deceptive addiction. One tablespoon of natural, unsweetened peanut butter contains 3 grams of carbohydrate, and will raise my blood sugar 15 mg/dl. Imagine the effect on blood sugar of downing 10 tablespoons.

Sugar-Free Gelatin

This is one of the few foods that in small amounts will have no effect upon blood sugar if you get the kind that is indeed sugar-free. I have found that in my area "sugar-free" Jell-O brand gelatin actually contains some maltodextrin, which is a mixture of sugars and will raise your blood sugar. The ready-to-eat Jell-O brand in plastic cups does not thus far contain maltodextrin—or at least that found on my grocery's shelves. Check the labels. Truly sugar-free Jell-O or other truly sugar-free brands of gelatin are fine for snacks and desserts. A ½-cup serving contains no carbohydrate, no fat, and only 1 gram of protein.* Just remember not to eat so much that you feel stuffed (see "The Chinese Restaurant Effect," page 101). You can enhance the taste by pouring a little heavy cream over your portion. One of my patients discovered that it becomes even tastier if you whip it in a blender with cream when it has cooled, just before it sets.

If the only "sugar-free" Jell-O you can find contains maltodextrin, try adding some liquid stevia or sucralose and DaVinci sugar-free syrup or Crystal Light powder to Knox unflavored gelatin as a tasty substitute.

Sugar-Free Jell-O Brand Puddings

Available in chocolate, vanilla, pistachio, butterscotch, banana cream, cheesecake, lemon, and white chocolate, these make a nice dessert

---

* In the United States, Walmart sells a flavored sugar-free product without maltodextrin.

treat. Unlike Jell-O brand gelatin, they contain a small amount of carbohydrate (about 6 grams per serving), which should be counted in your meal plan. Instead of mixing the powder with milk, use water or water plus cream. Every 2 tablespoons of cream will add 1 gram of carbohydrate.

Chewing Gum

Gum chewing can be a good substitute for snacking and can be of value to people with gastroparesis because it stimulates salivation, and saliva contains substances that facilitate stomach-emptying. The carbohydrate content of one stick of chewing gum varies from about 1 gram in a stick of sugar-free Trident or Orbit (tastes better) to about 7 grams per piece for some liquid-filled chewing gums. The 7-gram gum will rapidly raise my blood sugar by about 35 mg/dl. The carbohydrate content of a stick of chewing gum can usually be found on the package label. "Sugar-free" gums all contain small amounts of a sugar alcohol, usually xylitol—the primary ingredient of Trident "sugarless" gum is sorbitol, a corn-based sugar alcohol. It also includes mannitol and aspartame.

Very Low Carbohydrate Desserts

Part Three of this book consists of low-carbohydrate recipes, prepared and tested by chefs. It includes easy recipes for some low-carbohydrate desserts that are truly delicious. More low-carb desserts can be found in my book *The Diabetes Diet* (Little, Brown, 2005).

Coffee, Tea, Seltzer, Mineral Water, Club Soda, and Diet Soda

None of these products should have significant effect upon blood sugar. The coffee and tea may be sweetened with pure liquid or powdered stevia, or with *tablet* sweeteners such as saccharin, cyclamate, sucralose (Splenda), stevia, and aspartame (Equal). Remember to avoid the use of more than 2 teaspoons of cow's milk as a lightener. Try to use cream (which has much less carbohydrate, tastes better, and goes much further). Read the labels of "diet" sodas, as a few brands contain sugar in the form of fruit juices. Many *flavored* mineral waters, bottled "diet" teas, and seltzers also contain added carbohydrate or sugar, as do many powdered beverages. Again, read the labels. You can also try adding your flavor choice of or DaVinci sugar-free syrups to seltzer to create your own diet soda.

Frozen Diet Soda Pops

Many supermarkets and toy stores in the United States sell plastic molds for making your own ice pops. If these are filled with sugar-free sodas, you can create a tasty snack that has no effect upon blood sugar. Do not use the commercially made "sugar-free" or "diet" ice pops that are displayed in supermarket freezers. They contain fruit juices and other sources of carbohydrate. You might also try water flavored with the DaVinci or Fox's U-bet.

Alcohol, in Limited Amounts

Ethyl alcohol (distilled spirits), as we discussed on page 142, has no direct effect upon blood sugar. Moderate amounts, however, can have a rapid effect upon the liver, preventing the conversion of dietary protein to glucose. If you are following a regimen that includes insulin, a pancreas-stimulating oral hypoglycemic agent, or even an incretin mimetic (see page 214), you're dependent upon conversion of protein to glucose in order to maintain blood sugar at safe levels. The effects of *small* amounts of alcohol (i.e., 1½ ounces of spirits for a typical adult) are usually negligible. Most conventional American beers (light lagers), in spite of their carbohydrate content, don't seem to affect blood sugar when only one can or bottle is consumed. Darker beers, such as ales, stouts, and porters, can contain considerably more carbohydrate, and since beer does not have Nutrition Facts labeling, finding the true carbohydrate content can be difficult. "Lite" beers will generally have the least carbohydrate.

INCREASE YOUR AWARENESS OF FOOD CONTENTS

Read Labels

Virtually all packaged foods bear labels that reveal something about the contents. The FDA now requires that labels of packaged foods list the amount of carbohydrate, protein, fat, and fiber in a serving. Be sure, however, to note the size of the "serving." Sometimes the serving size is so small that you wouldn't want to be bothered eating it.

Beware of labels that say "lite," "light," "sugar-free," "dietetic," "diet," "reduced-calorie," "low-calorie," "net carbohydrate," et cetera. Counts of calories are only going to tell you so much, and "low-fat" is going to tell you nothing about carbohydrate content. "Fat-free" desserts may be the most dangerous of all. Even if you're losing weight, carbohydrate intake will impede your efforts much more than fat will (see Chapter 9, "The Basic Food Groups"). For example, I've found that it's impossible to put weight on very slim patients following low-carbohydrate diets by giving them *900 extra calories a day* in the form of 4 ounces of olive oil. Two studies support this—but only if carbohydrate is very limited. They showed that when carbohydrate is low, the fat is metabolized, not stored. "Low-fat" and "fat-free" foods frequently but not always contain more carbohydrate than the foods they replace. The only way you can determine the carbohydrate content is to read the amount stated on the label. But even this can be deceptive. For example, one popular brand of "sugar-free" strawberry preserves has a label that states, "Carbohydrate—0." Yet anyone can see the strawberries in the jar, and common sense would tell you that strawberries contain carbohydrate. So deceptive labeling occurs and, in my experience, is fairly prevalent in the "diet" food industry.

Use Food Value Manuals

In Chapter 3, three books are listed that show the carbohydrate content of various foods. These manuals are recommended but not essential tools for creating your meal plan. The guidelines and advice set forth in Chapters 9–11 of this book, plus perhaps the recipes in Part Three and in *The Diabetes Diet,* are all you really need to get started.

If you want the potential for considerable variety in your meals, get all the books listed in Chapter 3. The easiest of these to use is *The NutriBase Complete Book of Food Counts. Bowes & Church's Food Values of Portions Commonly Used* has been the dietitian's bible for more than sixty years. It is updated every few years. Be sure to use the index at the back to locate the foods of interest. Note that on every page in the main section, carbohydrate and fat content are listed in the same column. The carbohydrate content of a food always appears below the fat content. Do not get the two confused. Also, be sure to note the portion size in all these books.

The USDA's nutrient database is a very handy resource and offers software for use on PCs and handheld PDA computers that will enable you to find nutrition information on just about any food you choose. The Nutrient Data Laboratory home page can be found at www.ars .usda.gov/main/site_main.htm?modecode=12354500.

VITAMIN AND MINERAL SUPPLEMENTS

It is common practice to prescribe supplementary vitamins and minerals for diabetics. This is primarily because most diabetics have chronically high blood sugars and therefore urinate a lot. Excessive urination causes a loss of water-soluble vitamins and minerals. If you can keep your blood sugars low enough to avoid spilling glucose into the urine (you can test it with Diastix), and if you eat red meat at least once or twice a week, and a variety of vegetables, you should not require supplements, except for vitamin D-3, which is deficient in most people in the industrial world (see page 64). Note, however, that major dietary sources of B-complex vitamins include "fortified" or supplemented breads and grains in the United States. If you're following a low-carbohydrate diet and therefore exclude these from your meal plan, you should eat some bean sprouts, spinach, broccoli, brussels sprouts, or cauliflower each day. If you do not like vegetables, you might take a B-complex capsule or a multivitamin/ mineral capsule each day. See page 189 for a discussion of calcium supplementation for certain people who follow high-fiber or high-protein diets or use metformin. Note, however, that people who consume excessive amounts of calcium supplements (not food sources of calcium) have been shown to have a higher incidence of arterial calcification.

Supplemental vitamins and minerals should not ordinarily be used in excess of the FDA's recommended daily requirements. Large doses can inhibit the body's synthesis of some vitamins and intestinal absorption of certain minerals. Large doses are also potentially toxic. Doses of vitamin C in excess of 500 mg daily may interfere with the chemical reaction on your blood sugar strips. As a result, your blood sugar readings can appear erroneously low. Large doses of vitamin C can actually raise blood sugar and even impair nerve function (as can doses of vitamin B-6 in excess of 200 mg daily). Vitamin E has been shown to reduce one of the destructive effects of high blood sugars (glycosylation of the body's proteins), in a dose-dependent fashion — up to 1,200 IU (international units) per day. It has recently been shown to lower insulin resistance. I therefore recommend 400–1,200 IU per day to a few of my patients. Be sure to use the forms of vitamin E known as gamma tocopherol or mixed tocopherols, not the common alpha tocopherol, which can inhibit the absorption of essential gamma tocopherol from foods and at high doses has actually been shown to increase risk of cardiac death.

This advice may be inappropriate for people who exercise. A 2009 study of exercising type 2 diabetics, performed in Jena, in Germany, and at the Joslin Diabetes Center in Boston, showed that giving subjects 1,000 mg of vitamin C and 400 IU of vitamin E daily eliminated the benefit that exercise had in lowering insulin resistance. Furthermore, these vitamins acted on oxidants by opposing the natural antioxidant effect of exercise.

CHANGES IN BOWEL MOVEMENTS

A new diet often brings about changes in frequency and consistency of bowel movements. This is perfectly natural and should not cause concern unless you experience discomfort. Increasing the fiber content of meals, as with salads, bran crackers, and soybean products, can cause softer and more frequent stools. More dietary protein can cause less frequent and harder stools. One possible treatment for this that won't raise blood sugar is a soluble fiber product called Phloe. It is available on the Internet and at many health food stores. Calcium tablets can cause hard stools and constipation, but this may be offset if they contain magnesium. Normal frequency of bowel movements can range from 3 times per day to 3 times per week. If you notice any changes in your bowel habits more or less than these frequencies, discuss them with your physician.

If you continue to experience carbohydrate cravings after several weeks on our diet, don't feel lost. We can still cure it. Read the section titled "Incretin Mimetics" on page 214.

HOW DO PEOPLE REACT TO THE NEW DIET?

Most of my patients initially feel somewhat deprived, but also grateful because they feel more alert and healthier. (See the chapter "Before and After" for reactions of some patients to the new diet.) I fall into this category myself. My mouth waters whenever I pass a bakery shop and sniff the aroma of fresh bread, but I am also grateful simply to be alive and sniffing.

I will personally answer questions from readers for
one hour every month. This free service is available by
visiting www.askdrbernstein.net.

11

Creating a Customized Meal Plan

Now that you have the essentials of what you should eat and what you should avoid, it's time to take you through the steps of customizing a meal plan that will get you on your way to blood sugar normalization.

A NOTE BEFORE YOU EMBARK UPON THE DIET

If you found yourself thinking as you went through the No-No foods section of the prior chapter that all of this information goes against conventional thinking—you're right. No doubt as you embark upon a meal and treatment plan to normalize your blood sugars, well-meaning but ill-informed friends and relatives will urge you to try more "fun" foods, or to eat less fat and more "complex" carbohydrates. I suggest that you read Appendix A, which provides some possible explanations as to why conventional wisdom may have taken a wrong turn.

GENERAL PRINCIPLES FOR TAILORING A MEAL PLAN

If you use blood sugar–lowering medications such as insulin or oral agents, the first rule of meal planning is *don't change your diet unless your physician first reviews the new meal plan and reduces your medications accordingly.* Most diabetics who begin our low-carbohydrate diet show an immediate and dramatic drop in postprandial blood sugar levels, as compared to blood sugars on their prior, high-carbohydrate diets. *If at the same time your medications are not appropriately reduced, your blood sugars can drop to dangerously low levels.*

The initial meal plan should be geared toward blood sugar control, and also toward keeping you content with what you eat. So with those things in mind, if I were to sit down with you to "negotiate" your meal plan, I would need to have before me a GLUCOGRAF data sheet (see Chapter 5) showing blood sugar profiles and blood sugar–lowering medications (if any) taken during the preceding week or two. I also would ask for a list of what and when you eat on a typical day. This information would give me an idea of what you like to eat and what effect particular doses of blood sugar–lowering medications have on your blood sugars. I also must know your current weight and about any other factors—such as delayed stomach-emptying and medications for other ailments—that might affect your blood sugar. In negotiating the meal plan, I'd try wherever possible to incorporate foods you like.

We will discuss weight reduction in Chapter 12. Changes for this purpose can be made after observing the effects of the initial diet for a month or so.

If you've tried dieting to lose weight or to control your blood sugar, you may have found that simply cutting back on calories according to preprinted tables or fixed calculations can be frustrating and can even have the opposite effect. Say you have a supper that's too small to satisfy you. Later you're so hungry you feel you must have a snack. If you're like most people, your snack will likely be snack food, a bowl of cereal, or some fruit—that is, something loaded with carbohydrate—so you end up with high blood sugars and more calories than you would have consumed if you'd started with a sensible meal. My experience is that it's always best to start with a plan that allows you to get up from the table feeling comfortable but not stuffed.

If you've ever followed the old ADA "exchange" system for preparing diabetic meal plans, you'll find that keeping track of grams of carbohydrate and ounces of protein food (we always estimate carbohydrate in grams and protein food in ounces) requires considerably less effort. Not only is it easier than the exchange approach, it's also more effective, because it places the focus on the nutrients that actually affect blood sugar.

Since all of my patients bring me glucose profiles, over the years it has not been very difficult to develop guidelines for carbohydrate consumption that make blood sugar control relatively easy without causing too great a feeling of deprivation, even for those trying to lose weight.

My basic approach in negotiating a meal plan is that I first set carbohydrate amounts for each meal. Then I ask my patients to tell me how many ounces of protein we should add to make them feel satisfied. (I actually show them plastic samples of protein foods of various sizes, to help them estimate amounts.) For example, I usually advise adult patients to restrict their carbohydrate intake to no more than 6 grams of *slow-acting* carbohydrate at breakfast, 12 grams at lunch, and 12 grams at supper.* Few people would be willing to eat less than these amounts of carbohydrate. (Lower carbohydrate amounts apply to small children.) There is no such thing as an essential carbohydrate for normal development, despite what the popular press might have you believe, but there most certainly are essential amino acids (protein) and essential fatty acids. As mentioned in Chapter 9, the main reason I don't suggest that you avoid all carbohydrate is that there are many constituents of vegetables—such as vitamins and minerals, but also many other nonvitamin chemicals (phytochemicals)—that are only recently becoming understood but that are nonetheless crucial to diet and cannot be obtained through conventional vitamin supplements. This is particularly true for whole-plant and leaf varieties. Folic acid—so called because it is derived from foliage—is essential to all manner of development, but strictly speaking is neither vitamin nor mineral.

Ideally, your blood sugar should be the same after eating as it was before. If blood sugar increases by more than 10 mg/dl after a meal, even if it eventually drops to your target value, either the meal content should be changed or blood sugar–lowering medications should be used before you eat. Contrary to ADA guidelines, it has recently been shown that postprandial, or after-meal, blood sugars are more likely than fasting blood sugars to cause cardiovascular damage.

_____

* It's not at all necessary to consume carbohydrate of any type for breakfast. If you do, the only kind I recommend is in the form of acceptable vegetables (which can work well in, for example, an omelet) or the bran crackers mentioned in the previous chapter.

SLOW-ACTING CARBOHYDRATE

Distinctions are often made between "complex" and "simple" carbohydrates, with foods such as multigrain breads or pasta touted as "full of complex carbohydrates." This is essentially a meaningless distinction, if not a foolish one. There are fast-acting carbohydrates—starches and sugars that break down rapidly and have a consequent rapid effect on blood sugars—and there are slow-acting carbohydrates. Generally, slow-acting carbohydrate comes from whole-plant vegetables (and others listed on page 155). They are predominantly indigestible fiber accompanied by some small amount of digestible carbohydrate and vitamins, minerals, and other compounds, but have relatively little effect on blood sugars.

The foods in the following list are slow-acting carbohydrate foods. These can constitute the building blocks of the carbohydrate portion of each meal. Of course you needn't limit your foods to these—many other such building blocks can be created. Read labels on packaged foods, consult nutrition tables for carbohydrate values of foods you like, check your blood sugars, and find out which foods work for you.*

Equivalent in blood sugar effect to approximately 6 grams of carbohydrate per serving

- 6 Worthington Stripples or Morningstar Farms Breakfast Strips (meatless soy bacon) (also contains 1 ounce protein)
- 3 Morningstar Farms Breakfast Links (meatless soy sausage) (also contains 2 ounces protein)
- 2 GG Scandinavian Bran Crispbreads
- 1½ Wasa Crisp'n Light 7 Grain crackerbreads
- 7-ounce container Fage whole-milk yogurt (also contains 2½ ounces protein)
- 4½ ounces Brown Cow Farm or Stonyfield Farm whole-milk unflavored yogurt (8 ounces contains 11 grams carbohydrate and 2 ounces protein)
- 1 cup mixed salad with oil-and-vinegar (not balsamic) dressing

---

* These foods are listed because they contain small amounts of slow-acting carbohydrate. They do not have any special nutritional or health benefits.

- ⅔ cup cooked whole slow-acting carbohydrate vegetable (or ¼ cup mashed or ½ cup sliced or diced) from list on page 158
- 1 serving sugar-free Jell-O brand pudding made with water or with water and 1 tablespoon cream
- ½ small avocado (3 ounces)

Equivalent in blood sugar effect to approximately 12 grams of carbohydrate per serving

- 1 cup mixed salad with oil-and-vinegar (not balsamic) dressing, plus ⅔ cup cooked whole vegetables (or ¼ cup mashed or ½ cup sliced or diced) from list on page 158
- 8 ounces Brown Cow Farm or Stonyfield Farm whole-milk unflavored yogurt (contains 11 grams carbohydrate and 2 ounces protein)

These lists slightly exaggerate the carbohydrate content of salad and cooked vegetables, but because of their bulk and the Chinese restaurant effect, the net effect upon blood sugar is approximately equivalent to the amounts of carbohydrate shown. To this slow-acting carbohydrate, we'd add an amount of protein that, in your initial opinion, would allow you to leave the table feeling comfortable but not stuffed.

PROTEIN

As with carbohydrate, it is necessary to keep the size of the protein portion at a particular meal constant from one day to the next, so if you eat 6 ounces at lunch one day, you should have 6 ounces at lunch the next. This is especially important if you're taking blood sugar–lowering medications. If you're using tables of food values and need to convert grams of protein to ounces of a protein food, keep in mind that for these meal plans, 6 grams of protein is the equivalent of 1 ounce of an uncooked protein food. To estimate by eye, a portion the size of a deck of playing cards weighs about 3 ounces (red meats weigh about 3.7 ounces because of their greater density).

In order to maintain muscle mass, most physically active people should consume at least 1–1.2 grams of protein per kilogram of ideal body weight.* Athletes will require considerably more, as will growing children. A recent study reported that the average American adult eats about 1.5 grams of protein per 1 kilogram of body weight daily, in spite of the usual sedentary lifestyle.

Protein foods with virtually no carbohydrate (unless added in processing)

- Beef, lamb, veal
- Chicken, turkey, duck
- Eggs
- Most cold cuts (bologna, salami, et cetera)
- Fish and shellfish (fresh or canned)
- Most frankfurters
- Pork (ham, chops, bacon, et cetera)
- Most sausages

Protein foods with a small amount of carbohydrate (1 gram carbohydrate per ounce of protein)

- Cheeses (other than cottage cheese and feta cheese); the gram of carbohydrate per ounce found in most cheeses should usually be included when computing the carbohydrate portion of a meal

Soy products (up to 6 grams carbohydrate per ounce of protein—check Nutrition Facts label on package)

- Veggie burgers
- Tofu
- Meatless bacon
- Meatless sausage
- Other soy substitutes (for fish, chicken, et cetera)

If you have a rare disorder called familial dyslipidemia, where dietary fat actually can increase LDL, restrictions on certain types of dietary fats contained in some protein foods may be appropriate.

_____

≈ 98 grams

* This would amount to 11.7–14 ounces of protein daily for a nonathletic individual whose ideal body weight is 155 pounds.

Unfermented soy foods contain small amounts of phytoestrogens—female sex hormones. Amounts consumed should therefore be limited, especially for children.

THE TIMING OF MEALS AND SNACKS

Meals need not follow a rigidly fixed time schedule, provided, in most cases, that you do not begin eating within 4 hours of the end of the prior meal. This is so the effect of the first meal upon blood sugar won't significantly overlap that of the next meal. For those who inject insulin before meals, it's very important that meals be separated by at least 5 hours if you want to correct elevated blood sugars before eating (see Chapter 19, "Intensive Insulin Regimens"). This is also ideally but not always true of snacks covered by insulin.

Snacks are permitted for some diabetics but certainly not required. The carbohydrate content of snacks may in some cases duplicate but should not exceed that allocated for lunch or supper. So if you ate lunch at noon, you might tolerate a snack that didn't exceed 6 grams of carbohydrate at about 4 P.M. You would then eat supper at about 8 P.M. Snacks are discussed in greater detail later in the chapter.

If you do not take insulin, you need not be restricted to only three daily meals if you prefer four or more low-carbohydrate meals on a regular basis. The timing, again, should ideally be at least 4 hours after the end of the prior meal or snack. For most type 2 diabetics, it may be easier to control blood sugar, with or without medication, after eating several smaller meals than after eating only one or two large meals.

Remember that there are no diabetes-related prohibitions on coffee and tea, either plain or with limited cream (not milk) and/or tablet (not powdered, except for pure stevia) sweeteners.*

Now, let's attempt to translate our guidelines into some practical examples.

---

* Remember that the carbohydrate in 10 cups of coffee, each with 2 tablespoons cream, can raise the blood sugar of a 140-pound type 1 diabetic by 50 mg/dl.

BREAKFAST

With or without blood sugar–lowering medications it is usually more difficult to prevent a blood sugar rise after breakfast than after other meals. Therefore, for the reasons discussed under "The Dawn Phenomenon" (pages 97–98), I usually suggest half as much carbohydrate at breakfast as at other meals. Your body will probably not respond as well to either the insulin it makes or to injected insulin for about 3 hours after you get up in the morning because of the dawn phenomenon.

It is wise to eat breakfast every day, especially if you're overweight. In my experience, most obese people have a history of either skipping or eating very little breakfast. They then become hungry later in the day and overeat. Nevertheless, for most of us, any meal can be skipped without adverse outcomes, provided, of course, that insulin or any other blood sugar–lowering medication taken specifically to cover that meal is also skipped.

A typical breakfast on our meal plan would include up to 6 grams of carbohydrate and an amount of protein to be determined initially by you. There are numerous possible sources of appetizing ideas for the carbohydrate portion of your breakfast. The best place to start is with what you currently eat, as long as it's not on the No-No list (pages 160–161). You can also sample recipes from Part Three or from my book *The Diabetes Diet.* You can experiment with foods in "So What's Left to Eat?" (pages 157–158). There are many soybean products, such as the foods mentioned on pages 162 and 164. Despite restrictions, with a little creativity you can find any number of satisfying things to have for breakfast.

Suppose that, like many of my new patients, you've been eating for breakfast a bagel loaded with cream cheese and 2 cups of coffee with skim milk and Sweet'n Low powdered sweetener (totaling about 40 grams of rapid-acting carbohydrate altogether). As we negotiate, I might propose that you substitute other sweeteners for the Sweet'n Low and 1 ounce WestSoy soymilk (0.5 gram carbohydrate) for the skim milk in each cup of coffee (or use cream). Then I'd recommend that instead of a bagel you eat a Wasa Crisp'n Light 7 Grain crackerbread (2 grams carbohydrate) with 1 ounce of cream cheese (1 gram carbohydrate plus 1 ounce protein). This adds up to about 4 grams of carbohydrate. Finally, I'd suggest that you add a protein food to your meal to make up for the calories and "filling power" that disappeared with the bagel.

Let's say you decide you'll eat eggs for breakfast (or egg whites or Egg Beaters, although for most of us on a low-carbohydrate regimen, neither of these is necessary for cholesterol control). I'd ask how many eggs it would take to make you feel satisfied after giving up the bagel. You might want to make a vegetable omelet instead of eating one of the carbohydrate foods mentioned above. If you're unnecessarily afraid of egg yolks, you might use organic eggs or egg whites. If you find egg whites bland, you could add spices, soy or Tabasco sauce, some mushrooms, a small amount of onion or cheese, chili powder, or even cinnamon with pure stevia to enhance the taste. One of my current personal favorites for flavoring is a "chili sauce" made from Better Than Bouillon Chili Base. This packs a nice chili punch with very little carbohydrate (according to the label, 1 gram of carbohydrate per 2 teaspoons), and works quite well on eggs or other foods, depending on your taste. (I like to make chili burgers with it—which you could certainly have for breakfast.) This product, a kind of mushy paste, comes in a small glass jar and is available at most supermarkets or from Superior Quality Foods, 2355 E. Francis St., Ontario, CA 91761, (800) 300-4210, www.superiortouch.com.

Some years ago, I tried to help my patients who felt they had to have cold cereal include a small amount in their breakfast meal plan, but blood glucose profiles showed consistently that this just didn't work. Grain products, with the exception of the bran products I've mentioned, contain too much fast-acting carbohydrate to allow us to keep blood sugar under control, and so we've had to eliminate breakfast cereals entirely. An alternative might be GG Scandinavian FiberSprinkle.

The good news is that there are lots of other tasty, filling things to eat.

If you don't want eggs, you might try some smoked fish, tuna fish, or even a hamburger. I have one patient who eats two hot dogs for breakfast—her favorite food. The quantity of fish or hamburger would be up to you, but it would have to be kept constant from one day to the next. You can either weigh the protein portion on a food scale or estimate it by eye. The rule of thumb is, again, that a portion of poultry or fish the size of a standard deck of playing cards will weigh about 3 ounces (3.7 ounces for red meat). One egg has the approximate protein content of 1 ounce of meat, poultry, or fish plus up to 0.6 gram of carbohydrate (which we usually ignore).

You can take any of the foods in the 6 grams of carbohydrate list on page 179 and add protein to them (cheese, eggs, et cetera) to make a satisfying breakfast. You can have less than 6 grams of carbohydrate or even no carbohydrate, provided the amount is unchanged from day to day.

LUNCH

Follow the same guidelines for lunch as for breakfast, with the exception that the slow-acting carbohydrate content may be doubled, up to 12 grams.

Say, for example, that you and your friends go to lunch every day at the "greasy spoon" around the corner from work and are served only sandwiches. You might try discarding the bread and eating the filling—meat, turkey, cheese, or other protein food—with a knife and fork. (If you choose cheese, remember to count 1 gram carbohydrate per ounce.) You could also order a hamburger without the bun. And instead of ketchup, you could use mustard, soy sauce, or other carbohydrate-free condiments. You then might add 1⅓ cups of cooked whole vegetables from the list on page 158 (12 grams carbohydrate) or 2 cups of salad with vinegar-and-oil dressing, not balsamic (12 grams carbohydrate), to round out your meal.

If you want to create a lunch menu from scratch, use your food value books to look up foods that interest you. If you like sandwiches, one double cheese puff as described later in this chapter under the "Snacks" heading will be about the size of a large slice of bread. The cheese puffs are sturdy enough that you can make a sandwich from two of them. Just make sure to account for the protein and carbohydrate in the cheese.

The following building blocks may be helpful in giving you a start.

For the protein portion, one of the following

- A small can of tuna fish contains 3 ounces by weight in the United States. If you're packing your lunch, these can be quite convenient if you like tuna. The next larger size can contains 5 ounces. The tastiest canned tuna I've tried is made by Progresso, packed in olive oil.
- 4 standard slices of packaged pasteurized process American cheese (process cheddar in the U.K.) weigh about 2⅔ ounces. They will contain about 3 ounces of protein and 3 grams of carbohydrate.

For about 12 grams carbohydrate, one of the following

- 1⅓ cups cooked whole vegetables (from the list on page 158).
- 2 cups mixed green salad, with 1 slice tomato and vinegar-and-oil (not balsamic) dressing. Sprinkling bacon or soy bacon bits or grated cheese will have negligible additional blood sugar effect.
- 1½ cups salad, as above, but with 3 tablespoons commercial salad dressing (other than simple vinegar-and-oil) containing 1 gram carbohydrate per tablespoon. Check the label.

You might decide that 2 cups of salad with vinegar-and-oil dressing is fine for the carbohydrate portion of your lunch. You then should decide how much protein must be added to keep you satisfied. One person might be happy with a 3-ounce can of tuna fish, but another might require 2 large chicken drumsticks or a packet of lunch meat weighing 6 ounces. For dessert, you might want some cheese (in the European tradition) or perhaps some sugar-free Jell-O brand gelatin (if it contains no maltodextrin) covered with 2 tablespoons of heavy cream. You might consider some of the desserts described in Part Three or in *The Diabetes Diet.* The possible combinations are endless; just use your food value books or read labels for estimating protein and carbohydrate. Some people, after having routinely eaten the same thing for years, discover that their new meal plan opens up culinary possibilities they never knew existed. Our patients, as well as our readers, are always looking for recipes, so if you come up with a recipe that you think is particularly good, please feel free to share it on the website for this book, www.diabetes-book.com. Choose the "Recipes" link and follow the directions for submission. The simple recipe format used in Part Three must be followed precisely for it to be acceptable.

SUPPER

Supper should follow essentially the same approach as lunch. There is, however, one significant difference that will especially apply to those who are affected by delayed stomach-emptying (gastroparesis) and take insulin. As we've discussed briefly, this condition can cause unpredictable shifts in blood sugar levels because food doesn't always pass into the intestines at the same rate from meal to meal. The difficulty with supper is that you can end up with unpredictably high or low blood sugars while you are sleeping and unable to monitor and correct them. Sustained exposure to high blood sugars while sleeping—even if they are normalized during the day—can lead to long-term diabetic complications. For certain affected people, a viable approach to this problem is to facilitate stomach-emptying by replacing salads with cooked vegetables (from our list) that are low in insoluble fiber and reducing protein content. For these people, the amount of protein at supper would be less than that eaten at lunch—just the opposite of what has become customary for most Americans. A more complete analysis of this problem appears in Chapter 22.

If you like cooked vegetables (from our list) for supper, remember that most can be interchanged with salads as near equivalents—⅔ cup of cooked whole vegetables (or ¼ cup mashed or ½ cup sliced or diced) and 1 cup of salad each have the blood sugar effect of about 6 grams of carbohydrate.

If you like wine with dinner, choose a very dry variety and limit yourself to one 3-ounce glass (see page 142). As noted on page 171, one "lite" beer may actually turn out to have no effect upon your blood sugar. Still, don't drink more than one if you take insulin or use one of the oral agents that stimulate insulin secretion (sulfonylureas; remember that our program prohibits use of these agents).

SNACKS

For many people with diabetes, snacks should be neither mandatory nor forbidden. They do, however, pose a problem for people who take rapid-acting insulin before meals. Snacks should be a convenience, to relieve hunger if meals are delayed or spaced too far apart for comfort. If your diabetes is severe enough to warrant the use of rapid-acting blood sugar–lowering medication before meals, such medication may also be necessary before snacks.

The carbohydrate limit of 6 grams during the first few hours after arising and 12 grams thereafter that applies to meals also applies to snacks. Be sure that your prior meal has been fully digested before your snack starts (this usually means waiting 4–5 hours). This is so that the effects upon blood sugar will not add to one another. You needn't worry, however, if the snack is so sparse (say, a bit of toasted nori) as to have negligible effects on blood sugar. Sugar-free Jell-O brand gelatin (without maltodextrin) can be consumed pretty much whenever you like, provided you don't stuff yourself. As a rule, snacks limited to small amounts of protein will have less effect upon blood sugar than those containing carbohydrate. Thus 2–3 ounces of cheese or cold cuts might be reasonable snacks for some people.

Among my patients, a common favorite snack, which has a negligible amount of carbohydrate, is homemade microwave cheese puffs. They're simple and convenient to make. Get some freezer paper from the grocery—not waxed paper. It has a dull side and a shiny side. Place a slice of American cheese (process cheddar in the U.K.) on the shiny side of a piece of the freezer paper, then pop it into the microwave for 1–2 minutes, depending on how powerful your microwave is. The cheese will bubble up and puff quite nicely, but let it cool a little before attempting to remove it from the paper. Cooling can be accelerated by putting it into the freezer for 30 seconds.

Two slices side by side in the microwave will melt together to make a double cheese puff. Two of these are suitable for a sandwich. I have put mayonnaise on one and mustard on the other and ham or turkey and cheese in between. Cheese puffs can also be substituted for toast at breakfast.

If you're being treated with only longer-acting blood sugar–lowering agents, the question of random or even preplanned snacking is best answered by experimentation using blood sugar measurements.

OTHER CONSIDERATIONS

Meal and Medication Adjustments

Although your blood sugars will respond best if you adhere to our restrictions on carbohydrate, you'll find that you have considerable leeway when it comes to planning the amount of protein for each meal, provided that you don't have gastroparesis or another digestive disorder and inject insulin. At the initial meal-planning session with your physician or other health care provider, you may estimate that you will require perhaps 6 ounces of protein to satisfy your appetite at lunch. When you actually try eating such a lunch, you may conclude that this amount of protein is either too much or too little for your satisfaction. This can readily be changed, provided that you first advise your health care provider, so that dosage of any blood sugar–lowering medication you take may be adjusted accordingly. Once a comfortable amount of protein has been established for a meal, it should not change from day to day but, like the carbohydrate, be held constant. The predictability of blood sugar levels under this regimen depends, in part, upon the predictability of your eating pattern.

Carbohydrate or Protein Juggling

Many patients ask me if they can juggle carbohydrate or protein from one meal to another, keeping the totals for the day constant. Such an approach doesn't work, for reasons that should be obvious by now, and can be downright dangerous if you're taking medications that lower blood sugar. Some patients who visit me for the first time after reading this book have totally ignored this very important point and have found it impossible to achieve stable blood sugars.

Calcium Concerns

Some people who follow my dietary guidelines consume considerable amounts of fiber. Slow-acting carbohydrate foods that are especially high in fiber include salads, broccoli, cauliflower, bran, and soybean products. Fiber binds dietary calcium in the gut, causing a reduction of calcium absorption and potential depletion of bone mineral, which contains 99.5 percent of our calcium reserves. The phosphorus present in proteins also may bind calcium slightly. Since I discourage the use of milk and certain milk products (except cheese, yogurt, and cream), which are good sources of dietary calcium, the potential for bone mineral depletion may indeed be real. This is a special problem for women, who tend to lose bone mass at an increased rate after menopause. Since recent research targets calcium supplements as a risk factor for arterial disease, I recommend increased consumption of calcium-rich foods such as cheese, whole-milk yogurt, and cream. For women it also makes sense to build up calcium stores earlier in life, and to offset high-fiber and high-protein diets with extra calcium. This is most important for growing teenagers. Vitamin D replacement to bring blood levels to 50–80 mg/ml will make this more effective, as vitamin D aids calcium uptake by bone.

Calcium also facilitates weight loss by slightly elevating your metabolic rate, but that doesn't mean that the more you take, the more weight you'll lose. Nor does it mean that if you are in the minority of diabetics who are trying to gain weight you should avoid calcium.

Sedentary and thin people lose more bone calcium over a lifetime than do physically active people. Exercise builds bone just as it builds muscle.

SOME PROTOTYPE MEAL PLANS

The guidelines set forth in this chapter should be adequate for you to create your own meal plan, but I don't want to leave you with any uncertainty as to how it is done. I have, therefore, listed below 3 days' worth of breakfasts, lunches, and suppers to give you an idea of how I do it. These meals should serve as a starting point. You may want to overhaul them entirely to reflect your favorite foods. If, for example, you prefer canned salmon to frankfurters, just substitute a small can (3 ounces) of salmon for the two 1.7-ounce frankfurters in the lunch of Day One.

The carbohydrate content of each meal reflects our 6-12-12 guidelines. If you're going to maintain normal blood sugars, then whatever amounts of carbohydrate you use must remain rigid. (Small children should theoretically consume less, but this may pose problems of compliance.) That said, exceeding or diminishing carbohydrate allocations by 1–2 grams per meal for adults will not make a great difference in your blood sugars—remember the Laws of Small Numbers. Aside from these constraints, you are otherwise limited only by your imagination. The protein content of meals, on the other hand, is completely up to you, provided that you don't take insulin *and* have a digestive disorder. For the following examples, I've arbitrarily assumed certain amounts of protein that may be too much or too little to satisfy your desires; you will want to experiment to determine your own preferences. Remember, however, that protein, like carbohydrate, should be kept constant from one day to the next for any given meal.

Let's assume that you've negotiated a meal plan, and the amounts of assigned carbohydrate and amounts of protein that you think will satisfy you are as follows:

> **Breakfast:** 6 grams carbohydrate, 3 ounces protein
> **Lunch:** 12 grams carbohydrate, 4 ounces protein
> **Supper:** 12 grams carbohydrate, 5 ounces protein

Note that none of the nine meals that follow adds up precisely to these guidelines for total carbohydrate and protein, yet all of them are quite close and thus acceptable. Note also that I usually don't list beverages. This is simply because most acceptable beverages contain neither carbohydrate nor protein and may therefore be ignored in our computations. Remember, however, that every tablespoon of cream for your coffee or tea contains about 0.4 grams of carbohydrate.

I haven't made the protein and carbohydrate exactly equal for a given meal from one day to the next. That will be your job when you make your selections.

Day One

Breakfast	Carbohydrate (*grams*)	Protein (*ounces*)
Mushroom Omelet with Bacon (page 418)	3.1	2.8
1 Wasa Crisp'n Light 7 Grain crackerbread with butter	4.0	0.1
TOTAL	7.1	2.9

Lunch		
Green Cabbage Coleslaw with Lemon Zest (page 426), 1 serving	5.8	—
1 GG Scandinavian Bran Crispbread with mustard or butter	3.0	0.2
2 frankfurters	3.0	3.4
TOTAL	11.8	3.6

Supper		
⅔ cup mixed salad with oil, vinegar, and spices	4.0	—
2 tablespoons crumbled blue cheese on salad	0.4	0.7
Pan-Fried Swordfish with Ginger Scallion Butter (page 442)	7.6	4.8
TOTAL	12.0	5.5

Day Two

Breakfast	Carbohydrate (*grams*)	Protein (*ounces*)
Pancakes (page 420)	7.0	1.4
2 sausage patties, 1 ounce each	0.6	2.0
TOTAL	7.6	3.4

Lunch		
2 cups salad with vinegar-and-oil dressing, sprinkled with grated cheese	12.0	—
1 small can tuna (3 ounces) mixed with 1 tablespoon each mayonnaise and chopped celery	0.3	3.1
1 slice American cheese (place on top of tuna and heat in microwave for tuna melt)	0.67	0.67

12-ounce bottle "lite" beer	Assume 0	Assume 0*
TOTAL	12.97	3.772

Supper

Quiche Lorraine (page 456), ¾ serving	9.2	2.7
Chocolate Soufflé (page 459)	2.9	1.8
TOTAL	12.1	4.5

Day Three

Breakfast	Carbohydrate (*grams*)	Protein (*ounces*)
2 ounces smoked Nova Scotia salmon	—	2.0
2 Wasa Crisp'n Light 7 Grain crackerbreads	4.0	0.1
2 cheese puffs (page 188)	1.3	1.3
TOTAL	5.3	3.4

Lunch

Avocado Spread (page 454), 1 serving	6.6	0.4
½ red or green bell pepper, cut into strips	3.8	—
3½ ounces hamburger meat	—	3.5
1 tablespoon Bac-Os brand soy bacon bits	2.0	0.5
(knead into hamburger before cooking)		
TOTAL	12.4	4.4

Supper

1 medium artichoke, boiled, served with melted butter	12.4	0.5
4½ ounces any meat, fish, or poultry, cooked as you like	—	4.5
TOTAL	12.4	5.0

To any one of these meals you could add as a dessert a serving of sugar-free Jell-O brand gelatin (without maltodextrin), which would not appreciably affect your carbohydrate allocations. Again, you are limited only by your imagination, and there are countless different meals you could create that add up to no more than 6 or 12 grams of carbohydrate and 3, 4, 5, or more ounces of protein.

---

*Unless your blood sugars prove otherwise.

I will personally answer questions from readers for one hour every month. This free service is available by visiting www.askdrbernstein.net.

12

Weight Loss—If You're Overweight

Weight loss can significantly reduce your insulin resistance. You may recall from Chapter 1 that obesity, especially abdominal (truncal, or visceral) obesity, causes insulin resistance and thereby can play a major role in the development of both impaired glucose tolerance and type 2 diabetes. If you have type 2 diabetes and are overweight, it is important that weight loss become a goal of your treatment plan. Weight reduction can also slow down the process of beta cell burnout by making your tissues more sensitive to the insulin you still produce, allowing you to require (and therefore to produce or inject) less insulin.

It may even be possible, under certain circumstances, to completely reverse your glucose intolerance. Long before I studied medicine, I had a friend, Howie, who gained about 100 pounds over the course of a few years. He developed type 2 diabetes and had to take a large amount of insulin (100 units daily) to keep it under control. His physician pointed out to him the likely connection between his diabetes and his obesity. To my amazement, during the following year, he was able to lose 100 pounds. At the end of the year, he had normal glucose tolerance, no need for insulin, and a new wardrobe. This kind of success may only be possible if the diabetes is of short duration, but it is certainly worth keeping in mind—weight loss can sometimes work miracles.

Before we discuss weight loss, it makes sense to consider obesity, because if you don't understand why and how you are overweight or obese, it will be somewhat more difficult to reverse the condition.

THE THRIFTY GENOTYPE

When I see a very overweight person, I don't think, "He ought to control his eating." I think, "He has the thrifty genotype."

What is the thrifty genotype?

The hypothesis for the thrifty genotype was first proposed by the anthropologist James V. Neel in 1962 to explain the high incidence of obesity and type 2 diabetes among the Pima Indians of the southwestern United States. Evidence for a genetic determinant of obesity has increased over the years. Photographs of the Pimas from a century ago show a lean and wiry people. They did not know about obesity and in fact had no word for it in their vocabulary.

Their food supply diminished in the early part of the twentieth century, something that had occurred repeatedly throughout their history. Now, however, they weren't faced with famine. The Bureau of Indian Affairs provided them with flour and corn, and an astonishing thing happened. These lean and wiry people developed an astronomical incidence of obesity—close to 100 percent of adult Pima Indians today are grossly obese, with a staggering incidence of diabetes. Today more than half of adult Pimas in the United States are type 2 diabetics, and 95 percent of those are overweight. Since publication of the first edition of this book, many Pima children have become obese, type 2 diabetics. A similar scenario is now playing out across the country in the general population. The pace is accelerating and the result is similar.

What happened to the Pimas?* How did such apparently hardy and fit people become so grossly obese? Though their society was at least in part agrarian, they lived in the desert, where drought was frequent and harvests could easily fail. During periods of famine, those of their forebears whose bodies were not thrifty or capable of storing enough energy to survive without food died out. Those who survived were those who could survive long periods without food. How did they do it? Although it may be simplifying somewhat, the mechanism essentially works like this: Those who naturally craved carbohydrate and consumed it whenever it was available, even if they weren't hungry,

---

* For more information on the Pimas, visit http://diabetes.niddk.nih.gov/dm/pubs/pima/index.htm.

would have made more insulin and thereby stored more fat. Add to this the additional mechanism of the high insulin levels caused by inherited insulin resistance, and serum insulin levels would have become great enough to induce fat storage sufficient to enable them to live through famines. (See Figure 1-1, page 43.) Truly survival of the fittest—provided famines would continue.

A strain of chronically obese mice created in the early 1950s demonstrates quite vividly how valuable thrifty genes can be in famine. When these mice are allowed an unlimited food supply, they balloon and add as much as half again the body weight of normal mice. Yet deprived of food, these mice can survive 40 days, versus 7–10 days for normal mice.

More recent research on these chronically obese mice provides some tantalizingly direct evidence of the effect a thrifty genotype can have upon physiology. In normal mice, a hormone called leptin is produced in the fat cells (also a hormone human fat cells produce, with apparently similar effect). The hormone tends to inhibit overeating, speed metabolism, and act as a modulator of body fat. A genetic "flaw" causes the obese mice to make a less effective form of leptin. Experiments showed that when injected with the real thing they almost instantly slimmed down. Not only did they eat less but they lost as much as 40 percent of their body weight, their metabolism sped up, and they became much more active. Many were diabetic, but their loss of weight (and the change in the ratio of fat to lean body mass) reversed or even "cured" their diabetes. Normal mice injected with leptin also ate less, became more active, and lost weight, though not as much. Research on humans has now advanced sufficiently to provide evidence that the mechanism is the same in obese humans. Researchers believe it is at least equivalent and probably related to more than one gene, and to different gene clusters in different populations.

In a full-blown famine, the Pima Indian's ability to survive long enough to find food is nothing short of a blessing. But when satisfying carbohydrate craving is suddenly just a matter of going to the grocery or making bread, what was once an asset becomes a very serious liability.

Although current statistics estimate slightly more than 67 percent of the overall population of the United States as chronically overweight, there is even greater reason to be concerned, because the number has been increasing each year. Some researchers attribute rising obesity in the United States at least in part to increasing numbers of former smokers. Others attribute it to the recent increase in carbo-hydrate consumption by those trying to avoid dietary fat. Whatever the reasons, overweight and obesity can lead to diabetes.

The thrifty genotype has its most dramatic appearance in isolated populations like the Pimas who have recently been exposed to an unlimited food supply after millennia of intermittent famine. The Fiji Islanders, for example, were another lean, wiry people, accustomed to the rigors of paddling out into the Pacific to fish. Their diet, high in protein and low in carbohydrate, suited them perfectly. After the onset of the tourist economy that followed World War II, their diet changed to our high-carbohydrate Western diet, and they too began (and continue) to suffer from a high incidence of obesity and type 2 diabetes. The same was true of the Australian Aborigines after the Aboriginal Service began to provide them with grain. Ditto for South African blacks who migrated from the bush into the big cities. Inter-estingly, a study that paid obese, diabetic South African blacks to go back to the countryside and return to their traditional high-protein, low-carbohydrate diet found that they experienced dramatic weight loss and regression of their diabetes.

It's clear that thrifty genotypes work in isolated populations to make metabolism supremely energy-efficient, but what happens when the populations have unrestricted access to high-carbohydrate foods?

It would appear that the mechanism of the thrifty genotype works something like this: Some areas of the brain associated with satiety—that sensation of being physically and emotionally satisfied by the last meal—may have lower levels of certain brain chemicals known as neurotransmitters. A number of years ago, Drs. Richard and Judith Wurtman at the Massachusetts Institute of Technology (MIT) discov-ered that the level of the neurotransmitter serotonin is raised in cer-tain parts of the hypothalamus of the animal brain when the animal eats carbohydrate, especially fast-acting concentrated carbohydrate like bread. Serotonin is a neurotransmitter that seems to reduce anxi-ety as it produces satiety. Antidepressant medications such as Prozac, Celexa, and Zoloft work by increasing serotonin levels in the brain. Other neurotransmitters, such as amylin, dopamine, norepinephrine, and endorphins, can also affect our feelings of satiety and anxiety. There are now more than one hundred known neurotransmitters, and many more of them may affect mood in response to food in ways that are just beginning to be researched and understood.

In persons with the thrifty genotype, deficiencies of these neu-rotransmitters (or diminished sensitivity to them in the brain) cause both a feeling of hunger and a mild dysphoria—often a sensation of anxiety, the opposite of euphoria. Eating carbohydrates temporarily causes the individual to feel not only less hungry but also more at ease.

A frequent television sitcom scenario is the woman just dumped by her boyfriend who plops down on the couch with a pie or half a gallon of ice cream, a spoon, and the intention of eating the whole thing. She's not really hungry. She's depressed and trying to make herself feel better. She's indulging herself, we think, rewarding herself in a way for enduring one of life's traumas, and we laugh because we understand the feeling. But there is a very real biochemical mechanism at work here. She craves the sugar in the pie or the ice cream not because she's hungry but because she knows, consciously or not, that it really will make her feel better. It's the carbohydrate that will increase the level of certain neurotransmitters in her brain and make her feel better temporarily. The side effect of the carbohydrate is that it also causes her blood sugar to rise and her body to make more insulin; as she sits on the couch, the elevation in her serum insulin level will facilitate the storage of fat.

On television the actress may never get fat. But in real-life, high serum insulin levels caused by eating high-carbohydrate foods will cause people to crave carbohydrate again. A type 1 diabetic making no insulin will have to inject a lot of insulin to get his or her blood sugar down, with the same effect—more carbohydrate craving and building up of fat reserves.

GETTING IT OFF AND KEEPING IT OFF

There may be many mechanisms by which the thrifty genotype can cause obesity. The most common overt cause of obesity is overeating carbohydrate, usually over a period of years. Unfortunately, this can be a very difficult type of obesity to treat.

If you're overweight, you're probably unhappy with your appear-ance, and no less with your high blood sugars. Perhaps in the past you've tried to follow a restricted diet, without success. Generally, overeating follows two patterns, and frequently they overlap. First is overeating at meals. Second is normal eating at mealtime but with epi-sodic "grazing." Grazing can be anything from nibbling and snacking between meals to eating everything that does not walk away. Many of the people who follow our low-carbohydrate diet find that their carbohydrate craving ceases almost immediately, possibly because of a reduction in their serum insulin levels. The addition of strenuous exercise sometimes enhances this effect. Unfortunately, these interventions don't work for everyone.

Medications

If you're a compulsive overeater, if you just can't stop yourself from eating, and are addicted to carbohydrate, you may not be able to adhere to our diet without some sort of medical intervention (see Chapter 13, "How to Curb Carbohydrate Craving or Overeating"). Carbohydrate addiction is just as real as drug addiction, and in the case of the diabetic, it can likewise have disastrous results. (In actual fact, excess body weight kills more Americans annually from its related complications than all drugs of abuse combined, including alcohol.)

You need not despair of never losing weight, however. I have seen a number of "diet-proof" patients over the years get their weight down and blood sugars under control. Over the last several years, medical science has gained a much more sophisticated understanding of the interactions of brain chemicals (neurotransmitters) that contribute to emotional states such as hunger and mood. Many relatively benign medications have been successfully applied to the treatment of compulsive overeating. There is no doubt that when used properly, many appetite suppressants are quite effective in helping people to lose weight. If you simply cannot lose weight, it may be helpful to discuss with your physician medicines that may be of use to you. I have used more than 100 different medications with my patients and have found some of them to be of great value for treating carbohydrate addiction.

There is, however, a catch to this method. Over the years, I have found that none of these medications works continually for more than a few weeks to a few months at a time, a fact that many if not most medical and diet professionals may be unaware of.

I developed a reasonably successful method for prolonging the effectiveness of some by rotating them weekly, so that from one week to the next a different neurotransmitter would be called into action to provide the sensation of satiety. I found that about eight different medications, changed every week for eight weeks, and then repeating the cycle, would perpetuate the effect for as long as people continued to take them. At one point this looked to be a very promising means to help get weight off and keep it off. I even acquired a patent for the technique. Over time, however, I found several significant reasons not to continue pursuing this route. The most insurmountable of these was that it was just too difficult for most people to follow their normal regimen of diabetes medications while at the same time changing their regimen of appetite suppressants from week to week. Add to that the difficulty of working with a patient over a number of weeks just to find eight medications that worked for them and could be rotated.

What I did discover during all this trial and error were several effective natural medications for curbing overeating. The results my patients have had with them are so significant that I've devoted the whole next chapter to them.

Reducing Serum Insulin Levels

Another group of type 2 diabetics has a common story: "I was never fat until after my doctor started me on insulin." Usually these people have been following high-carbohydrate diets and so must inject large doses of insulin to effect a modicum of blood sugar control.

Insulin, remember, is the principal fat-building hormone of the body. Although a type 2 diabetic may be resistant to insulin-facilitated glucose transport (from blood to cells), that resistance doesn't diminish insulin's capacity for fat-building. In other words, insulin can be great at making you fat even though it may be, for those with insulin resistance, inefficient at lowering your blood sugar. Since excess insulin is a cause of insulin resistance, the more you take, the more you'll need, and the fatter you'll get. This is not an argument against the use of insulin; rather it supports our conclusion that high levels of dietary carbohydrate—which, in turn, require large amounts of insulin—usually make blood sugar control (and weight reduction) impossible.

I have witnessed, over and over, dramatic weight loss and blood sugar improvement in people who have merely been shown how to reduce their carbohydrate intake and therefore their insulin doses. Although this is contrary to common teaching, you need only visit the reader reviews of earlier editions of this book to read the similar experiences of many readers.*

An oral insulin-sensitizing agent, which we will discuss in detail in

---

* At www.amazon.com, www.amazon.co.uk, and www.diabetes-book.com.

Chapter 15, can also be valuable for facilitating weight loss. It works by making the body's tissues more sensitive to the blood sugar–lowering effect of injected or self-made insulin. As it then takes less insulin to accomplish our goal of blood sugar normalization, you'll have less of this fat-building hormone circulating in your body. I have formerly obese patients using this medication who are not diabetic. The body is more sensitive to insulin, so it needs to produce less, and there is, again, less of it present to build fat. One may also have less of a sense of hunger, and less loss of self-control.

Increasing Muscle Mass

The above suggests what we have been advocating all along—a low-carbohydrate diet. But what do you do if this plus the above medication does not result in significant weight loss? Another step is muscle-building exercise (Chapter 14). This is of value in weight reduction for several reasons. Increasing lean body mass (muscle mass) upgrades insulin sensitivity, enhancing glucose transport and reducing insulin requirements for blood sugar normalization. Lower insulin levels facilitate loss of stored fat. Chemicals produced during exercise (endorphins) tend to reduce appetite, as do lower serum insulin levels. People who have seen results from exercise tend to invest more effort in looking even better (e.g., by not overeating, and perhaps exercising more). They know it can be done.

HOW TO ESTIMATE YOUR REAL FOOD REQUIREMENTS

Now suppose you have been following our low-carbohydrate diet, have been conscientiously "pumping iron," and are, in effect, "doing everything right." What else can you do if you have not lost weight? Well, everyone has some level of caloric intake below which they will lose weight. Unfortunately, the "standard" formulas and tables commonly used by nutritionists set forth caloric guidelines for theoretical individuals of a certain age, height, and sex, but not for real people like us. The only way to find out how much food you need in order to maintain, gain, or lose weight is by experiment. Here is an experimental plan that your physician may find useful. This method usually works, and without counting calories.

Begin by setting an initial target weight and a reasonable time frame in which to achieve it. Using standard tables of "ideal body weight" is of little value, simply because they give a very wide target range. This is because some people have more muscle and bone mass for a given height than others. The high end of the ideal weight for a given height on the Metropolitan Life Insurance Company's table is 30 percent greater than the low end for the same height.

Instead, estimate your target weight by looking at your body in the mirror after weighing yourself. (It pays to do this in the presence of your health care provider, because he or she probably has more experience in estimating the weight of your body fat.) If you can grab handfuls of fat at the underside of your upper arms, around your thighs, around your waist, or over your belly, it is pretty clear that your body is set for the next famine. Your estimate at this point need not be terribly precise, because as you lose weight your target weight can be reestimated. Say, for example, that you weigh 200 pounds. You and your physician may agree that a reasonable target would be 150 pounds. By the time you reach 160 pounds, however, you may have lost your visible excess fat—so settle for 160 pounds. Alternatively, if you still have fat around your belly when you get down to 150 pounds, it won't hurt to shoot for 145 or 140 as your next target, before making another visual evaluation. Gradually you home in on your eventual target, using smaller and smaller steps.

Once your initial target weight has been agreed upon, a time frame for losing the weight should be established. Again, this need not be utterly precise. It's important, however, not to "crash diet." This may cause a yo-yo effect by slowing your metabolism and making it difficult to keep off the lost bulk. Bear in mind that if you starve yourself and lose 10 pounds without adequate dietary protein and an accompanying exercise regimen, you may lose 5 pounds of fat and 5 pounds of muscle. If you gain back that 10 pounds from eating carbohydrate and still are not exercising, it may be all fat. After crash dieting, once you've reached your target, you may go right back to overeating. I like to have my patients follow a gradual weight-reduction diet that matches as closely as possible what they'll probably be eating after the target has been reached. In other words, once your weight has leveled off at your target, you stay on the same diet you followed while losing weight—provided, of course, that you don't continue losing weight. This way you've gotten into the habit of eating a certain amount, and you stick to this amount, more or less, for life.

To achieve this, weight loss must be gradual. If you are targeted to lose 25 pounds or less, I suggest a reduction of 1 pound per week. If you're heavier, you may try for 2 pounds per week. If just cutting the carbohydrate results in a more rapid weight loss, don't worry—just enjoy your luck. This has happened to a number of my patients.

Weigh yourself once weekly—stripped, if possible, on the same scale, and before breakfast. Pick a convenient day, and weigh yourself on the same day each week at the same time of day. It's counterproductive and not very informative to weigh yourself more often. Small, normal variations in body weight occur from day to day and can be frustrating if you misinterpret them.* Generally speaking, you won't lose or gain a pound of body fat in a day. Continue on your low-carbohydrate diet, with enough protein foods to keep you comfortable.

Let's say that your goal is to lose 1 pound every week. Weigh yourself after one week. If you've lost the weight, don't change anything. If you haven't lost the pound, reduce the protein at any one meal by one-third. For example, if you've been eating 6 ounces of fish or meat at dinner, cut it to 4 ounces. You can pick which meal to cut. Check your weight one week later. If you have lost a pound, don't change anything. If you haven't, cut the protein at another meal by one-third. If you haven't lost the pound in the subsequent week, cut the protein by one-third in the one remaining meal. Keep doing this, week by week, until you are losing at the target rate. Never add back any protein that you have cut out, even if you subsequently lose 2 or 3 pounds in a week—unless you find that you've lost too much weight overall.†

If you've managed to lose at least 1 pound weekly for many weeks but then your weight levels off, this is a good time for your physician to prescribe the special insulin resistance–lowering agent described in Chapter 15. Alternatively you can just start cutting protein again. Continue this until you reach your initial target or until your visual evaluation of excess body fat tells you that further weight loss isn't

---

* This is especially true for many menstruating women, who retain more water during the week before their periods.
† This may not work for girls or women with polycystic ovarian syndrome (PCOS). They may fail to lose weight even on a near-starvation diet (see Appendix E). The same problem may occur if you are taking fat-building medications such as lithium or antipsychotic drugs.

necessary. The average nonpregnant, sedentary adult with an ideal body weight of 150 pounds requires about 11½ ounces of high-quality protein food (i.e., 69 grams of pure protein) daily to prevent protein malnutrition. It is therefore unwise to cut your protein intake much below this level (adjusted for your own ideal body weight). If you exercise strenuously and regularly, you may need much more than this in order to build your muscles. Growing children also need more protein per pound (or kilogram) of body weight. Once you've reached your target weight, you probably should not add back any food. You will likely have to stay on approximately this diet for many years, but you'll easily become accustomed to it. If you lose too much weight, add back a little protein. If you required one of the appetite-reducing approaches described in the next chapter, do not discontinue it.

SOME FINAL NOTES

Reduce Diabetes Medications While Cutting Protein or Losing Weight

While you're losing weight, keep checking blood sugars at least 4 times daily, at least 2 days a week. If they consistently drop below your target value for even a few days, advise your physician immediately. It will probably be necessary to reduce the doses of any blood sugar–lowering medications you may be taking. Keeping track of your blood sugar levels as you eat less and lose weight is essential for the prevention of excessively low blood sugars.

Increased Thrombotic Activity During Weight Loss

During weight loss, many people unknowingly experience increased clumping of the small particles in the blood (platelets) that form clots (thrombi). This can increase the risk of heart attack or stroke. Your physician may therefore want you to take an 80 mg chewable aspirin once daily during a meal to reduce this tendency. The aspirin should be chewed midway through a meal to reduce the possibility of irritation to the stomach or intestines. Rinse your mouth with water or diet soda after chewing aspirin to prevent inflammation of your gums. Alternatively, instead of aspirin you can use omega-3 fish oil capsules. The dosing would be one to six 1,000 mg capsules daily depending upon your size. It need not be taken during meals, as it won't irritate your gastrointestinal tract.

Elevated Serum Triglycerides During Weight Loss

When you're losing weight, fat is "mobilized" for oxidation — i.e., to be burned — and it will appear in the bloodstream as triglycerides. If you see elevated serum triglyceride levels as you're losing weight, it's not something to worry about. Your triglyceride levels will drop as soon as weight loss levels off.

Calcium May Help

There is evidence that dietary calcium and to a lesser degree calcium supplements (1,000–3,000 mg daily) may facilitate weight loss by inhibiting the accompanying slowdown in metabolism that may occur when you lose weight. If used for this purpose, the supplement should not contain vitamin D, as it will counteract the effect on weight loss. There is, however, a major problem with taking calcium supplements as opposed to just eating more cheese, yogurt, and cream. Supplements have been shown to increase the likelihood of developing atherosclerosis (arterial calcification).

Urinary Ketones During Weight Loss

Loss of body fat automatically generates by-products of fat oxidation — carbon dioxide, water, and ketones. Ketones can be detected in the urine with plastic dipsticks called Ketostix. In periods of famine, ketones enable humans to survive because the brain can use them as an energy source. Even without famine, many nonobese people will show positive tests for urinary ketones (ketonuria) after going without food all night.

Although we are taught in medical school that ketones are necessary for survival, physicians in training are subsequently traumatized by the sight of small children with very high blood sugars who are dying of dehydration, accompanied by high serum ketones. Thereafter they warn patients inappropriately that ketonuria with normal blood sugars is somehow hazardous.

At my monthly teleconferences, I repeatedly receive questions from listeners who were so warned by their physicians and are terrified because they find ketones in their urine when they awake in the morning or when they lose weight. My answer inevitably is "Don't test for ketones unless you have elevated blood sugars — usually more than 200 mg/dl." (See Chapter 21, "How to Cope with Dehydration, Dehydrating Illness, and Infection.")

How About a Low-Carbohydrate Diet for the Entire Family?

I once treated a slim teenager who came to me with very high blood sugars and severe complications of diabetes, including gastroparesis and kidney disease. Both of her parents were obese and sat in front of the television every night snacking on pretzels, cookies, and ice cream. Not only were they making it more difficult for her to stick to our meal plan, but they also were destroying their own health.

By contrast, I am currently treating a four-year-old who has five siblings. The entire family, including the parents, is following my dietary guidelines. Any further advice at this point would be superfluous.

I will personally answer questions from readers for one hour every month. This free service is available by visiting www.askdrbernstein.net.

13

How to Curb Carbohydrate Craving or Overeating

IF YOU ARE PLAGUED WITH CRAVINGS, THIS CHAPTER MAY CHANGE YOUR LIFE

The diet plan described in this book should make it possible for virtually any diabetic to achieve essentially normal blood sugars. There are, however, three exceptions.* The first, as I've mentioned, is the presence of gastroparesis, or the partial paralysis of the stomach, and other ailments that can impair stomach-emptying or digestion. These may include hiatal hernia, stomach or duodenal ulcers, a "tonic" (tight) stomach, gastritis, duodenitis, celiac disease, and scleroderma, among others. The next is infection. The third is the inability to control food intake, but especially carbohydrate intake. Because of the thrifty genotype, we should expect to find this condition in many type 2 diabetics. Indeed, about half of my type 2 patients find it extremely difficult to remain on a low-carbohydrate diet—or indeed any kind of structured diet. Typical scenarios include snacking when bored, eating bread in restaurants for no better reason than that it's on the table, and eating everything on your plate regardless of any actual hunger if you happen to be given a too-large portion, often at restaurants. Others may eat a whole pint, and some even a quart, of ice cream every night, often because they feel they have nothing else to do. At least 10 percent of my type 1 diabetic patients also have such problems, but their problems, when they occur, have a more devastating effect on blood sugars. These are the people who rapidly develop retinopathy, numb feet, kidney dysfunction, and so on.

---

* A fourth exception relates to the rare use of intravenous gamma globulin for treatment of an immune deficiency disorder, which causes random intermittent recovery of beta cells. (See page 360.)

Some years ago, I recalled how, in medical school, I had been taught a technique for self-hypnosis in order to avoid falling asleep when we had boring speakers and the lights were turned off. I wondered if perhaps the same technique might be helpful to those patients who just couldn't seem to stick to a low-carbohydrate diet or any other. I decided to get in touch with the physician, Herbert Spiegel, MD, who had taught me autohypnosis.

Remarkably, he was still in the same office at the same telephone number as more than twenty years before. To my amazement, he told me that he routinely used this technique to treat people with eating problems. Put this under the category of reasonably important discoveries I had missed. In fact, with his son, David, he had even written a book, *Trance and Treatment: Clinical Uses of Hypnosis*. It includes a chapter on just this subject. I subsequently referred many patients to him to learn this technique, with success in helping people break the cycle of carbohydrate addiction. (Dr. Spiegel used this method for altering a number of different behaviors, not just weight loss or the propensity of elderly medical students to snore during soporific lectures.)*

The whole cycle of going into a hypnotic state, giving yourself a message, and coming out of the state takes initially about 1 minute. Once you have some experience, *it takes only about 20 seconds to complete.* The technique only works if you're hypnotizable. A qualified medical hypnotist quite readily can determine whether you are a suitable subject. One of the things the specialist looks for is how high you can roll up your eyes as you attempt to look toward the top of your head. Additionally, the technique will only work if you perform autohypnosis *at least* 10 times daily (for a total of about 3½ minutes per day). The section below, which is adapted with permission from Dr. Spiegel's book, is the handout that our eminent consultant gave to his patients with eating problems. This handout is a reminder of what they were taught in his office.

---

* Dr. Spiegel passed away in 2009, but his widow, Marcia Greenleaf, PhD, was a student of his and still teaches autohypnosis to curb overeating. She practices in New York City. You can contact her at (212) 534-8877.

A METHOD OF SELF-HYPNOSIS*

Sit or lie down. At first, being in a quiet place can help. To yourself, count to three. At *one* you are going to do one thing, at *two,* you will do two things, at *three,* you will do three things.

1. Without moving your head, look upward toward your eyebrows, all the way up.
2. Close your eyelids and take a deep breath.
3. Exhale; let your eyes relax and let your body float.

As you feel yourself floating, you permit one hand or the other to feel like a buoyant balloon and allow it to float upward. As it does, your elbow bends and your forearm floats into a vertical position. Sometimes you may get a feeling of magnetic pull on your hand as it goes up. When your hand reaches this vertical position, it becomes a signal for you to enter a state of meditation and increase your receptivity.

In this state of meditation, you concentrate on this feeling of imaginary floating and at the same time concentrate on these three messages:

1. For my body, overeating is a poison.
2. I need my body to live.
3. I owe my body this respect and protection.

In the beginning, do these exercises as often as 10 different times a day,[†] preferably every 1–2 hours. At first, the exercise should take about a minute, but it will come more rapidly with practice.[‡]

As you meditate, reflect on the implications of these critical points and then bring yourself out of this state of concentration by counting backwards in this manner: *Three,* get ready; *two,*

---

* Reproduced (with minor modifications by me) from *Trance and Treatment: Clinical Uses of Hypnosis,* by Herbert Spiegel, MD, and David Spiegel, MD, American Psychiatric Press, 1987.
[†] I have some patients who must do this 15 times daily, including once before each meal.
[‡] Requiring only about 20 seconds each time.

with your eyelids closed, roll up your eyes (do it now); and *one,* let your eyelids open slowly. Then, when your eyes are back into focus, slowly make a fist with the hand that is up and, as you open the fist slowly, your usual sensation and control returns. Let your hand float downward. This is the end of the exercise, but you retain a general, overall feeling of floating.

By doing this exercise (at least) 10 different times each day, you can float into this state of buoyant repose. Give yourself an island of time. Twenty seconds, 10 times a day, in which to use this state of extra receptivity to reimprint these three points. Reflect upon it, then float back to your usual state of awareness and get on with what you ordinarily do.

Camouflage

Now, suppose an hour or two passes and you want to do the exercise. You don't have the privacy and you don't want to attract attention. Here's the way to camouflage. There are two changes. First, you close your eyes and *then* roll your eyes up, so that the eye roll is private. Second, instead of your hand coming up as done in the hypnosis session [with the hypnotist], let it come up and touch your forehead. To an outsider, the exercise looks as though you are in deep thought. In 20 seconds you can shift gears, establish this extra receptivity, reimprint the critical points, and shift back out again.

You might be sitting at a desk, a table, or maybe in a conference, in which case you lean over on your elbow with your hand already on your forehead, you close your eyes, roll them up, and shift into the brief meditative state.

By doing this basic or camouflaged exercise every day, every one or two hours, you establish a private signal system so that you are ever alert to the messages you are sending yourself and the commitment you are making to yourself and your good health.

HOW TO DO IT

It is possible but unlikely that you will be able to master this technique without training from a professional medical hypnotist. Sufficient training should be possible to accomplish in a single office visit with a doctor trained in medical hypnotism. I stress the necessity of using the services of a doctor because I have had patients who, upon visiting nonphysician hypnotherapists, were convinced (you might even say conned) that many office visits were necessary, and spent considerable sums but failed to learn the technique. (If the word "hypnotism" automatically conjures up images of charlatans and carnival sideshows in your mind, this may be a reason.)

You should be able to locate a competent medical hypnotist by phoning the department of psychiatry at the nearest medical school or teaching hospital. Ask for the secretary/assistant to the chairman of the department, and then ask who their top MD hypnotherapist is. Your insurance may or may not cover the visit, depending on your plan, but it almost certainly will not pay for a nonphysician hypnotherapist.

When you visit the MD hypnotherapist, bring either this book or a photocopy of the above paragraphs so that he or she will know exactly what you are seeking.

In *Trance and Treatment* Dr. Spiegel is very emphatic on the following:

> Accept responsibility for Your Eating Behavior. It is very tempting to blame your eating behavior on your parents, your wife, the mayor, Watergate, the moon, the tides. As soon as you see the absurdity of that you will realize that of all the things you do in life, there is nothing in which you are more clearly 100 percent responsible than your eating behavior. Reflect on the fact that most of the things you do in life have to take into account other considerations or other people, but in your eating behavior you are in business for yourself.

I should note that Dr. Spiegel's three points, or messages, were developed for the treatment of obese overeaters, not necessarily diabetics but certainly people at higher risk for developing type 2 diabetes. For many of my patients, his three points hit the mark. For others, the points they want to stress are more closely attuned to their personal situations, and you can customize your approach as well. I have one patient who is simultaneously losing vision and kidney function. This patient's personal points are to curb overeating in order to preserve eyesight and to stay off dialysis. Another tells herself that she doesn't want to be like the lady who lived across the street from her when she was a kid — the woman was diabetic and had both her arms and legs amputated. Another patient is a fund-raiser — his points are attuned to the greater likelihood of people making donations to someone who is slim and trim rather than obese. Makes sense.

Some people have a difficult time remembering to hypnotize themselves every 1–2 hours, so for these people, I recommend an alarm watch (which you can purchase quite reasonably) that can be set to go off every hour. Get one that has a vibration mode if you don't want to be beeping regularly.* Alternatively, you can set the alarm on your cell phone.

For those who learn how to hypnotize themselves and do it 10–15 times a day, I've found that the success rate for curbing carbohydrate craving is about 80 percent. For those who self-hypnotize fewer than 10 times a day, the success rate is essentially zero. I cannot overemphasize the value of engaging in autohypnosis when you sit down at a table for a meal, especially if you're in a restaurant and have not yet ordered. I have patients who are walking around with normal blood sugars *only* because they have been successful in using this technique. It has the added benefit of having no toxicity whatsoever, and it might be used to change other behaviors (smoking, biting fingernails, and so on).

There is, however, a major problem with autohypnosis. I find that many patients either refuse to try it or eventually stop doing it, even when it works. The following section offers a solution to overeating that people have been more than willing to pursue and continue to use.

WHAT IF YOU CANNOT BE HYPNOTIZED OR OBJECT TO AUTOHYPNOSIS?

I have a simple, patented technique that has had success for a few of my patients who otherwise have great difficulty controlling carbohydrate intake. It relates to the "runner's high" that people often experience during and after exercise, but it doesn't require running.

You may already know that very strenuous, prolonged physical exercise and climactic sexual activity cause the brain to produce

---

* An excellent source for such products is e-Pill, LLC, 70 Walnut Street, Wellesley, MA 02481, (800) 549-0095, www.medicalwatches.com. I recommend their 12 Alarm Vibrating Pager ($75.95). It will give as many alarms as you desire if used in the "repeat countdown" mode. The website displays a number of other alarms that you may prefer.

endorphins, also known as the body's own opiates because they are produced internally (or endogenously — so they're known in medical circles as "endogenous opiates") and bind to receptors in the brain that also bind actual opiates, such as morphine and codeine. Endorphins cause a pleasant, relaxed feeling, similar to that created by narcotics, but to a milder degree and without producing a tolerance.* You may have noticed that serious runners and many professional athletes tend to prefer protein foods, don't crave carbohydrate, and don't become fat as long as they continue their sport. It would seem that their endorphins prevent overeating and carbohydrate craving without losing their effect over time as do traditional appetite suppressants.

This technique involves a medication called naltrexone, which was originally introduced as a treatment for narcotics addicts because of its ability, in large doses, to prevent addicts from getting high on narcotics. In large doses, naltrexone will block the brain's receptor sites for endorphins, rendering them ineffective. However, when taken in small doses, it also appears to raise endorphin levels in the brain.

A very small dose of naltrexone taken at bedtime seems to block endorphin receptors for about 8 hours. The brain may then compensate for this by making more endorphins than usual that then keep working throughout the following day, when receptors are no longer blocked.

I've found that a small dose of naltrexone used in this way is effective in controlling carbohydrate addiction and overeating in general for a few of those who have tried it. Furthermore, just like the endorphins made by athletes, naltrexone, thus far in my experience, seems to work for a prolonged period — perhaps indefinitely.

I've had only five patients who discontinued naltrexone because of uncomfortable side effects. These effects included tiredness, headache, and difficulty concentrating on complex tasks. Such problems always occur after the first dose. When they occur, I must discontinue the medication.

One patient who snacked between dinner and bedtime also had insomnia. Since naltrexone made him tired, we were able to use it to treat his insomnia and his snacking simultaneously.

---

* In medical terms, "tolerance" refers to declining efficacy over time, so that higher and higher doses are required to produce the same results.

Naltrexone is supplied in 50 mg tablets. For the low dose that I prescribe, I use a compounding chemist to put naltrexone powder into
small capsules—usually about 4.5 mg.*

Although in the past I've prescribed naltrexone at various doses
and at different times of the day, I changed this to 4.5 mg at bedtime
at the suggestion of Dr. Bernard Bihari, who has prescribed it for ailments other than overeating. This dosing method indeed appears to
be the most effective.

As with the other suggestions in this book, ask your physician to give
low-dose naltrexone a try. He should pay particular attention to the
package insert warnings against overdosing. For other remarkable uses
for low-dose naltrexone, visit the website www.lowdosenaltrexone.org.

I patented this mode of using naltrexone, in order to encourage its
distribution by pharmaceutical companies in low doses. Unfortunately, I allowed the patent to lapse shortly before a drug company
released a mixture of naltrexone and Wellbutrin.

Another product has curbed overeating in many of the patients for
whom I've recommended it. This is hoodia, a nonprescription extract
of a South African cactus. The brand I prefer is HoodiaXtra 1,000 mg.
It is available online at www.diabetes911.net. Other brands, usually
in smaller doses, may be purchased at health food stores, www
.rx4betterhealth.com, and other websites. Since hoodia begins working within 30–60 minutes, it should be taken about 1 hour before an
anticipated need. Thus, if you usually overeat at dinner and then
snack thereafter, you might take 1–3 capsules before dinner and
another 1–3 after dinner. Some sources of hoodia supply a timed-
release version. It is most effective when taken on arising and again
6–8 hours later.

I have seen no adverse side effects from this product, but I have
never used it in children.

Because the demand for hoodia now exceeds the supply, many
phony formulations are being marketed, especially on the Internet. To

---

* The compounding chemist that most of my patients use is Rockwell Compounding Associates, (800) 829-1493. (Compounding chemists are pharmacists with special training in the precise mixing of pharmaceuticals and
over-the-counter medications. They can prepare capsules, powders, liquids,
and even ointments, just as all pharmacists did when I was a child. There are
many compounding chemists in the United States and elsewhere. Most require
a physician's prescription.)

secure a reliable product, you would be wise to use a known brand supplier and a product without additives that may dilute its strength.

I believe that carbohydrate craving is truly an addiction. This addiction can be reinforced by the consumption of foods on our No-No list (pages 160–161). So once you have discontinued them, I recommend never trying them again or you will likely relapse. Even a small taste can cause you to fall off the wagon—just as for smokers, alcoholics, and other drug addicts.

INCRETIN MIMETICS: AN EXCITING NEW CLASS OF DRUGS TO FIGHT OVEREATING

You may recall from our discussion of the Chinese restaurant effect (see pages 101–102) that intact pancreatic beta cells make a hormone called amylin. Amylin release into the bloodstream is brought about in response to a meal, by gut hormones called incretins. Since diabetics do not have beta cells that function adequately, they make little or no amylin and therefore may not experience the degree of satiety that nondiabetics do. As a result, they are more likely to remain hungry after a meal and thus to overeat at meals and snack between meals.

Perhaps the most exciting class of drugs to hit the market in many years actually solves this problem. Products in this category are called incretin mimetics (IMs)—that is, they imitate the effects of incretins or of amylin. What is so special about them is that in my experience they really work, and they do so for about 90 percent of users, a very high degree of success. At present these products are sold to lower blood sugar after meals. Our application to overeating is therefore considered "off-label" but is permitted by the FDA if prescribed by a physician. Field trials of IMs to prevent overeating by the general population are now progressing. If IMs are tested in combination with low-carbohydrate diets (unlikely), the stocks of several drug companies will go through the roof.

The most effective IMs, at this writing, must be administered by injection one or more times daily. The good news is that the needles are tiny, so these injections are painless if you follow our injection technique, described in Chapter 16. A once-weekly version may become available, and four oral versions (Januvia, Onglyza, Tradjenta, and Galvus) are now on the market. But start with the injections, because they are much more likely to work.

For example, I saw a new patient who weighed 286 pounds (130 kg) and had an $HgbA_{1C}$ of 6.9 percent when we first met. I started her on an IM, and over a period of slightly less than a month and a half (44 days), her weight came down to 258 pounds (117.3 kg) and her $HgbA_{1C}$ dropped to 5.2 percent. Thus she lost an average of nearly ¾ pound per day and her three-month moving average blood sugars dropped from 176 mg/dl to 108 mg/dl. Her highest blood sugar of the final week of this period was 95 mg/dl. Since the first dose of the new medication, she has been able to follow our low-carbohydrate meal plan without hunger, cravings, or any snacking.

The incretin mimetics fall into three categories:

Amylin analogs. The only one being marketed in 2011 is Symlin (pramlintide). It is marketed by Amylin Pharmaceuticals, Inc. It is chemically similar to amylin and performs the same functions in the body. It is only available for injection.

GLP-1 mimetics. GLP-1 is one of the hormones secreted into the bloodstream by the intestines that tell the beta cells of the pancreas to secrete amylin, insulin, and glucagon. GLP is an abbreviation for "glucagon-like peptide." The two versions currently on the market are Victoza (liraglutide), sold by Novo Nordisk, and Byetta (exenatide), jointly marketed by Amylin Pharmaceuticals, Inc., and Eli Lilly and Company. Both are available only for injection. Human GLP-1 has a half-life in the bloodstream of less than 2 minutes, so in nondiabetics it is secreted continuously for as long as it is needed. The GLP-1 analogs have been modified to last several hours (Byetta) and an entire day (Victoza). A GLP-1 analog that lasts an entire week is being tested, but it is not as potent as Victoza. Additional GLP-1 agonists may become available in the future.

DPP-4 inhibitors. DPP-4 is an abbreviation for dipeptidyl peptidase-IV, the enzyme that the body uses to destroy GLP-1. Administration of its inhibitor opposes the destruction of naturally produced GLP-1. This, in theory, circumvents the need for injecting a GLP-1 mimetic. As of 2011, four oral products are being marketed in this category:

Januvia (sitagliptin), Merck and Company—sold in United States
Onglyza (saxagliptin), Bristol-Myers Squibb—sold in United States
Tradjenta (linagliptin), Boehringer Ingelheim—sold in United States
Galvus (vildagliptin), Novartis—sold in European Union

Several similar products may be released over the next few years. All of the above oral products are meant to be taken once daily.

◂ THE STRANGE MISUSE OF INCRETIN MIMETICS

The FDA and the reigning powers in diabetes care have approved the use of IMs solely for lowering blood sugar. In clinical trials, they were shown to lower $HgbA_{1C}$ by a marginal amount — about 0.5–1 percent. They also caused a small amount of weight loss in some users. Had the patients in these trials been taught to avoid the high-carbohydrate foods commonly advocated for diabetes, the satiety effects of the IMs would have generated dramatic drops in both blood sugar and weight among obese overeaters. These are the effects that I seek when I prescribe them.

The conventional use of the GLP-1 agonists is to stimulate insulin production in type 2 diabetics. This small effect rarely justifies their use. Because type 1s don't make insulin, nor amylin in response to GLP-1, the reigning powers do not support GLP-1 agonists for their treatment. Yet I find that many type 1s, like type 2s, benefit from the satiety effects of these agents. I cannot explain why they work for type 1s who theoretically cannot make amylin in response to GLP-1.

The reigning powers do permit the use of the amylin analog Symlin for type 1s because it reduces the blood sugar by inhibiting the effect of glucagon at mealtime. Again, I use it for its commonly ignored satiety effect.

HOW DO WE USE INCRETIN MIMETICS?

There is one catch when using IMs for type 1s. Most type 1s have had high blood sugars for more than five years and are therefore likely to have at least some degree of gastroparesis, or delayed stomach-emptying. Since one of the actions of amylin (and therefore the other incretin mimetics) is to slow stomach-emptying, gastroparesis is likely to worsen. As explained in Chapter 22, severe gastroparesis can make blood sugar control impossible. If I am faced with a type 1 diabetic who has mild to moderate gastroparesis but who also snacks on carbohydrate or overeats, I must then decide which will disturb his blood sugars more, the eating behavior or the gastroparesis. This can be a tough call, but the decision can be facilitated with the help of the R-R interval study described in Chapter 22. Any physician contemplating this problem should certainly read that chapter.

Because these hormones will naturally slow stomach-emptying, they may cause nausea — even in people without gastroparesis. For this reason, we usually start at the lowest reasonable dose and increase it over time (days to weeks) until the full satiety effect is reached. Fortunately, nausea is the only adverse effect my patients have had over the past five years. It usually goes away at lower doses and after time has elapsed for adaptation.

I have one very obese patient who only overeats at restaurants and parties. He has moderate gastroparesis. I therefore have him taking Symlin only before eating out. Fortunately, this strategy is working.

Virtually any prescription medication has a potential for adverse side effects, and the IMs are no exception. Since they do slow stomach-emptying, their most common adverse effect is gastrointestinal disturbances such as nausea, constipation, stomachaches, and even diarrhea. It is therefore wise to start all of them at a low dose and work up slowly if necessary.

Manufacturers of Symlin and Byetta say they must be injected about 1 hour before breakfast and supper. Instead, I prescribe these IMs about 1 hour before the overeating or snacking usually occurs. For those who snack only in the late afternoon and otherwise stick to our meal plan, I prescribe it for use about 1 hour before the usual time of afternoon snacking. Strangely, some users find that Symlin must be injected 2–3 hours before the targeted time for it to be effective. Therefore timing of injections is a matter of trial and error.

Recall that amylin also reduces the body's production of or sensitivity to glucagon — the major culprit in the Chinese restaurant effect. Between the reduced overeating and the reduced glucagon effect, blood sugars can be much lower after meals — even dangerously low if you take blood sugar–lowering medications of any kind. It is therefore necessary that your physician lower your doses of these agents at the time you start any incretin mimetic.

How much should doses be lowered? To some extent it comes down to experimentation. I usually start by lowering premeal medications by about 20 percent. I then may look at blood sugars the next day to see if dosing of these medications should be increased or decreased.

THE INJECTABLE INCRETIN MIMETICS

Byetta, Symlin, and Victoza are all supplied in prefilled pen injectors. Each pen comes with an instruction sheet that should be followed carefully. Future injectable IMs will likely also be in pen injectors. Tiny needles for the pens are sold in boxes of 100 and must be ordered with a separate prescription. The needles may be reused until they become dull or bent.

All pens must be primed before the first use. This is achieved by squirting the first dose into a sink or basin in order to fill the needle. Subsequent doses do not require repriming. Once the pen is fired by pressing a trigger button, it takes about 5 seconds for the full dose to be expelled, so slowly count at least 5 seconds before removing the needle from your skin. Read about our painless injection technique on pages 265–267.

The pen cases can usually be pried open to expose the vial of medication, making it possible to use an ordinary insulin syringe to withdraw doses smaller than those set by the manufacturer. The following specifications for these pens include the dose one would get by injecting ½ unit from an insulin syringe (see page 268).

Byetta. Two pens are available:

- The 5 mcg pen dispenses 60 doses of 5 mcg each and has a total volume of 1.2 ml (0.02 ml per dose).
- The 10 mcg pen dispenses double the volume of liquid, or 0.04 ml per dose.

The concentration of the IM in each syringe is the same, but the volume each pen injects is different. If using a standard insulin syringe, ½ unit will contain only 1.25 mcg.

Symlin. One pen is provided that can be set for two different doses: 60 mcg or 120 mcg. The total volume of 2.7 ml will dispense 45–60 mcg doses or 22–120 mcg doses.

It appears to me that Symlin is more potent than Byetta, so there may be an advantage for some individuals to use an insulin syringe to dispense very small doses. One-half unit in an insulin syringe will contain only 5 mcg.

Victoza. One pen is provided that has numbered settings with detents at 0.6 mg, 1.2 mg, and 1.8 mg. Intermediate doses can be set by using 10 audible clicks between each pair of numbers. This 3 ml pen will dispense thirty 0.6 mg doses, fifteen 1.2 mg doses, or ten 0.18 mg doses. When using an insulin syringe for very small doses, ½ unit will contain only 0.03 mg.

Adjusting Doses of Symlin

I usually start patients who weigh less than 150 pounds on 2–4 units from an insulin syringe (see Figure 16-4, page 268), taken 30–60 minutes before their usual episodes of overeating or snacking. So if someone overeats only at supper, she would inject about 1 hour before supper. If someone else snacks between 9 P.M. and midnight, he'd inject at 8 P.M. and, if necessary, again at 10 P.M. If a person overeats only when eating out, he'd inject about 1 hour before he anticipates arriving at the restaurant and not on other days. If another person snacks all day long, she might inject on arising and every 3–4 hours thereafter.

If someone gets adverse side effects (I've seen only nausea), we'd cut back to a lower dose until the side effects diminish, then increase each dose ½ unit per week until either cravings vanish or side effects reappear. If no adverse effects appear initially, each dose might be increased by 2 or 4 units until cravings cease. Heavier people might start at higher doses, with larger increases, and use the pen instead of a syringe.

If doses total 600 mcg over the course of a day without a major effect on appetite, I would assume that the medication is ineffective.

Adjusting Doses of Byetta

Until we have a once-weekly dose of Byetta (which seems unlikely), it will be necessary to focus dosing on the times of day when overeating or snacking occurs. This means starting with the 5 mcg prefilled syringe (orange label) and injecting about 1–2 hours before times of snacking or overeating occur.

If you overeat only at one meal, inject about 1–2 hours before that meal. If 5 mcg helps partially, the dose can be increased to 10 mcg by either injecting two 5 mcg doses or 1 dose from the 10 mcg (blue label) pen. If the eating problem occurs several times daily, 5–10 mcg should be injected 1 hour prior to each time of the day when the problem eating usually occurs. The theoretical maximum daily dosage of Byetta is 20 mcg, but very obese people may need higher doses. For type 1 diabetics, Symlin may be more likely to work than Byetta.

THE ORAL INCRETIN MIMETICS

Januvia, Onglyza, Tradjenta, and Galvus are oral DPP-4 inhibitors that are meant to be taken once daily. In my experience, they have had no effect upon satiety and a slight effect upon blood sugar. They all have relatively benign adverse effect profiles. I have used them for patients who cannot quite achieve normal blood sugars with maximum doses of Glucophage (see page 253) plus Actos and need to add another medication but don't want to use insulin. These products would likely get an average blood sugar of 95 mg/dl down to our usual target of 83 mg/dl. I doubt that they would be effective for type 1 diabetics.

Another potential application of the DPP-4 analogs is to prolong the effects of the injected GLP-1 analogs. I've tried this, but with only marginal effectiveness.

MY PREFERENCE — VICTOZA

I apologize for saving the best for last in order to appropriately emphasize the value of this injectable medication in curbing overeating, snacking, and carbohydrate craving. Victoza is a once-daily (long-acting) GLP-1 agonist, marketed initially in 2010. It is very effective and usually lasts the 24 hours claimed by the manufacturer. This means that it can usually be taken at any time of the day. Nevertheless, if somebody has problems only after dinner, I would prescribe it to be taken an hour or two before the eating problem usually begins. A brief guide to using the Victoza pen appears on page 219. I have seen only one case of nausea, when a patient took two 1.2 mg doses by mistake when first using it. I'm sure that sooner or later I'll see more instances of reversible nausea.

Although the manufacturer recommends a maximum dose of 1 full pen (1.8 mg) daily, I've used as much as two 1.8 mg doses per day without any problems.

CAN ANY OF THESE TREATMENTS PERMANENTLY STOP OVEREATING?

I have seen patients using autohypnosis, low-dose naltrexone, and even just low-carbohydrate diets who, after one year, found that they no longer had cravings for carbohydrates or excess food, even when they discontinued hypnosis or naltrexone. This is probably akin to some studies of depressed patients treated with certain antidepressants: after a period of time, the antidepressants may no longer be needed. Metabolic brain scans sometimes show an apparently permanent normalization of brain function in selected regions. For all we know, this may apply as well to the incretin mimetics.

One of my Symlin patients found that it ceased working after two months of use. She discontinued it for one week and restarted at a lower dose. The lower dose is still working after two and a half months.

A number of my patients found that their injectable IM lost effectiveness after several months, but that they were able to prolong satiety by switching agents every few months.

In any event, the improvement in blood sugars and concomitant weight loss are major incentives to give these methods a try.

POTENTIAL ADVERSE AND BENEFICIAL EFFECTS OF INCRETIN MIMETICS

The manufacturers of these products have reported that animal studies show regeneration of the pancreatic beta cells that make insulin and amylin. Whether this occurs in humans has not yet been demonstrated in the scientific literature. Animal studies over many years have shown small increases in the incidence or progression of rare thyroid C-cell cancers. This problem has rarely been reported in humans. On the other hand, substantially increased risk of twenty-four different cancers has been observed in poorly controlled diabetics before the advent of these products. A possible slight increase in the incidence of reversible pancreatitis in humans at high risk (such as alcoholics) has been reported for IMs. A sign of pancreatitis would be sudden, severe, unexplained abdominal pain extending through the body from back to front. Although pancreatitis is very rare, you should take any abdominal pain seriously. Stop the IM immediately and advise your physician of the situation. He or she can confirm pancreatitis by testing your blood for pancreatic amylase and lipase.

Another rare adverse effect is possible kidney failure in those who already have kidney deterioration. On the other hand, IMs have also been found to reverse early diabetic kidney disease. I recommend that IMs not be used for those with elevated serum creatinine or significant protein in the urine.

GASTRIC SURGERY

This is the latest fad to prevent overeating and even partially reverse diabetes. Many procedures are in use, from the adjustable Lap-Band to total removal of the stomach. Although surgical mortality at many centers is less than 1 percent, the subsequent complications of gastric surgery are legion. Several grossly obese people have come to my office as a last resort before surgery, and one patient came in after failed Lap-Band surgery. In all these cases, overeating was terminated with incretin mimetics. It is interesting that the ADA recommends gastric surgery as a treatment for obesity but has not embraced the combination of a low-carbohydrate diet and IMs.

UPDATES ON FORTHCOMING APPETITE SUPPRESSANTS

Anyone can purchase a subscription to Obesity-news at www.obesity-news.com or by faxing an order to (703) 960-7462. This is the best update source that I know of for news on upcoming and newly approved medications. Keep an eye out for reports of another natural appetite suppressant called PYY.

I will personally answer questions from readers for one hour every month. This free service is available by visiting www.askdrbernstein.net.

14

Using Exercise to Enhance Insulin Sensitivity and Slow Aging

S trenuous, prolonged exercise is the next level of our treatment plan after diet, and should ideally accompany any weight-loss program or treatment for insulin resistance (as in type 2 diabetes). Before we go into our specific recommendations for exercise, all of which should be approved by your physician prior to putting them into practice, it's important that you understand the benefits exercise can bring.

WHY EXERCISE?

While many people may begin exercising out of a sense of responsibility—the way children eat vegetables they don't like—the main reason they keep exercising is that it feels good. Whether it's the intense competition of a fast and furious basketball game, or cycling alone in the countryside, exercise brings many rewards—physical, psychological, and social.

The genes of all our cells contain at their tail ends a sequence of identical groups of nucleic acids called telomeres. Every time a cell replicates, it loses a telomere. After the last telomere is gone, that cell line dies off. Thus the lifetime of every cell and, in turn, of the whole person, depends upon the lengths of telomere chains. *Intense exercise generates new telomeres and thereby prolongs life.* This discovery is very new and obviously very important.

People who aren't diabetic and exercise strenuously and regularly tend to live longer, are healthier, look healthier and younger, and have lower rates of debilitating and incapacitating illnesses such as osteoporosis, heart disease, high blood pressure, memory loss as a result of aging—and the list goes on. Overall, people who exercise regularly are better equipped to carry on day-to-day activities as they age.

Many type 1 diabetics have been ill for so long with the debilitating effects of roller-coaster blood sugars that they are often depressed about their physical health. Numerous studies have established a link between good health and a positive mental attitude. If you're a type 1 diabetic, as I am, strenuous exercise will not improve your blood sugar control as it will for type 2s (which we'll discuss shortly), but it can have a profound effect on your self-image. It's possible, if you keep your blood sugars normal and exercise regularly and strenuously, to be in better health than your nondiabetic friends. Also, it's been my experience that type 1 diabetics who engage in a regular exercise program tend to take better care of their blood sugars and diet.

Think of exercise as money in the bank—every 30 minutes you put into keeping in shape today will not only leave you better off right now, it will pay continuing dividends in the future. If going up the stairs yesterday left you huffing and puffing, in a while you'll bound up the steps. Your strength will likely make you feel younger and possibly more confident. There is evidence that exercise actually does make you look younger; even the skin of those who exercise regularly tends not to age as rapidly.

After working out for a few months, you'll look better, and people will mention it. With this kind of encouragement, you may be more likely to stick to other aspects of our regimen.

Although most of us who engage in bodybuilding exercise can experience increases in muscle mass and strength, the degree to which we respond is in part genetically determined. With very similar exercise regimens, some people will show dramatic increases in both muscle mass and strength; others will show neither. Most of us lie between these two extremes. There are even people who gain strength but not large muscles, and others who build large muscles without getting much stronger. Unlike men, women who engage in strength training are much more likely to develop muscular definition than bulk. They don't become "muscle-bound." If you don't develop big muscles or great strength, you will still enjoy the other benefits from the weight training described here.

It has long been known that strenuous exercise raises the levels of serum HDL (good cholesterol) and lowers triglycerides in the bloodstream. Recent studies suggest that bodybuilding exercise (anaerobic rather than aerobic exercise) also lowers serum levels of LDL (bad cholesterol). There is even evidence that atherosclerosis (hardening of the arteries) may be reversible in some individuals. I'm nearly eighty years old, I exercise strenuously on a daily basis, I don't eat fruit, I've had type 1 diabetes for sixty-five years, and I have eggs for breakfast every day. Where's my cholesterol? It's in a very healthy range that nondiabetics one-third my age rarely attain (see page 137). Part of that is due to my low-carbohydrate diet, but part of it is due to my daily exercise program.

Frequent strenuous exercise has been shown to reduce significantly the likelihood of heart attack, stroke, and blockage of blood vessels by lowering serum fibrinogen levels. Long-term strenuous exercise lowers resting heart rate and blood pressure, further reducing the risk of heart attack and stroke.

Weight-bearing, resistance, and impact exercise slow the loss of bone mineral associated with aging. Ever hear the slogan "Use it or lose it"? In a very real sense, if we don't use our bones, we lose them.

Although exercise does make weight control easier, it does not directly — at least not as much as we may wish — "burn fat." Unless you work out at very strenuous levels for several hours each day, exercise isn't going to have a significant direct effect upon your body fat. The effects of exercise are broader and more indirect. One of the great benefits is that many people find that when they exercise, they have less desire to overeat and are more likely to crave proteins than carbohydrates. The reasons for this are probably related to the release in the brain of neurotransmitters such as endorphins. (As noted in the previous chapter, endorphins are "endogenous opiates" manufactured in the brain. They can elevate mood, reduce pain, and reduce carbohydrate craving. Brain levels of endorphins are reduced in poorly controlled diabetes.)* It might be said that in the same way that obesity leads to further obesity, fitness leads to further fitness.

Even though your fat won't "melt away," exercise, particularly if you're a type 2 diabetic, is still of value in a weight-reduction program because muscle building reduces insulin resistance. Insulin resistance,

---

* Plasma endorphin levels can be measured by most commercial laboratories. If you are curious about your level, just ask your physician to order plasma beta endorphin prior to starting an exercise program or a regimen of naltrexone and again a few weeks or months later.

remember, is linked to your ratio of abdominal fat to lean body mass. The higher your ratio of abdominal fat to muscle mass, the more insulin-resistant you're likely to be. As you increase your muscle mass, your insulin needs will be reduced — and having less insulin present in your bloodstream will reduce the amount of fat you pack away. If you remember my old friend Howie from Chapter 12, his insulin resistance dropped dramatically when he lost 100 pounds and radically changed his ratio of abdominal fat to lean body mass.

Long-term, regular, strenuous exercise also reduces insulin resistance independently of its effect upon muscle mass. This makes you more sensitive to your own and injected insulin. As a result, your insulin gradually becomes more effective at lowering blood sugar. If you inject insulin, your dosage requirements will drop, and the fat-building effects of large amounts of insulin will likewise drop. In my experience, daily strenuous exercise will, over time, bring about a steady, increased level of insulin sensitivity. This effect continues for about two weeks after stopping an exercise program. Awareness of this is especially important for those of us who inject insulin and must increase our doses after two weeks without our usual exercise. If you go out of town for only a week and cannot exercise, your increased insulin sensitivity will probably not suffer.

Although increased muscle mass also increases insulin sensitivity independently of the above effect, this is very gradual and may require many months of bodybuilding before its separate blood sugar effects become noticeable.

HOW DOES EXERCISE DIRECTLY AFFECT BLOOD SUGAR?

Exercise does affect blood sugar, and for that reason it can make your efforts at blood sugar control slightly more difficult if you're taking insulin or sulfonylurea blood sugar–lowering medications.* The benefits, however, are so great that if you're a type 2 diabetic, you'd be foolish not to get involved in an exercise program.

For years, guidelines for the treatment of diabetes have repeated the

---

* As I will explain in Chapter 15, I recommend not using sulfonylureas and similar medications.

half-truth that exercise always lowers blood sugar levels. In reality, physical exertion can indeed lower blood sugar via increased number and mobilization of glucose transporters in muscle cells. Certain conditions, however, must be present: exertion must be adequately prolonged, serum insulin levels must be adequate, blood sugar must not be too high, and for most of us, exercise should not be performed within 3 hours of arising in the morning (see page 228).

Moderate to strenuous exercise, such as swimming, running, weight lifting, or tennis—as opposed to more casual exercise, such as walking—causes an immediate release of "stress," or counterregulatory, hormones (epinephrine, cortisol, et cetera). These signal the liver and muscles to return glucose to the bloodstream by converting stored glycogen into glucose. The nondiabetic response to the additional glucose is to release small amounts of stored insulin to keep blood sugars from rising. Blood sugar therefore will not increase. If a type 2 diabetic without phase I insulin response were to exercise for a few minutes, his blood sugar might increase for a while, but eventually it would return to normal, thanks to phase II insulin response. Thus, *brief* strenuous exercise can *raise* blood sugar, while *prolonged* exercise can *lower* it. For this reason, Dr. Elliott P. Joslin told a group of us (in 1947): "Don't run a block for a bus, run a mile."

When insulin is nearly absent in the blood, the glucose released in response to stress hormones cannot readily enter muscle and liver cells. As a result, blood sugar continues to rise, and the muscles must rely upon stored fat for energy. On the other hand, suppose that you have injected just enough long-acting insulin within the previous 12 hours to keep your blood sugar on target without exercise, and then you run a few miles. You will have a higher serum insulin level than needed, because exercise facilitates the action of the insulin already present. Blood sugar may therefore drop too low. The same effect may occur if you are using sulfonylureas, a class of oral hypoglycemic agents. Furthermore, if you have injected insulin into tissue that overlies the muscle being exercised, or perhaps into the muscle itself, the rate of release of insulin into the bloodstream may be so great as to cause serious hypoglycemia. Nondiabetics and type 2s not on insulin or sulfonylureas can automatically turn down their insulin in response to exercise.

It may be unwise for you to exercise if your blood sugar exceeds about 170 mg/dl. This number varies with the individual and the medications taken. This is because elevated blood sugars will tend to rise even further with exercise. This effect will be less dramatic if you're making a lot of insulin, and is most dramatic for a type 1 diabetic who doesn't take extra insulin to prevent the blood sugar elevation. I have one type 1 patient who keeps her blood sugars essentially normal. She still makes a little insulin and dislikes insulin injections so much that she works out every day after lunch to save herself a shot to cover the lunch. In her case, the exercise plus the small amount of insulin she still makes together work very well.

One great benefit of regular, strenuous exercise in type 2 diabetes, as mentioned earlier, is that it can bring about a long-term reduction of insulin resistance, by increasing muscle mass. Long-term muscle development, therefore, can facilitate blood sugar control and weight loss. It also reduces the rate of beta cell burnout, because the increased ratio of muscle mass to abdominal fat reduces insulin resistance and thus reduces the demand for insulin production.

THE DAWN PHENOMENON AND EXERCISE

Several of my type 1 patients must take additional rapid-acting insulin when they exercise in the morning, but not when they exercise in the afternoon. This is a dramatic example of how the dawn phenomenon reduces even injected serum insulin levels. In the afternoon these patients' blood sugar drops with exercise, but in the morning it actually goes up if they do not first inject some rapid-acting insulin.

RESTRICTIONS ON EXERCISE

Despite the benefits that exercise can have, an exercise program that isn't sensibly put together can have disastrous results. Even if you think you're perfectly fit, your physician should be consulted before you proceed. Keep in mind that there are certain physical conditions that may restrict the type and intensity of exercise you should attempt. Your current age, your cardiac and muscle fitness, the number of years you've had diabetes, the average level of your blood sugars, whether or not—and how much—you're overweight, and what sort of diabetic complications you have developed: all these must be considered to determine what kind of exercise you should undertake, and at what intensity.

Before You Start

Following are several different aspects of your health you should consider and discuss with your physician before embarking upon an exercise program.

Heart. Everyone over the age of forty, and diabetics over the age of thirty, should be tested for significant coronary artery disease before beginning a new exercise program. At the very least, an exercising electrocardiogram, stress echocardiogram, or stress thallium scan is usually advised. A recent report published in the *Journal of the American Medical Association* demonstrated that the best test for predicting a heart attack within the next ten years is the coronary artery calcium score as displayed by high-speed electron beam tomography. I require that this test be performed on adults with type 1 diabetes and all diabetics over the age of forty before I prescribe cardiovascular exercise (see page 223). This test actually counts the number and volume of calcified plaques in the coronary arteries. If the results are abnormal, I ask the patient to see a cardiologist, who will recommend a maximum heart rate during exercise. If he permits, we will slowly increase the target exercise heart rate over a period of months or years. An abnormal test may not necessarily rule out exercise, but it may suggest restraint or close supervision while exercising. Again, seek your doctor's advice before starting any new exercise program.

High blood pressure. Although long-term exercise helps to lower resting blood pressure, your blood pressure can rise while you are exercising. If you're subject to wide pressure swings, there may be a risk of stroke and retinal hemorrhages during strenuous exercise. Again, first contact your physician.

Eyes. Before beginning any exercise program, you should have your eyes checked by a physician, ophthalmologist, or, ideally, a retinologist experienced in evaluating diabetic retinal disease (retinopathy). Certain types of retinopathy are characterized by the presence of neovascularization, or very fragile new blood vessels growing from the retina into the vitreous gel that overlies it. If you strain too much, assume a head-down position, or land hard on your feet, these vessels can rupture and hemorrhage, causing blindness. If your physician or ophthalmologist identifies such vessels, you'll probably be warned to avoid exercises requiring exertion of strong forces (e.g., weight lifting, chinning, push-ups, or sit-ups) and sudden changes of motion (e.g., running, jumping, falling, or diving). Bicycling and surface swimming are usually acceptable alternatives, but first check with your physician.

Fainting. A form of nerve damage called vascular autonomic neuropathy (caused by chronically high blood sugars) can lead to light-headedness and even fainting during certain types of exertion (see page 376), such as weight lifting and sit-ups. Such activities should therefore be embarked upon gradually and only after instruction by your physician.

If you take blood sugar–lowering medications. If you take insulin or oral hypoglycemic agents, it is wise to make sure your blood sugars are stabilized before you begin a strenuous exercise program. As previously noted, exercise can have significant effects upon blood sugars and introduce another variable that can confuse anyone reviewing your blood sugar data. It's much easier to readjust your diet and/or medications to accommodate physical activity *after* blood sugars are under control.

Sympathetic autonomic neuropathy. If you're unable to sweat below your waist, there is a possibility that prolonged exercise may cause undue elevation of your body temperature.

Proteinuria. Elevated levels of urinary protein are usually exacerbated by strenuous exercise. This in turn can accelerate the kidney damage that you may already have. Blood and urine tests for kidney function can render false abnormal results for 2–3 days after strenuous exercise.

Ongoing Concerns for Exercising Diabetics

Following is a list of aspects of health you should consider on an ongoing basis as you pursue your exercise program. Also postpone such exercise if you are scheduled for kidney, blood, or urine tests.

Recent surgery. A history of recent surgery usually warrants restraint or abstinence until you receive clearance from your surgeon.

Blood sugar changes. Even after blood sugars are reasonably well controlled, illness, dehydration, and even transient blood sugar values over 170 mg/dl are reasons for you to refrain from exercise. For many people, blood sugars above 170 mg/dl will increase further with exercise, due to the production of the stress hormones that we discussed previously.

Blood sugars below target values. If you take blood sugar–lowering medications, do not exercise if blood sugar is below your target value. Bring it up to target first with glucose (see the next section and Chapter 20, "How to Prevent and Correct Low Blood Sugars").

Possible foot injury. If you've had diabetes for a number of years, there is a good chance that your feet are especially susceptible to injury while exercising. There are several reasons for this:

- The circulation to your feet may be impaired. With a poor blood supply, the skin is readily damaged and heals poorly. It also is more likely to be injured by freezing temperatures.
- Injury to nerves in the feet caused by chronically high blood sugars leads to sensory neuropathy, or diminished ability to perceive pain, pressure, heat, cold, and so on. This enables blisters, burns, abrasions, and the like to occur and continue without pain.
- The skin of the feet can become dry and cracked from another form of neuropathy that prevents sweating. Cracks in heels are potential sites of ulcers.
- A third form of neuropathy, called motor neuropathy, leads to wasting of certain muscles in the feet. The imbalance between stronger and weaker muscles leads to a foot deformity very common among diabetics which includes flexed or claw-shaped toes, high arches, and bumps on the sole of the foot due to prominence of the heads of the long metatarsal bones that lead to the toes. These prominent metatarsal heads are subject to high pressure during certain types of weight-bearing exercise. This can lead to calluses and even skin breakdown or ulcers. The knuckles of the claw-shaped toes are subject to pressure from the tops of your shoes or sneakers. The overlying skin can therefore blister and ulcerate.
- Another form of neuropathy makes it difficult to perceive joint position in the feet. This, in turn, can lead to orthopedic injuries (e.g., bone fractures) while running, jogging, or jumping.

All of this implies that the feet must be carefully protected during exercise. Your physician or podiatrist should be consulted before you start any new exercise, as some restrictions may be necessary. Even prolonged swimming can cause maceration of the skin. You should also be thoroughly trained in foot care (see Appendix D, "Foot Care for Diabetics").

You or a family member should examine your feet daily for any changes, abrasions, pressure points, pink spots, blisters, and so on. Be sure to check the soles of your feet, using a hand mirror if necessary. If you find any changes, see your physician immediately. Bring with you all the shoes and sneakers that you currently wear, so that he can track down the cause of the problem. At the very least he may recommend the use of flexible orthotic inserts and sneakers with a wide, deep toe box while exercising. No attempt should ever be made by anyone (including a podiatrist) to remove calluses, as this is probably the most common cause of foot ulceration and amputation.

FOR DIABETICS WHO USE BLOOD SUGAR–LOWERING MEDICATIONS: COVERING EXERCISE WITH CARBOHYDRATE

People who do not take medications that lower blood sugar are usually able to "turn off" their insulin secretion in response to a drop in blood sugar brought about by exercising. You cannot, however, turn off sulfonylurea hypoglycemic agents or injected insulin once you've taken them. (This is one of the reasons I never prescribe sulfonylureas and similar products.) To prevent the occurrence of dangerously low blood sugars, it is wise to cover the exercise with glucose tablets (e.g., Dex4 tablets; see page 343) in *advance* of a drop in blood sugar.

Some type 1 diabetics try to use "treats," such as fruit or candy, to cover an anticipated blood sugar drop. I don't ordinarily recommend this approach, because it's not as precise as using glucose tablets, and the timing of their effects may be too slow. My experience with patients who've taken raisins or grapes or candies to cover their exercise has been that they suffer subsequent elevated blood sugars. Say you eat an apple. It will contain some fast-acting sugars that enter the bloodstream almost immediately. It will also contain other, slower-acting sugars that may take several hours to have their full effect upon blood sugar. On the other hand, as we will discuss below, certain sustained activities—such as cross-country skiing or physical labor for many hours—can keep your blood sugar dropping all day. For those, you'll need something longer-acting to help keep you from becoming hypoglycemic.

To discover how much carbohydrate you should take for a given exercise session requires some experimentation and the help of your blood sugar meter. One valuable guideline is that 1 gram of carbohydrate will raise blood sugar about 5 mg/dl for people with body weights in the vicinity of 140 pounds. A child weighing 70 pounds would experience double the increase, or 10 mg/dl per gram, and an adult weighing 280 pounds would probably experience only half this increase (2.5 mg/dl).

My own preference is Dex4 tablets, each of which contains 4 grams of glucose.* If you weigh 150 pounds, ½ Dex4 will raise your blood sugar about 10 mg/dl. Since these glucose tablets start raising blood sugar in about 3 minutes and finish in about 40 minutes, they're ideal for relatively brief exercise periods.

Let's run through a hypothetical example to demonstrate how you'd go about determining how many tablets you ought to take. Let's assume you weigh 170 pounds and ½ Dex4 will likely raise your blood sugar about 8 mg/dl. You've decided to swim (or play tennis) for an hour.

- First, check your blood sugar before starting (you should *always* check blood sugar before starting to exercise). If it's below your target value, take enough tablets to bring it up to target. Wait 40 minutes for them to finish working. If you don't come up to your target, you may be too weak to exercise effectively. Record your blood sugar level upon starting. (I urge the use of GLUCO-GRAF data sheets for recording all exercise-related blood sugars.)
- When you begin such an activity — the first time you exercise after beginning our regimen — take ½ Dex4, and then ½ again every 15 minutes thereafter.
- Halfway into your activity, check your blood sugar again, just to make sure it's not too low. If it is, take enough tablets to bring it back up, and continue the exercise. If it's too high, you may need to skip the next few tablets, depending upon how high the value.
- Continue the exercise and the tablets (depending upon blood sugar levels).

---

* Alternatively, you may prefer Dex4 bits, which contain only 1 gram of glucose per bit.

- At the end of the exercise period, measure blood sugar again. Correct it with glucose tablets if necessary. Remember to write down all blood sugar values and the time when each tablet was taken.
- About an hour after finishing your workout, check blood sugar again. This is necessary because it may continue to drop for at least 1 hour after finishing. Bring it back up with glucose tablets if necessary. (Very intense or prolonged exercise may keep blood sugars dropping for as long as 6 hours.)
- If you required, say, a total of 8 tablets altogether, this suggests that in the future you should take 8 tablets spread out over the course of your workout. If you only required 4 tablets, then you'd take 4 tablets the next time. And so on. For some exercise programs you may need no tablets.
- Repeat this experiment on occasion, because your activity level is rarely exactly the same for every exercise period. If you required 3 tablets the first time and 5 tablets the second time, take the average, or 4 tablets, the next time. If your activity level increases — say you've been playing with a slow tennis partner and you find another who makes you sweat your butt off — you may find it necessary to increase the number of glucose tablets.

There are some activities where coverage with a slower-acting form of carbohydrate may be appropriate, and it's here, perhaps, that you could use the "treats" I would normally discourage. For example, I have two patients, both on insulin, who are housepainters. Neither works every day, and the hours of work vary from day to day. They rarely work for less than 4 hours at a time. The painter in Massachusetts finds that half a blueberry muffin every hour keeps his blood sugars level, while the painter in New York eats a chocolate chip cookie every hour.

Some patients find that their blood sugars drop when they spend a few hours in a shopping mall. I tell them to eat a slice of bread (12 grams carbohydrate) when they leave their car. The bread will start to raise blood sugar in about 10 minutes, and will continue to do so for about 3 hours. The cookies and blueberry muffins contain mixtures of simple and complex sugars, so they start working rapidly but also continue to raise blood sugar for about 3 hours. I discourage the use of fruits, which can raise blood sugar less predictably. If your exercise is not going to continue for many hours, cover it with glucose — not a fun food — if you want predictable results.

Beware, however, if you have a history of craving carbohydrate. Fun foods are likely to exacerbate the problem, making the addiction impossible to control.

Whatever your plan for covering exercise with carbohydrate, *always carry glucose tablets with you!* If you have gastroparesis, you may do better with a liquid glucose solution (see pages 396–397).

WHAT FORM OF EXERCISE IS BEST FOR YOU?

As you are by now aware, insulin resistance, which is the hallmark of type 2 diabetes, is enhanced in proportion to the ratio of abdominal fat to lean body mass. One of the best ways to improve this ratio in order to lower your insulin resistance is to increase your lean body mass. Therefore, for most type 2 diabetics, the most valuable type of exercise is muscle-building exercise. (It's good for type 1s too, because it makes you feel better, look better, and can improve your self-image.) There also is cardiovascular exercise, which benefits the heart and circulatory system, and will be discussed later in the chapter.

First, what is muscle-building exercise? Resistance training, weight training (weight lifting), or gymnastics would all qualify. If done properly, weight lifting has many attributes that make it superior to the so-called aerobic exercises. Aerobic exercise is exercise mild enough that your muscles are not deprived of oxygen. When muscles exercise aerobically, they don't increase much in mass and they don't require as much glucose for energy. Anaerobic exercise deprives the muscles of oxygen; it tires them quickly and requires nineteen times as much glucose to do the same amount of work as aerobic exercise. When you perform anaerobic exercise, your muscles break down for the first 24 hours, but then they build up over the next 24 hours. I have little old ladies performing weight-lifting exercise. They're never going to look like Arnold Schwarzenegger — it's physically impossible because women don't have the hormones for it — but they feel much better and are certainly stronger and younger-looking because of it. They also build enough muscle to reduce their insulin resistance.

But what about aerobic exercise, such as jogging or outdoor biking? I don't think it's as uniquely valuable for diabetics — or for anyone really, for reasons we shall discuss. Still, I usually suggest that my patients engage in activities that they will enjoy and will continue to pursue in a progressive fashion. Progressive exercise is exercise that intensifies over a period of weeks, months, or years. Below are listed various characteristics of an appropriate exercise program:

- It should comply with any restrictions imposed by your physician.
- The cost should not exceed your financial limitations.
- It should maintain your interest, so that you'll continue to pursue it indefinitely.
- The location should be convenient, and you should have the time to work out at least every other day. Daily activity is very desirable.
- It should be of a progressive nature.
- It should ideally build muscle mass, strength, and endurance.
- The same muscle groups should not be exercised anaerobically 2 days in a row.

AEROBIC AND ANAEROBIC EXERCISE

You've often heard of aerobics, and now you've seen me mention "anaerobic" several times. What makes one of these types of exercise better for diabetics than the other?

Our muscles consist of long fibers that shorten, or contract, when they perform work like lifting a load or moving the body. All muscle fibers require high-energy compounds derived from glucose or fatty acids in order to contract. Some muscle fibers utilize a process called aerobic metabolism to derive high-energy compounds from small amounts of glucose and large amounts of oxygen. These fibers can move light loads for prolonged periods of time, and are most effective for "aerobic" pursuits, such as jogging, racewalking, aerobic dancing, tennis, nonsprint swimming, moderate-speed bicycling, and similar activities. Other muscle fibers can move heavy loads but only for brief periods. They demand energy at a very rapid rate, and so must be able to produce high-energy compounds faster than the heart can pump blood to deliver oxygen. They achieve this by a process called anaerobic metabolism, which requires large amounts of glucose and virtually no oxygen (anaerobic = without oxygen).

This is of interest to diabetics for two reasons. First, the blood sugar drop during and after nearly continuous anaerobic exercise will be much greater than after a similar period of aerobic exercise because of this requirement for large amounts of glucose. Second, as your body becomes accustomed to this requirement, it will adjust to the stresses you put on it and more efficiently transport glucose into your muscle cells. As muscle strength and bulk develop, glucose transporters in these cells will increase greatly in number. Glucose transporters also multiply in tissues other than muscle, including the liver. As a result, the efficiency of your own (or injected) insulin in transporting glucose and in suppressing glucose output by the liver becomes considerably greater when anaerobic exercise is incorporated into your program.

In relatively short order, you will develop greater insulin sensitivity for lowering blood sugar. Similarly, your requirements for insulin (that which you create or inject) will diminish. The overall drop in insulin in your bloodstream will reduce your body's ability to hold on to stored fat, thus further lowering insulin resistance.

Think here of the Pimas. Not only did they gain access to an almost unlimited carbohydrate food supply, they also went from a strenuous existence, one that naturally incorporated both aerobic and anaerobic activity, to one that was almost entirely sedentary. Thus their circumstances were changed utterly from what you might call the biological expectations of their bodies. Of course, it's not just the Pimas who are sedentary. When you understand how to meet your body's evolutionary expectations, you can begin to bring it back into balance.

Anaerobic metabolism produces metabolic by-products that accumulate in the active muscles, causing pain and transient paralysis—for a few seconds, you just can't contract that muscle again. Since these by-products are cleared almost immediately when the muscles relax, the pain likewise vanishes upon relaxation, as does the paralysis. You can identify anaerobic exercise by the local pain and the accompanying weakness. This pain is limited to the muscles being exercised, goes away quickly when the activity stops, and does not refer to agonizing muscle cramps or to cardiac pain in the chest. Anaerobic activities can include weight lifting, sit-ups, chinning, push-ups, running up a steep incline, uphill cycling, gymnastics, using a stair-climber, and so forth, provided that these activities are performed with adequate loads and at enough velocity to cause noncardiac pain or transient discomfort (not heart attack, but the pain of "no pain, no gain").

BODYBUILDING: NEARLY CONTINUOUS ANAEROBIC EXERCISE

Continuous anaerobic activity, as you can well imagine, is really impossible. The pain in the involved muscles becomes intolerable, and the weakness that develops with extreme exertion leaves you unable to continue.

Bodybuilding, or resistance exercise—which includes weight lifting, sit-ups, chinning, and push-ups—may focus on one muscle group at a time and then shift the focus to another muscle group. After you finish exercising certain of your abdominal muscles by doing sit-ups, for instance, you switch to push-ups, which focus on various arm and shoulder muscles. From there, you go to chinning. Similarly, different weight-lifting exercises also focus on different muscle groups. Anaerobic exercise also can increase the benefits of exercise by stimulating heart rate and thereby exercising the heart. To maintain an elevated heart rate, you switch immediately from one anaerobic exercise to another, without resting in between.*

I personally prefer anaerobic activity for type 2 or obese diabetics because—as I have said before and will say again—the buildup of muscle mass lowers insulin resistance and thereby facilitates both blood sugar control and weight loss. A number of my patients engage in bodybuilding exercises, including men and women over seventy years of age. They are all very pleased with the results.†

Since the publication of the first edition of this book, there has been a change in our society in the recognition of the importance of this kind of exercise. A significant benefit is its ability to help increase bone density. Bones, like muscles, tend to be only as strong as they need to be. When you strengthen your muscles, you're also exercising your bones—your muscles, after all, are attached to your bones; when they contract, your bones move on their joints. If

---

* This type of cardiac exercise is not nearly as effective in raising heart rate as those described under "Cardiovascular Exercise," page 242.
† A number of years ago, a report from the human physiology lab at Tufts University reported that only twelve weeks of weight training tripled the strength of male subjects ages 60–96. This was believed to improve their quality of life significantly. Subsequent studies showed similar effects in women.

your bones weren't as strong as the muscles attached to them, they'd snap.

Some Suggestions for a Bodybuilding Routine

Please refer back to "Restrictions on Exercise," page 229. These restrictions and cautions apply especially to bodybuilding.

Even if you have room in your home, and the finances, to equip your own private gym, I usually recommend that people go to an outside gym or health club to learn the different exercises before beginning an anaerobic exercise program. Then, if you want to buy dumbbells or a weight-lifting machine for use at home, that's fine. But it's important to learn good technique and good form first. You can also consult books on the subject, but attending at least a few sessions supervised by an experienced instructor is best.

Equipment. For your upper body, you're going to have to use weights. I don't recommend that you lift barbells—they can be dangerous, and you therefore must have assistance if you're using them—but I do recommend dumbbells and weight-lifting machines, which for the most part are quite safe to use.* Whether you're using dumbbells at home or in the gym, they should be solid cast iron, usually painted black enamel or gray. They're inexpensive—usually 50–75 cents a pound, so a 10-pound dumbbell costs about $5–$7.50. Don't use dumbbells consisting of a bar with plates on either end that can be added or removed. These can be dangerous—the plates frequently slide off.

Exercises. If you're going to a health club or gym to learn the ropes, I suggest that you learn fifteen upper body exercises, and as many lower body exercises as are available. Upper body would be for the arms, hands, shoulders, flanks, chest, abdomen, and back. If you're going to the gym every day, which I recommend, you'd do your upper body exercises on one day and your lower body exercises on the next. Why alternate days? Because of the muscle breakdown over the first 24

---

* A number of inexpensive multiexercise machines on the market utilize thick rubber bands instead of weights. Beware of these: since you have to stop and change the bands to change the resistance, they do not permit true anaerobic training. Hydraulic and pneumatic machines that utilize rotary knobs to adjust settings are usually excellent but often quite costly.

hours after exercise and the need for time to rebuild. So on the second day, while you're doing your lower body exercises, your upper body muscles are rebuilding.

As you can guess, there are more muscle groups that work in more ways in the upper body than in the lower body, so there are fewer sensible lower body exercises. If you're using a treadmill, a stair-climber, a bike, and a cross-country ski machine all in the same day, you're exercising more or less the same lower body muscles with each apparatus, which isn't sensible. The other types of lower body exercises that involve weight lifting are few in number: leg presses, knee curls, toe presses, and knee extensions. In all, there are at most six leg exercises commonly available.*

As a consequence, I always add some other exercises on the days I do lower body exercises: grip strengthening, side bends (which exercise the side muscles), and sit-ups or crunches, as well as what's called cardiovascular exercise (see page 242). The instructor at your health club will be able to help you with all of these.

Form. To get the most out of your weight-lifting exercises, it's important to have as close to perfect form as possible. This means that you isolate and use only the muscles targeted by a particular exercise. You shouldn't, for example, use your back muscles to help perform an arm exercise. You should also lift slowly, say gradually over about 10–15 seconds, and let the weight down very slowly over about 15–20 seconds, so that the entire individual repetition takes about 25–35 seconds—or as long as you can tolerate. This tends to be much easier on joints and has been shown to be a higher quality of exercise. It also makes the weights easier to control. Do not fully flex or extend your muscles while weight lifting. Instead, stop just before you would reach the end point of any motion. This is where having good instruction can pay off. Your instructor can critique your form and help you select the right equipment for each exercise. I usually use a weight that is just heavy enough to give me about 2 minutes (on a RadioShack or West Bend timer) until my muscles are exhausted. Frequently, my

---

* Some gyms have a machine that strengthens the adductor muscles of the legs by having you squeeze them together against resistance. I got a double hernia when I used this machine improperly, so I recommend that you avoid it.

entire body vibrates as I near the point of exhaustion. I keep a record of the weight and time for each exercise and try to increase them slowly from session to session.

Many weight lifters follow a regimen that requires 10 repetitions ("reps") of a lift, followed by a rest, another 10 reps, another rest, and another 10 reps. The rest between each set of reps allows the heart to slow, replenishes oxygen to the muscles, and thereby defeats our central goals. Anaerobically, you must continually keep your muscles deprived of oxygen and force them to develop new metabolic pathways that demand less oxygen. The idea is quality, not quantity, and it's my belief that you can accomplish a more thorough and sensible workout in 30 minutes than you can in an hour and a half of conventional, less strenuous aerobic activity.

Once you've done your reps for a particular muscle group, you don't need to do that exercise again until the day after tomorrow. You immediately go on to the next exercise. In this way, you can accomplish considerably more in a shorter time frame.

The same system applies to sit-ups, whether you're doing them with your legs straight or bent, or with one of those sit-up boards. Initially, it may be too difficult for you to sit up slowly, so do it rapidly and record your total time. Eventually, you will be able to do it slower and slower. When you find yourself doing dozens of slow sit-ups, you can get an inclined board or a Roman chair, which is like a sit-up board but is raised about four feet off the ground and permits you to begin with your head below your waist. Again, you follow the same tactic. You can also get an abdominal crunch machine with variable resistance (not those with removable weights that take time to change). They're the best, but they're expensive. Use the same technique as you would with any other weight-lifting machine.

THE PLANK

There is an amazing yoga exercise called "the plank"—also "the right plank" and "the left plank." You put your forearms on a mat and lift your straight body off the floor, so that it is supported by your forearms and your feet. The right or left plank uses only the right or left forearm and is more difficult. You can see this exercise illustrated on the Internet if you search for "yoga exercises the plank."

CARDIOVASCULAR EXERCISE

Cardiovascular exercise is widely associated in the public mind with what the popular press calls aerobic exercise. However, aerobic exercise as many people practice it—a leisurely jog, a relaxing bike ride, mild calisthenics, even a brisk walk—is really of only limited benefit to your cardiovascular system, doesn't build muscles, and has relatively little impact on your stamina and capacity. The kind of cardiovascular exercise I recommend to my patients (and follow myself) is very strenuous, operates intermittently in the anaerobic range, and accomplishes tremendous things. For example, many years ago, before I became a physician, I used to go to diabetes conventions. There was always a group of doctors who would get up in the morning, don their running togs, and go running. These were people who ran every day. I'm not a runner; I work out in the gym every day. But I do a particular cardiovascular workout on a recumbent exercise bicycle that I will explain. I would go out with these mostly younger doctors on their runs. After a few miles, people would start dropping out. Eventually, I'd be the only one left—and then I'd go another five miles and come back. Clearly, although I was older than most of these people, and not a runner, I had much more stamina. The stamina was created by this anaerobic cardiovascular exercise.

Exercise Harder, Exercise Better
Cardiovascular workouts can be performed on a treadmill, stair-climber, or bicycle. If you're female, I'd recommend a treadmill, because running impacts your feet and thus helps increase bone density in your legs. However, if done to excess or with inadequate arch supports, the impact can injure your knees. If you're male, I recommend a recumbent bicycle rather than the standard upright bike; it's much more comfortable for men because the seat is like an ordinary chair.

Ideally, your machine should have a meter that reads the amount of work that you're doing in calories (or joules) per minute as well as total calories (or joules), but certainly you can get a good workout with just a mileage meter. It is important to wear a pulse meter. The brand that I like best is the Timex Personal Trainer; it costs about $50, and you wear a sensor around your chest with a wristwatch-type readout. If you belong to a health club that has a treadmill with a pulse meter in the handlebars, you won't have to put one on your chest, but some sort of pulse meter is essential. The degree of workout you're getting is measured by how fast your heart beats. If you get evaluated by a cardiologist before you start your exercise program, you should ask him or her what your initial target pulse rate ought to be. Over time, you can increase it.

There's a formula that we use to specify a theoretical maximum attainable pulse rate: we take 220 and subtract from it your age. So if you're sixty years old, you'd have a theoretical maximum pulse rate of 160 — that is, in theory, you shouldn't be able to exercise at a faster pulse rate. Your doctor will decide based on your overall health and fitness level what percentage of this would be a good initial target rate for you — say, 75–80 percent of maximum. Rarely would a doctor start you out at 85 percent of maximum or higher if you were not in shape. I insist that most of my patients get a coronary artery calcium test (discussed earlier in this chapter) before starting cardiovascular exercise, so that their physicians will know if they have coronary artery disease and how severe it is. Eventually, you may find that you can get up to and beyond your theoretical maximum — I can exercise at 155 even though my theoretical maximum is 143. I can do this without having a heart attack in part because I've been exercising strenuously for forty-four years. Don't expect — even after years of this kind of exercise — to get your heart rate up to or even near your theoretical maximum, or to your target, right after you begin this kind of workout. It takes time. I get to my target pulse rate at the end of about 10 minutes of trying.

To do a really effective nearly anaerobic/cardiovascular workout, start out by selecting a slow speed and setting the resistance of your machine to the point where your muscles are so tired after about 2 minutes that you can't go any further. As soon as you reach this point, either slow down slightly or lower the resistance setting slightly and keep going. For treadmills, the resistance will be the angle at which you're running uphill. So if you're using a treadmill, you need to be able to set the incline of your treadmill from the handle-bars — you don't want to get off, reset the angle, then get back on. You'll lose your rhythm, regain some of the oxygen in your muscles and heart, and defeat the point of the workout.

Lower your speed or the resistance a little at a time, and only if absolutely necessary. Each time you lower it, continue until you can't go anymore. Nearly from the beginning you're almost wiped out, yet you keep doing it at a lower and lower speed or resistance. *This* is a real workout.

Your goal will be to get your heart rate up to (but not above) the training level recommended by your physician. If you can't reach the recommended rate when you have lowered the resistance of your machine to the point where you can barely notice it, increase the resistance and use a lower speed until you get to your target pulse. Try to maintain this rate for up to 5 minutes, or until you decide that you have had enough. Although I'm pretty wiped out when I reach 155, I have one patient who can continue at his target for 45 minutes.

A major goal of cardiovascular exercise is to enhance your heart rate recovery time—that is, to shorten it. (Cardiologists now believe that the faster your heart rate slows from your target to your resting rate, the better your cardiac fitness.) A minimal test of recovery would be to slow your heart rate by 42 beats per minute from your maximum within 2 minutes of stopping.

I recommend that rather than timing your workout, you look at the calorie counter on the machine, if it has one, and decide on a particular number of calories that you want to shoot for. Calories are a measure of work done and therefore a reasonable gauge of your workout. Minutes or even miles don't take effort into account. When I was seventy years old, I aimed for about 200 calories. Now I shoot for 100 calories. When it gets up to that range, I call it quits. But the point of this kind of exercise isn't weight loss, so don't start looking at the calorie counter thinking that if you burn 200 more calories you'll lose another pound—exercise just doesn't work that way. Incidentally, I have a retired patient who actually has the time and the stamina to continue intermittent sprinting for an hour.

There is a neat trick that will enable you to more easily reach your target heart rate. My goal is to exceed 150 beats per minute. On the first try, I feel tired at about 130, so I stop for 2 minutes. Then I try again and easily get to 147 before feeling tired. I again stop for 2 minutes. On the third try, I easily exceed 150 and continue until I feel I've had enough.

AN IMPORTANT CAUTION

If you're doing cardiovascular exercise of this type, you have to be very careful, especially if you're a long-term diabetic, or a recent-onset diabetic over the age of forty, or you have a family history of coronary disease. One rule is that you *never finish a cardiovascular workout and stop cold* if you are using a standard bicycle or a treadmill. I had an overweight nondiabetic cousin who started jogging when he was about fifty years old. He was in his second month of exercising, not doing anything more than jogging with friends. One day, after they stopped jogging, he dropped dead of a heart attack. He and his jogging buddies were in the habit of stopping cold after their run to chat. Stopping cold is an extremely bad idea—if someone is going to drop dead of a heart attack from running or biking, it's most likely to happen immediately after the exercise. Why?

While you're exercising, your heart is beating very rapidly because it and your legs require a lot of blood. By pumping your legs up and down, you're pumping blood from your legs back to your heart. The muscles that are demanding a lot of blood are both in your legs and in your heart, but the blood's getting pumped back to your heart by running. If you stop cold, your muscles are still going to demand a lot of blood—they've been depleted of oxygen and glucose—and gravity is going to help them get the blood. The problem is, they're no longer pumping the blood back to the heart. Suddenly your heart is deprived and, if your coronary arteries are narrowed by atherosclerosis, you're set up for a heart attack.

Whether you're on a treadmill, standard bike, or stair-climber, cut the resistance setting to zero and proceed at a very slow pace after your workout until your heart rate slowly comes down to no higher than about 30 percent above your initial starting rate. If your resting pulse is 78, you don't want to stop your biking, walking, or stair-climbing until your heart rate is 101 or below. This protocol can be safely avoided if you use a recumbent bicycle, as I do. Here your legs are level with your heart, and blood will not drain from your heart to your legs.

PROGRESSIVE EXERCISE

As your strength and endurance increase for any exercise, it will become progressively easier to perform. If it becomes too easy, you won't get any stronger. The key to getting progressively more strength and endurance is to make the exercise progressively more difficult. This can be done for almost any activity.

If you are lifting weights, for example, every few weeks (or months) you can add a very small weight (say a separate 2½-pound plate) to the weight stack for any exercise. You can also increase the exercise time for a given set. When doing a cardiovascular exercise, you might try to increase your maximum heart rate by, say, 2 beats per minute every 2 months, preferably by increasing your resistance setting. A swimmer can assign a fixed time period, say 30 minutes, for doing laps. The goal would be to gradually increase the number of laps. Thus, after a month you might increase your speed to get 15½ laps instead of 15 laps in 30 minutes, and so on. Of course, a waterproof wristwatch would be helpful.

Even walking can evolve into both an endurance and a bodybuilding activity. All you need is a wristwatch, a few lightweight dumbbells, and a pedometer. The pedometer is a small gadget from a sporting goods store that you clip onto your belt. It measures distance by counting your steps. Suppose you wish to set aside 30 minutes per session for walking. You begin by walking at a leisurely pace for 15 minutes and then returning at the same pace. Record your distance from the pedometer. Thereafter, try to walk at least that distance in the same time period. After five to ten sessions, you might try to increase distance by 5 percent over the same time. If you increase distance by this amount every five or ten sessions, you'll eventually find yourself running. You can then gradually increase your running speed in the same fashion.

Suppose your doctor has told you not to run because of a bad knee or fragile retinal blood vessels. Limit your speed to a fast walk, but start swinging your arms a little bit. Over time, try swinging them higher and higher. When you think they are going so high that you look silly, start with the dumbbells. You might begin with a pair of 1-pound dumbbells and short swings of the arms. Wear gloves if the dumbbells feel cold. Again, gradually increase the distance you swing. When you eventually feel you look silly, try 2-pound dumbbells. After a year or two, you may be going at a very fast walk, swinging 5-pound (or even heavier) dumbbells. Imagine what your physique will look like then. You'll also probably feel younger and healthier.

The exercises I've mentioned above are by no means the only ones. There are countless different ways you can exercise—volleyball, snowboarding, surf-kayaking, cross-country skiing, you name it. The most important considerations are keeping within the restrictions your physician might place on your activity, and discovering what you like best to do—and sticking with it. After that, all you have to do is monitor and correct your blood sugars, record the exercise on your GLUCOGRAF form, and keep exercising in a progressive fashion. The payoff — longer life, lower stress, weight loss if you're overweight, and better overall health — is usually worth the time and effort.

I will personally answer questions from readers for one hour every month. This free service is available by visiting www.askdrbernstein.net.

15

Oral Insulin-Sensitizing Agents, Insulin-Mimetic Agents, and Other Options

If diet and exercise are not adequate to bring your blood sugars under control, the next level of treatment to consider is oral blood sugar–lowering medication, commonly known as oral hypoglycemic agents (OHAs).

There are three categories of OHAs—those that increase sensitivity to insulin, those whose action resembles that of insulin, and those that provoke your pancreas to produce more insulin. The first group is known as insulin sensitizers or insulin-sensitizing agents (ISAs); the second group is called insulin mimetics, which act like insulin but do not build fat. Finally, there are the original OHAs, like sulfonylureas and similar newer agents that push beta cells to make more insulin.

I recommend only insulin sensitizers and insulin mimetics, for reasons that will become plain in short order. (Some drug companies have combined pancreas-provoking OHAs with insulin sensitizers, a move I strongly challenge. Tell your doctor you do not want any product containing an agent that works by causing the pancreas to make more insulin. This includes the old sulfonylureas and the new, similar drugs called meglitinides and phenylalanine derivatives.)*

For people who still have sufficient insulin-producing capacity,

---

* In addition to eventually impairing beta cell insulin production, sulfonylureas also impair circulation in the heart and elsewhere by closing ATP-sensitive potassium channels that relax blood vessels. They have been shown to increase all causes of mortality, including deaths from heart disease and cancer.

insulin sensitizers alone may provide the extra help they need to reach their blood sugar targets. Some insulin-resistant individuals who produce little or no insulin on their own may find a combination of insulin sensitizers and insulin mimetics useful in reducing their doses of injected insulin.

There are four ISAs currently on the market—metformin (Glucophage), rosiglitazone (Avandia), pioglitazone (Actos), and bromocriptine mesylate (Cycloset)—but at this writing I prescribe only two of them, Glucophage and Actos. Avandia and Actos have similar effects upon blood sugar, so it serves no purpose for one individual to use both. Furthermore, the FDA has imposed severe restrictions on the use of Avandia, so it is now impractical to use it.

Metformin has the additional beneficial effect of reducing cancer incidence and suppressing the hunger hormone ghrelin, thereby reducing the tendency to overeat. In my experience, however, ***not all generic metformins match the effectiveness of Glucophage,*** so I prescribe only Glucophage, even though it is more expensive than other versions.

Some of the OHAs on the market are not insulin-sensitizing or insulin-mimetic. Instead, they provoke the pancreas to produce more insulin. For several reasons, this is considerably less desirable than taking a medication that sensitizes you to insulin. First, the pancreas-provoking OHAs can cause dangerously low blood sugar levels (hypoglycemia) if used improperly or if meals are skipped or delayed. Furthermore, forcing an already overworked pancreas to produce yet more insulin can lead to the impairment of remaining beta cells. These products also facilitate beta cell destruction by increasing levels of a toxic substance called amyloid. Finally, it has been repeatedly shown in experiments—and I have seen it in my own patients—that controlling diabetes through blood sugar normalization can help restore weakened or damaged beta cells. It makes absolutely no sense to prescribe or recommend agents that will cause them renewed damage. In a nutshell, pancreas-provoking drugs are counterproductive and no longer have any place in the sensible treatment of diabetes.

As it's far more productive to talk about good medicine, I will leave pancreas-provoking OHAs in the past, where even the newer ones belong, and from here on out discuss only insulin sensitizers and insulin mimetics. Then, at the end of the chapter, I will look at possible new treatment options for three special circumstances.

INSULIN-SENSITIZING AGENTS

The great advantage of insulin sensitizers is that they help to reduce blood sugar by making the body's tissues more sensitive to insulin, whether it's the body's own or injected. This is a benefit that can't be underestimated. Not only is it a boon to those trying to get their blood sugars under control, but it's also quite useful to those who are obese and simultaneously trying to get their weight down. By helping to reduce the amount of extra insulin in the bloodstream at any given time, these drugs can help alleviate the powerful fat-building properties of insulin. I have patients who are not diabetic but have come to me for treatment of their obesity. Insulin sensitizers have been a real plus to the weight-loss efforts of some because of their ability to curtail insulin resistance. Their major shortcoming is that they're rather slow to act—for example, they will not prevent a blood sugar rise from a meal if taken an hour before eating, as some of the beta cell–pushing medications will. As you will learn, however, this can be circumvented.

Some obese diabetic patients who come to me (including many type 1s) are injecting very large doses of insulin because their obesity makes them highly insulin-resistant. These high doses of insulin facilitate fat storage, and weight loss becomes more difficult. Insulin sensitizers make these patients more sensitive to the insulin they're injecting. In a typical case I had a patient taking 27 units of insulin at bedtime, even though he was on our low-carbohydrate diet. After he started on Glucophage, he was able to cut the dose to about 20 units. This is still a high dose, but the Glucophage facilitated the reduction.

Insulin sensitizers have also been shown to improve a number of measurable cardiac risk factors, including blood-clotting tendency, lipid profile, lipoprotein(a), serum fibrinogen, blood pressure, C-reactive protein, and even abnormal thickening of the heart muscle. In addition, Glucophage has been found to inhibit the destructive binding of glucose to proteins throughout the body—independent of its effect upon blood sugar. It has been shown to reduce absorption of dietary glucose, and also improves circulation, reduces oxidative stress, reduces blood vessel leakage—in the eyes and kidneys—and reduces the growth of fragile new blood vessels in the eyes. It has also been shown to improve satiety in women near menopause and, as indicated in the previous section, reduces cancer incidence. Thiazolidinediones such as rosiglitazone (Avandia) and pioglitazone (Actos) can slow the progression of diabetic kidney disease, independent of their effects on blood sugars. These medications can also down-regulate the genes that cause fat storage, and they have been found to delay or prevent the onset of diabetes in some high-risk individuals. On the other hand, Actos and Avandia have been shown to increase the risk of bone fractures in postmenopausal women. Both of these drugs can cause water retention, and people with congestive heart failure are already overloaded with fluid. Avandia users have been shown to have a higher incidence of heart attacks than Actos users. I therefore no longer prescribe Avandia.

Cycloset lowers insulin resistance by an unknown mechanism. Its active ingredient, bromocriptine, is used to treat Parkinson's disease and thus can affect the brain. I will not prescribe it until it's been on the market without adverse consequences for five years.

This leaves me with Glucophage as my principal insulin sensitizer, with Actos as a backup.

INSULIN-MIMETIC AGENTS

In addition to the insulin sensitizers, there are some substances sold in the United States as dietary supplements that are sometimes effective for helping to control blood sugars. Many studies in Germany have demonstrated this effect from R-alpha lipoic acid, or R-ALA. A 2001 study showed it to work in muscle and fat cells by mobilizing and activating glucose transporters—in other words, it works like insulin, or is an insulin mimetic. German studies have also shown that its effectiveness in mimicking the effects of insulin is greatly enhanced when used with equivalent amounts of evening primrose oil, another dietary supplement. R-ALA can reduce the body's natural levels of biotin, so it should be taken in a preparation that contains biotin (see footnote, page 252). R-ALA and evening primrose oil are no substitute, however, for injected insulin—they are at best a fraction as potent. Still, their combined effectiveness is significant for some people, though not for everyone.

Additionally, R-ALA is perhaps the most potent antioxidant on the market and has certain cardiovascular benefits similar to those claimed for fish oil. Many of the cardiologists who were taking vitamin E for its antioxidant properties fifteen years ago are now taking

R-ALA. I've been taking it myself for about twelve years. When I began, I promptly found that I had to lower my insulin doses by about one-third. R-ALA and evening primrose oil do not appear to mimic one important property of insulin—they don't appear to facilitate fat storage. They are both available without a prescription from some health food stores and pharmacies.* The products have the potential to cause hypoglycemia in diabetics who inject insulin if they don't adjust their insulin dosages accordingly. I have never seen them cause hypoglycemia when they are not used with injected insulin, however.

Other German studies have shown dramatic improvements in diabetic neuropathy (nerve damage) when alpha lipoic acid is administered intravenously in large doses over several weeks. Given its antioxidant and likely anti-inflammatory properties, this isn't that surprising. But it falls under the category of "Don't Try This at Home."

R-alpha lipoic acid, like high-dose vitamin E (the form called gamma tocopherol) and Glucophage, can impede glycosylation and glycation of proteins, both of which cause many diabetic complications when blood sugars are elevated.

When I use it, I recommend two 100 mg tablets every 8 hours or so, with one 500 mg capsule of evening primrose oil at the same time. I prescribe Insulow because it contains biotin. If an insulin-resistant patient is already taking insulin, I will start her on half this dose once daily and observe blood glucose profiles, then lower the insulin dose as I raise the R-alpha lipoic acid and evening primrose oil. Again, it's all trial and error. The same can be said for whether R-ALA will work at all. It appears to lower blood sugars for some people, but not for everyone.

WARNING: Cancer cells can thrive on antioxidants. If you have a family or personal history of any form of cancer, it would be wise to steer clear of R-ALA and other antioxidants.

---

* Note that ALA has two molecular forms—a right (R) enantiomer and a left (L) enantiomer. For many years, commercial ALA was a mixture of the two called alpha lipoic acid (ALA). Then it was discovered that the active form is the R enantiomer. R-ALA is twice as potent as the R-L mixture (ALA), and this is the form usually marketed today. Although conventional ALA is widely available, R-ALA is more effective. As of this writing, the principal manufacturer in the United States is Glucorell, Inc., of Orlando, Florida, phone (866) 467-8569, www.insulow.com. Their product, Insulow, contains 100 mg of R-ALA per capsule, plus 750 mcg (0.75 mg) biotin. Insulow is available from Rosedale Pharmacy, (888) 796-3348, and www.Rx4betterhealth.com.

WHO IS A LIKELY CANDIDATE FOR INSULIN-SENSITIZING OR INSULIN-MIMETIC AGENTS?

Generally speaking, these agents are natural choices for a type 2 diabetic who despite a low-carbohydrate diet cannot get his weight down or his blood sugars into normal ranges. The blood sugar elevation may be limited to a particular time of the day, it may be during the night, or it may entail a slight elevation all day. We base our prescription on the individual's blood sugar profiles. If even on our diet, blood sugar exceeds 160 mg/dl at any time of the day, I'll immediately prescribe insulin and won't even attempt to use these agents, except perhaps to eventually reduce doses of injected insulin. If your blood sugar is higher upon arising than at bedtime, we'd give you the sustained-release version of Glucophage (Glucophage XR) at bedtime. If your blood sugar goes up after a particular meal, we'd give you rapid-acting Glucophage about 2 hours before that meal. Since food reduces the possibility of diarrhea from this agent, we might give it with the meal. If blood sugars are slightly elevated all day long, we might use alpha lipoic acid and evening primrose oil on arising, postlunch, and postdinner. It should be noted, however, that the ISAs are considerably more effective than insulin mimetics in lowering blood sugars.

GETTING STARTED: SOME TYPICAL PROTOCOLS

Let's say you're a type 2 diabetic and through weight loss, exercise, and diet, you pretty much have your blood sugars within your target range. Still, your blood sugar profiles show a regular elevation in the mornings after a low-carbohydrate breakfast, probably due in part to the dawn phenomenon (see page 97).

My first attempt to resolve the dawn phenomenon would be to try a small dose (500 mg) of Glucophage XR before you go to bed. This will achieve its peak blood level after about 7 hours. If this still doesn't get your blood sugars into target range, then you could increase the dose gradually, perhaps by one more tablet at bedtime for a week and so on, until you reach a maximum of 4 tablets a night or you hit your target. I always recommend the least possible dosage — partly due to the

Laws of Small Numbers, but also because of the reduction of likelihood for potential side effects. With metformin, if you build up your
dosage slowly, it lessens the possibility of gastrointestinal discomfort
that about one-third of users of the older, more-rapid-acting version
experience.

Another option would be to use Actos at bedtime either instead of
Glucophage XR or in addition to it, if necessary. We could start with
15 mg and increase the dose to a maximum of 45 mg.

In some cases, blood sugar levels either increase overnight or
increase during the first 2 hours after you arise. The latter situation is
most likely due to the dawn phenomenon. Either situation may
respond to the above treatment.

Another possibility that would warrant oral medication would be if
your blood sugar levels increased after lunch or dinner. Some potential

TABLE 15-1

RECOMMENDED ORAL AGENTS FOR
BLOOD SUGAR CONTROL

Agent	Type	U.S. brand name	Available dosages	Maximum (effective) daily dosage
Metformin	Insulin sensitizer	Glucophage, not generic	500, 850, 1,000 mg	2,500 mg
Metformin extended release	Insulin sensitizer	Glucophage XR, not generic	500 mg	2,000 mg*
Pioglitazone	Insulin sensitizer	Actos	15, 30, 45 mg	45 mg
R-alpha lipoic acid (R-ALA) with biotin	Insulin mimetic	Insulow	100 mg	1,800 mg
Evening primrose oil (EPO)	Insulin mimetic booster for every 300 mg of R-ALA	Many	500 mg recommended	3,000 mg

* For reasons not apparent to me, the manufacturer's recommendation for
maximum daily dosing is less for extended-release Glucophage XR than for
the standard version.

solutions include taking rapid-acting Glucophage 1–2 hours before eating or rapid-acting insulin 0–30 minutes before eating if the Glucophage is inadequate.

All of the incretin mimetics described in Chapter 13 can be used to prevent blood sugar increase after meals. I prefer to use them for appetite control.

WILL THESE MEDICATIONS CAUSE HYPOGLYCEMIA?

Sulfonylureas and the newer glitazar OHAs carry the very real possibility of causing dangerously low blood sugars, which is one of the reasons I never prescribe them. However, this is only remotely likely with the insulin-sensitizing and insulin-mimetic agents listed above. None of them interferes with the self-regulating system of a pancreas that can still make its own insulin. If your blood sugar drops too low, your body will most likely just stop making insulin automatically. Sulfonylureas and similar drugs, on the other hand, because they stimulate insulin production whether the body needs it or not, can cause hypoglycemia.

Although the manufacturers and the scientific literature claim that Glucophage does not cause hypoglycemia, I did have a patient who experienced hypoglycemia. She was very obese but only very mildly diabetic, and I was giving her Glucophage to reduce insulin resistance to facilitate weight loss. When I put her on Glucophage, her blood sugars went too low (but not dangerously)—down into the 60s.

So there may be some very slight risk of hypoglycemia with the insulin sensitizers or insulin mimetics, but this is not at all comparable to the great risk with the sulfonylureas and similar medications. *One warning, however: the body cannot turn off injected insulin, so if you are taking insulin plus an insulin sensitizer, hypoglycemia is very possible.* (See Chapter 20, "How to Prevent and Correct Low Blood Sugars.")

WHAT IF THESE AGENTS DON'T BRING BLOOD SUGARS INTO LINE?

If oral agents are not adequate to normalize blood sugars completely, there may be something awry in the diet or exercise portion of your treatment program. The most likely culprit for continued elevated blood sugars is that the carbohydrate portion of your diet is not properly controlled. So the first step is to examine your diet again to see if that's where the problem lies. With many patients, this is a matter of carbohydrate craving or snacking on nuts. If this is the case and your carbohydrate craving is overwhelming, I'd recommend that you reread Chapter 13, "How to Curb Carbohydrate Craving or Overeating," and consider pursuing one of the techniques described there. If diet is not the culprit, then the next thing—no matter how obese or resistant to exercise you might be—would be to try to get you started on a strenuous exercise program. If even this doesn't do the trick, you probably have lost enough beta cell function to require injected insulin.

It's also worth keeping in mind that infection or illness can seriously impair your efforts at blood sugar normalization. If your blood sugar levels are way out of line even with the use of insulin, you might also consider talking to your physician about potential underlying infection, especially in the mouth (see page 105).

DISADVANTAGES OF INSULIN SENSITIZERS AND INSULIN MIMETICS

Although insulin mimetics and insulin-sensitizing agents are some of the best tools we have for controlling blood sugars, they are not without their difficulties. Since R-alpha lipoic acid and evening primrose oil are not prescription drugs in most countries (Germany is a notable exception), they are not covered by most health insurance. R-alpha lipoic acid is not inexpensive; at this writing, a supply of 180 Insulow 100 mg tablets costs about $30.

R-ALA reduces body stores of biotin, a substance that aids in the utilization of protein and a variety of other nutrients, so when you take R-alpha lipoic acid, you might be wise to take biotin supplements also—unless you are taking Insulow, which already contains biotin. Your biotin intake should theoretically equal about 1 percent of your R-alpha lipoic acid intake, so if you are taking 1,800 mg R-ALA per day, in theory you would take about 18 mg of biotin. Most of my patients who use R-alpha lipoic acid don't take more than about 15 mg biotin per day, and they experience no apparent adverse effects. Most biotin preparations come only in 1 mg strengths.

Glucophage has a very low side-effects profile, with the exception of gastrointestinal distress—queasiness, nausea, diarrhea, or a slight bellyache—in as many as a third of the people who try the non–extended-release version. Most people who experience such discomfort, however, find that it diminishes as they become accustomed to the medication. Only a very few patients can't tolerate it at all. (Some patients, particularly obese people who are anxious to achieve the weight loss that metformin can facilitate, will ignore any initial gastrointestinal distress and use an antacid drug such as Pepcid or Tagamet for relief. Others, who may experience only relatively mild discomfort, are willing to tolerate it for a few weeks just to get things rolling. These adverse effects are much less common with Glucophage XR.) Rare cases of diarrhea have been reported long after the start of Glucophage therapy. They have been reversed by discontinuation of the medication. I have not observed gastrointestinal side effects associated with the use of thiazolidinediones.

Rare individuals find that gastrointestinal distress (e.g., diarrhea) from Glucophage XR continues even at low doses. These people can try Actos or metformin gel.* The gel is applied to the skin, so gastrointestinal effects don't occur. I haven't prescribed it yet, but it's worth a try.

Metformin's predecessor, phenformin, was, in the 1950s, associated with a potentially life-threatening condition called lactic acidosis. This occurred in a small number of patients who were already suffering from heart failure or advanced liver or kidney disease. Although I have read of only a few instances of lactic acidosis associated with metformin, the FDA advises against using it in individuals with these conditions. A recent retrospective study found a lower frequency of lactic acidosis among metformin users than among non-users. Metformin has also been reported to block vitamin B-12 absorption in about one-third of users. This effect can be prevented by increasing your intake of dietary calcium (see page 189).†

The one thiazolidinedione readily available in the United States, Actos, has the potential for minor problems. Actos is cleared from the

---

* Available from Med Specialties Compounding Pharmacy, Yorba Linda, California, (877) 373-2272.
† A deficit of vitamin B-12 can increase serum levels of the renal disease risk factor homocysteine. It would therefore be wise for your physician to check your serum homocysteine every six months while you are using metformin.

bloodstream by the liver, utilizing the same enzyme used to clear many other common medications. The competition for this enzyme can leave dangerously elevated blood levels of some of these medicines. If you are taking one or more of these competing medications, such as some antidepressants, antifungal agents, certain antibiotics, and others, you should likely not be using Actos. You should check the package insert for potential drug interactions and talk to your physician and pharmacist.

Actos can cause a small amount of fluid retention in some people. The consequence of this is a dilution of red blood cell count and swelling in the legs. I've seen a number of such cases. There can also be a small weight gain due to the retained water, not to fat. This water retention has been associated with a few instances of heart failure in individuals taking Actos plus insulin. In the United States, the FDA has therefore recommended that doses not exceed 30 mg per day for people who inject insulin. I have treated many insulin users with them and have seen slight swelling of the legs in some cases. When this occurred, I discontinued the Actos immediately. There also have been very rare cases of reversible liver damage associated with Actos.* On the other hand, it has been shown to improve lipid profiles (LDL, HDL, and triglycerides).

Because of the possibility of fluid retention, Actos should not be used by patients with significant cardiac, lung, or kidney disease, or with any degree of heart failure.†

USING MULTIPLE AGENTS

Glucophage works principally by lowering insulin resistance in the liver. It also impairs, somewhat, the absorption of carbohydrate by the intestine. Actos principally affects muscle and fat, and less so the liver. Thus, if Glucophage does not fully normalize blood sugars, it makes sense to add Actos—and vice versa. The FDA suggests that doses of Actos not exceed 30 mg daily when taken with Glucophage.

---

* Even though reports of liver toxicity are far fewer than with some commonly used medications such as niacin and the so-called statins, it's a good idea for users of Actos to have their blood tested for liver enzymes annually.
† The FDA may restrict the use of Actos because of a weak association with bladder cancer.

Since R-ALA and evening primrose oil work as insulin mimetics, it is certainly appropriate to add these to any combination of the other agents. Whether they will make a difference depends on individual responses.

OTHER CONSIDERATIONS

Actos does not have full blood sugar–lowering effects on the day it is started. It achieves its full potency after a few weeks.

When blood sugars are *much higher* than the targets that I set, both Glucophage and Actos can cause the pancreas to increase its insulin production in response to glucose. Because of the lower blood sugars that we see, this effect becomes insignificant.

Vitamin A supplementation has been shown to lower insulin resistance (as do vitamins D and E)* in doses of about 25,000 IU daily. Since slightly higher doses of vitamin A are potentially *very* toxic, and doses as low as 5,000 IU can cause calcium loss from bone, I would consider only moderate doses of its nontoxic precursor, beta carotene, for this purpose.

Studies have shown that magnesium deficiency can cause insulin resistance. It would therefore be a sensible idea for physicians to test type 2 diabetics for red blood cell magnesium (not serum magnesium) levels. If the level is low, magnesium supplementation should help. I recommend magnesium orate in small doses that can be increased if the test remains low after three months. Since red blood cell magnesium is not a perfect indicator of the body's magnesium stores, and since magnesium supplements are benign to people with normal kidneys (except for diarrhea), it is appropriate to use magnesium supplements as a test to see if blood sugars decline. Doses as high as 700 mg daily are common for adults. Since diseased kidneys are less able to clear excess magnesium from the blood, magnesium supplements should not be used in the presence of kidney impairment.

Similarly, zinc deficiency can cause diminished production of

---

* Vitamin E should only be used in the forms called gamma tocopherol or mixed tocopherols. Remember, however, that high doses of the common alpha tocopherol form, which can inhibit the absorption of essential gamma tocopherol from foods, has been shown to increase the risk of cardiac death.

leptin, a hormone that impedes overeating and weight gain. Such deficiency can also impair functioning of the thyroid gland. It is thus wise for all type 2 patients to ask their physicians to test their serum zinc levels and to prescribe zinc supplementation if warranted. Follow-up serum zinc levels should be measured to ensure that normal levels are not exceeded, because high blood levels can cause adverse effects, such as increased risk of prostate cancer.

Compounds of the heavy metal vanadium have been shown to lower insulin resistance, reduce appetite, and possibly also act as insulin-mimetic agents. They are quite potent in lowering blood sugars, but there's a catch. Vanadium compounds work by inhibiting the enzyme tyrosine phosphatase, which is essential to many vital biochemical processes in the body. The possibility is quite real that this inhibition can be damaging. Since clinical trials in humans have not exceeded three weeks in duration, long-term freedom from adverse effects has yet to be documented. Some users of vanadium compounds have experienced GI irritation. Although vanadyl sulfate is widely available in health food stores as a dietary supplement and has been used for years without any reports of adverse effects in medical journals, I tentatively recommend that it be avoided until more is known.*

ACARBOSE: FOR PEOPLE WHOSE CARBOHYDRATE CRAVING CANNOT BE CONTROLLED

In theory at least, there are individuals who do not respond to any of the measures recommended in Chapter 13 for the control of carbohydrate craving and overeating. These people can be helped *slightly* by a product called acarbose (Precose). Acarbose is available as 25 mg, 50 mg, and 100 mg tablets to inhibit the action of enzymes that digest starches and table sugar,† thereby slowing or reducing the effects of these no-no foods upon blood sugars. It is interesting that the ADA recommends eating starches and sugars and then the simultaneous use of acarbose to prevent their digestion.

---

* Except by commercial pilots, who must avoid insulin (see page 261).
† The enzymes are alpha-glucosidase and pancreatic amylase.

The maximum recommended daily dose of acarbose is 300 mg. It is usually taken at the time of carbohydrate consumption. Its major adverse effect, in about 75 percent of users, is flatulence (predictably), so it is wise to increase the dose gradually. It should not be used for patients with any intestinal disorders (e.g., gastroparesis). Since Victoza became available, I have had to prescribe acarbose for only one patient.

SELENIUM MAY SET YOU UP FOR TYPE 2 DIABETES

A recent study in the U.K. showed that excess selenium supplementation increased the risk of type 2 diabetes by nearly 50 percent. On the other hand, low serum selenium levels can increase the risk of hypothyroidism. If you are taking selenium supplementation, have your blood levels checked. If necessary, adjust your dose so that your blood level is around the middle of the normal range.

PHLEBOTOMY: A LAST RESORT FOR SOME, BUT IT MAY WORK

Commercial airline pilots with diabetes are currently faced with regulations in the United States that threaten loss of license (and livelihood) if they inject insulin. Certainly these people should try all of the oral agents recommended above, as well as a low-carbohydrate diet and strenuous exercise. They should also consider vanadyl sulfate, magnesium, and the other supplements listed earlier in this chapter under "Other Considerations."

There is yet another potentially powerful way of lowering insulin resistance for people with this problem. It's been demonstrated that men whose body iron stores placed them in the top 20 percent of the nonanemic population had much greater insulin resistance than those in the bottom 20 percent. Furthermore, their insulin resistance dropped dramatically when they donated enough blood every two months to keep them in the bottom 20 percent. I've actually seen this work on my own patients. A good measure of total body iron is the serum ferritin test. Since some blood banks will not accept blood donations from diabetics, it may be necessary to visit a hematologist for a phlebotomy (removal of blood from a vein) every two months. It is likely that most insurance plans will pay the hematologist's fee.

Women are much less likely than men to have high normal ferritin levels.

AND ONE MORE OPTION

The availability of DPP-4 inhibitors such as Januvia, Onglyza, Tradjenta, and Galvus (see Chapter 13, "How to Curb Carbohydrate Craving or Overeating") provides one more option for those who refuse to take injections. Although their effect upon overeating is at best trivial, they will significantly reduce the effect of glucagon upon blood sugar during and after meals (the Chinese restaurant effect). They can be used as part of a three-way combination with Glucophage and Actos.

AVOID PREMADE MIXTURES OF MEDICATIONS

When a patent expires on a popular drug, the manufacturer may try to get one up on the competition by patenting a mixture of that drug with another drug. This is rarely beneficial to patients, increases costs, and may result in untoward effects. This applies to both oral and injected drugs.

I will personally answer questions from readers for one hour every month. This free service is available by visiting www.askdrbernstein.net.

16

Insulin: The Basics of Self-Injection

As you may have learned from the preceding chapter, certain oral agents, such as ISAs and insulin mimetics, are valuable for controlling blood sugars but can only go so far. If you're taking the maximum effective doses of oral agents and your blood sugars remain elevated—in spite of diet, exercise (where feasible), and weight loss—injected insulin will be essential to bringing your blood sugars down to your target range.*

Although many patients initially balk at the idea of injecting insulin, you should look at this as an opportunity, not a curse, *because insulin injections will increase the likelihood that you can bring about a partial recovery of your pancreatic beta cell function.* This is especially true if you are a slim type 2 or a recently diagnosed type 1.

If you're afraid of insulin because you imagine that once you start, you'll never be able to stop, you've fallen victim to a common myth.

---

* Investigators in Buffalo, New York, have demonstrated that injected insulin appears to lower the production of inflammatory substances and increase levels of anti-inflammatory agents in obese individuals. Since inflammation increases the likelihood of atherosclerosis, chronic use of insulin injections can lower the risk of cardiac disease, peripheral vascular disease, and stroke, independent of its effects upon blood sugar. Injected insulin also facilitates the dilation (opening) of coronary and other arteries that may be constricted in many diabetics and even in nondiabetics. It also has been found to improve the absorption of oxygen by blood flowing through the lungs. On the other hand, the industrial doses of insulin used to cover high carbohydrate diets have pretty much the opposite of these effects.

In reality, injected insulin is the best means we have at this writing for preventing beta cell burnout.

The Biostator GCIIS, an "artificial pancreas," was a device developed in the 1970s when the average insulin-using diabetic took a single, daily, industrial dose of insulin. The device may still be available. In any case, its initials stood for "glucose-controlled insulin infusion system." That's exactly what it aimed to do—infuse insulin as a pancreas would, based on blood glucose levels. It attached to the patient through two intravenous connections, one that measured blood sugars constantly and another that delivered glucose or insulin to correct blood sugars to 90 mg/dl virtually instantaneously. Although it was not practical for home use (it had a staff of two—one to operate the machine and one to service it—and rented for tens of thousands of dollars a month), it did useful research, the most important element of which was that it showed that beta cell burnout could be reversed or halted, even by relatively short exposure to normalized blood sugars. How?

Many years ago, Gerald Reaven, MD, author of *Syndrome X,* conducted a study with thirty-two diabetics, half of them female, half of them male. One at a time, he put them into the hospital and had them attached to the Biostator for two weeks. His staff checked HgbA$_{1C}$ on arrival, at discharge, and every three months thereafter. They found that HgbA$_{1C}$ plummeted during the two-week treatment period, but the most important thing they found was that when the subjects went back to their ordinary lives and their poor diets, their HgbA$_{1C}$ measures took an average of two years to return to their high, pretreatment values.

Considerable beta cell recovery clearly occurred after just *two weeks* of normal blood sugars. In fact, it took *two years* to undo those two weeks of healing. I'm not inviting you to normalize your blood sugars for two weeks and then go back to your old diet. My intent is to demonstrate the value of using insulin, and the value of normalized blood sugars. We might envision that a mild diabetic still has three types of beta cells, active, dying, and dead. My own beta cells may be all of the last variety—dead. I've mentioned it previously, but if I'd had the kind of treatment upon my diagnosis sixty-five years ago that I advocate today, I might still have a significant number of working beta cells. If you have some beta cell function left, you can probably increase it by normalizing your blood sugars.

If the prospect of injecting yourself horrifies you, don't let it. Many people assume injections must be painful, but they needn't be. If you've already been using insulin for years and find the shots painful, the likelihood is you were taught to inject improperly.

HOW TO GIVE A PAINLESS INJECTION

If you have type 2 diabetes, sooner or later you may require insulin injections, either temporarily (as during infections) or permanently. This is nothing to be afraid of, even though many people with long-standing type 2 diabetes spend literally years worrying about it. I usually teach all my patients how to inject themselves at our first or second meeting, before there's any urgency. Once they give themselves a sample injection of sterile saline (salt water), they find out how easy and painless it can be, and they are spared years of anxiety. If you're anxious about injections, after you read this section please ask your physician or diabetes educator to allow you to try a self-administered injection (without the insulin).

Insulin is usually injected subcutaneously. This means into a layer of fat under the skin. The regions of the body that are likely to contain appropriate deposits of fat are illustrated in Figure 16-1. Examine your body to see if you have enough fat at the illustrated sites to comfortably grab a big hunk between your thumb and first finger.

Most diabetics are erroneously taught to inject into their thighs in spite of the obvious: most thighs have inadequate fat for satisfactory

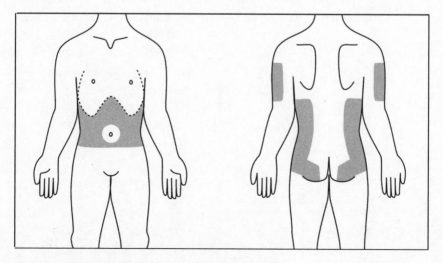

Fig. 16-1. *Potential sites for subcutaneous injections.*

injections. The net result is that the injection ends up going into muscle instead of fat and the timing of the insulin is sped up inappropriately. This intramuscular injection usually hurts.

To show you how painless a shot can be, your teacher should
self-administer a shot to illustrate that no pain is felt. Your teacher
should next give you a shot of saline or "throw" the needle into your
skin to prove the point. Now it's time for you to give yourself an injection, using a syringe that's already empty or has been partly filled for
you with about 5 "units" of saline.

1. First, with your "nonshooting" hand, grab as big a chunk of
   skin plus underlying fat as you can hold comfortably. If you
   have a nice roll of fat around your waist, use this site. If not,
   select another site from those illustrated in Figure 16-1. Nearly
   everyone has enough subcutaneous buttocks fat to inject there
   without grabbing any flesh. Just locate a fatty site by feel. To
   inject into your arm, use the top of a chair, the outside corner
   of two walls, or the edge of a doorway to push the loose flesh
   from the back of your arm to a forward position that you can
   easily see and reach with the needle.
2. Hold the syringe like a dart, with the thumb and first two or
   three fingers of either hand.
3. Now comes the most important part. *Penetration must be rapid.*
   Never *put the needle against the skin and push.* That's the
   method still taught in many hospitals, and it's often painful. If
   you can find only a small amount of flesh to hold, the needle
   should pierce the skin at a 45-degree angle, as in Figure 16-2, or

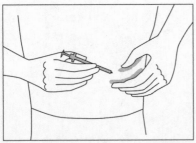

Terry Eppridge

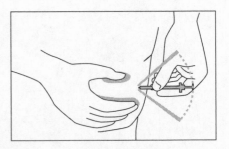

Fig. 16-2. *If you are skinny, pierce*
the skin at a 45-degree angle, or use a
short (⁵⁄₁₆-inch) needle.

Fig. 16-3. *If you're chunky, pierce the*
skin at any angle between 45 degrees
and 90 degrees.

even better, use one of the new insulin syringes with a short needle (5/16 inch, or 8 mm). If you can grab a hefty handful, you should plunge the needle straight in, perpendicular to the skin surface, or at any angle between 45 degrees and 90 degrees, as shown in Figure 16-3.

4. The stroke should begin about 4 inches from your target to give the moving needle a chance to pick up speed. Pretend you're throwing a dart—but don't let go of the syringe. Move your entire forearm and give the wrist a flick at the end of the motion. You shouldn't get hurt. The needle should penetrate the skin for its entire length.

5. As soon as it's in, rapidly push the plunger all the way down to inject the fluid. If the demonstration syringe is empty, then don't bother to push the plunger. Now promptly remove the needle from the skin.

There's no need to practice injecting oranges, as has been taught in the past. If you're going to practice anything, you might first practice "throwing" a syringe, with the needle cover on, at your skin.

All you need do is experience one rapid stick to realize that speed makes it painless. Never has it taken more than a moment for me to get a patient to self-inject. I've had grown men in tears at the prospect of injecting insulin who soon discover that it's easy and painless and of considerable value in treatment. It doesn't demand much skill, and certainly doesn't require bravery.

HOW TO SELECT AN INSULIN SYRINGE

In recent years, a number of new insulin syringes have appeared on the market in the United States. Although they are all sterile, plastic, and disposable, some are better than others. The important features to consider are described below. Refer to Figure 16-4, which identifies the parts of a typical insulin syringe that you might find at your local pharmacy.

The Scale

When selecting a syringe, the printed scale is the most important feature, because the spacing of the markings determines how accurately you can measure a dose. Think Laws of Small Numbers: accuracy and consistency of dose are both highly important.

Insulin doses are measured in "units." One unit of our most-rapid-acting insulin will lower my blood sugar by 100 mg/dl. One unit will lower the blood sugar of a 45-pound child by about 255 mg/dl. Some of my slim adult patients with mild type 2 diabetes find that 1 unit will drop them by 150 mg/dl. Clearly, an error of only ¼ unit can make the difference between a normal blood sugar and hypoglycemia for many of us. My insulin-using patients never inject as much as 8 units in a single dose. It would therefore be ideal to have a long, slender syringe with a total capacity of 10 units and markings for every ¼ unit spaced far enough apart that ⅛ unit can be accurately estimated visually. The numbers on the scale should be easy to read. The lines should be dark, but no thicker than 1/12 unit. Such a syringe, unfortunately, does not exist quite yet.*

A currently available preferred syringe is illustrated in Figure 16-4. Note that the scale line nearest to the needle is longer than the other lines. This is the zero line. It overlies the end of the gasket when the plunger is pushed in fully. It is *not* the 1-unit line. The upper scale in the figure displays whole units; the lower scale shows half units.

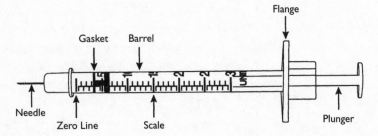

Fig. 16-4. *A preferred insulin syringe, calibrated in half-unit increments (enlarged image).*

The Rubber Gasket

This is the dark-colored piece of synthetic rubber at the end of the plunger nearest the needle. It indicates a given dose by its position along the scale. The best gasket has a surface that's flat and not conical, as some are, so that doses can be read without confusion. Note: the end of the gasket that is nearest the needle is the end that should be set at the dose.

---

* For obvious reasons, many of my patients, including myself, must use diluted insulin for precise measurement (see pages 287–290).

The Needle

The needle should be ¼–⅝ inch (about 8 mm) long. Longer needles may go too deeply into thin people. Until 1996 all disposable insulin syringes sold in the United States had ½-inch (12 mm) needles. Syringes with shorter (⁵⁄₁₆-inch) needles are now available. With these syringes you do not always need to "grab a hunk of flesh" or inject at a 45-degree angle unless, like me, you have very little fat at the injection site. Just throw it in. Do not, however, use short needles for intramuscular injection, as described on page 326.

Needle thickness is specified by gauge number, just as for nails and wire. The higher the gauge number, the thinner the needle. With a very thin gauge, even penetrating the skin too slowly may not hurt. With too thin a gauge, the needle might bend or break when puncturing tough skin. The ideal compromise between thinness and strength is probably 31 gauge, which is now widely available.

The Point

The needle points of disposable insulin syringes currently sold in the United States are quite sharp. Advertising that claims special sharpness for a particular brand is usually exaggerated.

FILLING THE SYRINGE

My technique for filling a syringe with insulin differs from what is usually taught, but it has the advantage of preventing the development of air bubbles in the syringe. Although it is not harmful to inject air bubbles below your skin, their presence in the syringe interferes with accurate measurement of small doses.

General Technique

This step-by-step approach may be followed for all clear insulins. Only one insulin now on the market is cloudy. It is called NPH in the United States and isophane overseas. If you use cloudy insulin, read Filling a Syringe with Cloudy Insulin, page 271, before proceeding.

1. Take the cap off your needle and the second cap off the end of the plunger.
2. Draw room air into the syringe by pulling the plunger back until

the end of the rubber gasket nearest the needle is set close to the dose you intend to inject. If the gasket has a dome or conical shape, the dose should be set at the widest part of the gasket, not at its tip.

3. Puncture the midpoint of the insulin vial's rubber stopper with the needle and inject the air into the vial. This seemingly useless step has a purpose. If you were not to inject air to replace the insulin you withdrew, after many fillings a vacuum would eventually develop in the vial, which would make subsequent fillings difficult.

4. Invert the syringe and vial and hold them vertically, as shown in Figure 16-5. Press the syringe barrel against your palm with the little finger of the hand that holds the vial to ensure that the needle remains in the stopper, then *rapidly* pull back on the plunger until the barrel is filled with insulin well beyond your dose (e.g., to about 15 units if your dose is to be 5 units).

5. Slowly push the plunger in, still holding vertically, until the appropriate part of the rubber gasket reaches the desired dose.

6. Continue to hold the syringe and vial vertically as you remove the filled syringe and needle from the vial.

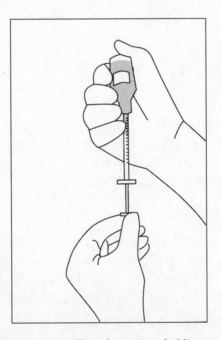

Fig. 16-5. *Filling the syringe, holding the vial and syringe vertically.*

Filling a Syringe with Cloudy Insulin

The one intermediate-acting insulin (NPH) sold today comes in vials that contain a clear liquid and a gray precipitate. The gray particles tend to settle rapidly from the liquid when the vial is left undisturbed. They must be resuspended uniformly in the liquid immediately prior to every use. Failure to do this will result in inconsistent effects upon blood sugars from one shot to another. The way to secure a uniform suspension is to shake the vial. Many years ago, egg white–based vaccines were of a syrupy consistency and tended to form a permanent foam when shaken. This is not the case with today's water-based insulins. Yet most textbooks—and even the American Diabetes Association—still tell nurses and doctors to roll the vial between the hands and not to shake it. This misinformation is unfortunate, because we don't get consistent results when vials are rolled.

When filling a syringe with a cloudy insulin, observe the following procedure to ensure an even suspension.

1–3. Remove the cap(s) from the syringe, draw air into it, and inject the air into the vial as described in steps 1–3 on pages 269–270.
   4. Before drawing out any insulin, while still holding the vial and syringe in one hand, *vigorously* shake them back and forth 6–10 times as shown in Figure 16-6. Holding the upward-pointing syringe and vial vertically, rapidly draw

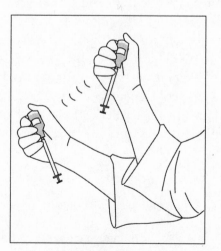

Fig. 16-6. *Shaking a vial of cloudy insulin before drawing out the dose.*

back the plunger immediately after shaking to fill the syringe with insulin well beyond your dose. Do not delay, as the gray particles will settle very rapidly.

5–6. Still holding vertically, slowly push the plunger in until the desired dose is reached, then remove the needle and filled syringe from the vial (see steps 5–6, page 270).

ON THE REUSE OF DISPOSABLE INSULIN SYRINGES

The annual cost of sterile disposable insulin syringes can be considerable, especially if you take multiple daily injections. You may become tempted to reuse your syringes, especially if your medical insurance doesn't fully reimburse you for the cost. (Many medical insurance policies in the United States do at least partially cover this expense.) Although I haven't encountered any infection caused by a single person reusing his own syringes, I have encountered the problem of polymerization of insulin.*

Many of my patients pass through a stage when they routinely reuse their syringes several times, to save money or to enable them to travel with only a small supply. These patients never use the same syringe for two different types of insulin, so we can't say that one insulin is contaminating another. Inevitably, I get a telephone call with the message, "My blood sugars are high and I can't get them down." I ask, "Bring your clear insulin to the phone. Is it crystal clear, like water?" Inevitably the reply is, "No, it's slightly hazy." Insulin that becomes hazy has been partially deactivated by polymerization and will not adequately control blood sugars. This is not found by people who do not reuse their syringes.† Of course, I advise such patients to immediately replace all insulin vials, whether long- or short-acting, that have been used to fill reused syringes. Replacement of the vials always

---

* A polymer is a large molecule made up of identical smaller molecules bound together.
† The reason for this is that the minute amount of insulin remaining in a used needle will become polymerized (inactivated) within a few hours. If it is injected back into the vial, it will eventually act as a seed for the polymerization of much of the insulin in the vial.

cures the problem. Naturally, syringes should not subsequently be reused.

What if you encounter a situation where you have only one syringe to last for a week and have no way of getting new ones? Flush the syringe with air several times after each use to clear out any remaining insulin. When filling the syringe, do not inject air into the insulin vial (step 3), and don't inject the excess insulin back into the vial (step 5). Just draw the needle from the vial and squirt the excess into the air. This way, you won't contaminate your vial with the minute amount of old insulin that may remain in the needle or syringe. If you have a second unused syringe, you can use it just to inject air into your vials, making certain the needle does not come into contact with the insulin in the vials.

If for financial reasons you really must reuse your syringes, the following procedure should help minimize contamination with polymerized insulin. You will, at the minimum, need three syringes, but four would be better.

- Use your insulin vials for a week without injecting air into them. Squirt any excess insulin from each filling into a sink or wastebasket, not back into the vial.
- At the end of a week, remove the plunger from an unused syringe. Stand the vial stopper up on a flat surface and push the needle of the unused syringe into the stopper of the vial. Within seconds, the vacuum in the vial will suck in enough air through the needle to replace the vacuum.
- Pull the needle out of the stopper, reinsert the plunger, and recap the "air" syringe for use the next week. Since my insurance will not fully pay for insulin syringes, this is the method that I use.

WHEN TO DISCARD A REUSED SYRINGE

The needle will not last forever, so discard a syringe:

- When the needle doesn't go through your skin as if it were butter.
- When, on pulling the needle out, you feel it briefly catch, as from a hook.

WHAT IF YOU INJECT SEVERAL DIFFERENT INSULINS AT THE SAME TIME?

As discussed in Chapter 19, "Intensive Insulin Regimens," you might have to inject several different insulins at the same time. For example, when you arise in the morning, you might inject a most-rapid-acting insulin (e.g., Humalog) to bring down a slightly elevated blood sugar, then a rapid-acting insulin (regular) to cover your breakfast, then a long-acting (basal) insulin (Levemir). Take the most-rapid-acting (Humalog), then the less-rapid-acting (regular), and last the long-acting, one injection after another, all using the same syringe. Use different sites for each injection. You can safely do this because the insulin has not had enough time to polymerize in the needle (this takes several hours). If your long-acting insulin is Lantus,* however, don't use the same syringe. Just a small amount of Humalog or regular in the needle may inactivate some of the Lantus. This is very important.

Don't mix different insulins together, either in the same syringe or in the same vial, as this will result in a new insulin with new, inappropriate timing. The only exception would be to use NPH to slow down the action of regular insulin before a meal when dealing with gastroparesis.

MUST YOUR SKIN BE WIPED WITH ALCOHOL?

Most textbooks and instruction sheets that teach insulin injection or finger sticking advise that the skin should be "sterilized" with alcohol before puncturing with a needle. Alcohol will not sterilize your skin. At best it will clean off dirt. My patients and I have given millions of injections and finger sticks without using alcohol. None of us has become infected as a result. Certainly it's a sensible idea to clean off visible dirt first, but you can do this with simple soap and water on the rare occasions that it may be necessary. I often inject myself right through my shirt.

---

* I do not recommend Lantus for most patients.

HOW DO YOU KNOW IF YOU'VE LOST SOME INSULIN?

After I inject, I wipe my hand over the injection site, then smell my hand. If some insulin has leaked out of the site, my hand will smell of a preservative called metacresol. Whenever this occurs, I write on my GLUCOGRAF form "lost some." This will explain an elevated blood sugar later on.

DISPOSAL OF USED SYRINGES

A Cost-Free Method

I recommend the following cost-free, safe method for disposing of used syringes. Again, this is contrary to the recommendations of the ADA.

1. Recap the needle.
2. Put the capped syringe into a large plastic bottle such as that used for bleach, bottled water, seltzer, or soft drinks. Alternatively use a large coffee can.
3. When the container is full, replace the cover or cap and discourage its removal by applying duct tape.
4. Put the container into your trash* or take it to your physician, hospital, or pharmacy for pickup by the special disposal service that they might use.
5. If you are in a hotel or restaurant, don't put used syringes in the trash containers unless you first put them with the needle recapped in an opaque plastic bag, sealed with tape or knotted closed.† The cleaning people will not appreciate seeing loose syringes. In an airplane, recap the needle and put the syringe in the trash bin in the lavatory.

---

* Some communities forbid the disposal of such containers in local garbage. It is wise to contact your garbage collection department for advice. You can also visit www.safeneedledisposal.org to access a national database of local regulations in the United States.
† I save plastic grocery bags for this purpose and always pack a few empty ones when I travel.

6. Do not clip needles off your used syringes. This poses serious hazards to others and should be outlawed, even though it is promoted by the ADA.

A High-Tech Method

It's now possible to melt needles off insulin syringes. If you are especially conscientious about our environment or would enjoy using a brilliant technological device, you might try the Disintegrator Plus. This is a small device in a plastic box measuring about 6 × 3½ × 2½ inches (15.24 × 8.9 × 6.35 cm) and powered by a built-in rechargeable battery. It sells for $99 at Amazon.com.

To operate the device you merely insert the needle into a hole and press on the activating button for 3 seconds. The needle will disappear, melted into a tiny metal blob that is stored inside the instrument. You can then drop the plastic syringe into your ordinary trash container.

The stored metal blobs can be removed after a month or so by unscrewing a small screw in a hatch on the bottom and pouring them out. This may take 30 seconds.

Disintegrator Plus is distributed by Perfecta Products, Inc., of North Lima, Ohio, phone (800) 319-2225, www.perfectaproducts .com. It's fun to use and keeps needles off our beaches.

REMOVING BLOODSTAINS FROM CLOTHING

Nowadays, most of us will inject through a thin shirt when it's inconvenient to undress. This can cause a problem on the rare occasion that the needle encounters a small blood vessel. A drop of blood can appear at the puncture site and stain your clothing. Finger punctures sometimes bleed more freely than you expect, so that upon squeezing you may get a squirt in the eye, or blood on your tie, if you're not careful.

The answer to bloodstains on clothing is hydrogen peroxide solution. Hydrogen peroxide is very inexpensive and is sold in all pharmacies. Purchase several small bottles. Keep a bottle of peroxide handy at every location where you measure blood sugars. Put 2 ounces into a small brown medicine bottle when you travel. Once a bottle has been opened and closed, the solution will remain stable for perhaps six months, so you might want to have a backup bottle available.

You can make bloodstains disappear very simply without bleaching the dyes in your clothing. It's best if you treat the stain while the blood is still wet, as dried blood bleaches very slowly. If you allow the blood to dry, it may take 20 minutes of rubbing to get rid of the stain. Pour some peroxide on a handkerchief and rub it into the stain. The peroxide will foam when it contacts blood. Keep applying and rubbing until the stain has vanished.

If you don't have any peroxide handy, try milk or saliva—they work almost as well. Do not put hydrogen peroxide on wounds. It will destroy fibroblasts and thereby impede healing.

SPECIAL DEVICES FOR "PAINLESS" INJECTIONS

Many devices have been advertised with the claim that they inject insulin "without pain." Since most diabetics have not been taught the high-speed painless injection technique described in this chapter, many of these special, spring-driven devices are sold every year. I found that they add to the "pain" by slowing the insulin delivery. If your injections are already painless, it makes little sense to use them.

Other "painless" devices, called jet injectors, use very precise construction to inject a high-pressure jet of insulin, penetrating the skin without a needle. These injectors do not require a separate syringe since they must be loaded directly with insulin, using special adapters that plug into the insulin vial. Although the concept is very enticing, spray injectors pose some problems. First, they're very expensive, costing from $300 to $600 in the United States. Although this is a substantial initial investment, the cost can be recovered over the course of a year or two if you're discarding lots of disposable syringes.

They're not as convenient as disposable syringes because they must be taken apart and sterilized in boiling, deionized water every one to two weeks. Also, the adapters for the insulin vials sometimes leak when the vials are carried in a purse or bag.

You will require considerable training and experimentation with pressure settings in order to give yourself a proper jet injection. This can delay getting your blood sugars normalized. You will likely experience *slightly more pain* than you would with a speedily injected shot from a conventional syringe, and there's a high incidence of black-and-blue marks on the skin, minor bleeding, and even loss of small amounts of insulin at the puncture sites.

Despite these drawbacks, jet injectors do have two unique advantages, aside from reducing the number of syringes you must dispose of. First is that you will require about one-third less insulin, since the shots are better absorbed. Second, if you use rapid-acting insulin to lower elevated blood sugars, it will work even faster. But not faster than an intramuscular injection (see page 324). Finally, jet injectors should not be used for longer-acting insulins.

My conclusion: don't use jet injectors.

INSULIN PENS

Several manufacturers are advertising "insulin pens." These are syringes into which small cartridges of insulin can be loaded. They are intended to relieve you of the burden of carrying a vial of insulin if you have to inject away from home. None of those marketed as of this writing can be set at estimated quarter-unit increments, and only one of those sold in the United States can be set at half-unit increments. Most therefore cannot provide the fine-tuning of blood sugars that our regimens require. Stay away from them unless you are very obese and require large doses of insulin. With large doses, an error of ½ or ¼ unit is insignificant.

The cartridges used for insulin pens are less than one-third the size of standard insulin vials and are consequently more convenient to carry in a pocket or purse. To remove the cartridge from a pen, merely remove the plastic cover first. You can puncture the cap with the needle of a standard insulin syringe and slowly draw out insulin. ***Do not*** inject air or reinject insulin into these cartridges.

Pens used for the incretin mimetics Byetta and Victoza (see Chapter 13) do not pose the problems found with insulin pens.

I will personally answer questions from readers for
one hour every month. This free service is available by
visiting www.askdrbernstein.net.

17

Important Information About Various Insulins

If you start using insulin, you ought to understand how its effects can be controlled. It can do some remarkable things, but it must be handled with respect and knowledge. Much of the information in this chapter is based upon my experience with my own insulin needs and with those of my patients. As in much of this book, you will likely note that some statements contradict traditional teachings and manufacturers' literature.

FOR ROUTINE USE, AVOID INSULINS THAT CONTAIN PROTAMINE

There are a confusing number of brands and types of insulins being marketed today—and even more are on the way. Insulins may be categorized by how long they continue to affect blood sugars after injection. There are most-rapid-acting, rapid-acting, intermediate-acting, and long-acting insulins. Until recently, the rapid-acting insulins appeared clear, like water, and the other insulins appeared cloudy. The cloudiness is caused by an additive that combines with the insulin to form particles that slowly dissolve under the skin. The one remaining intermediate-acting insulin, called NPH, is modified with an animal protein called protamine. Insulins that contain protamine may stimulate the immune system to make antibodies to insulin. These antibodies can temporarily bind to some of the insulin, rendering it inactive. Then, unpredictably, they can release the insulin at a time when it's not necessarily needed. This effect, although small, impairs the meticulous control of blood sugars that we seek. Protamine can present another, more serious problem if you ever require coronary angiography for the study of arteries that feed your heart (a common procedure nowadays). Just before such a study, you would be given an injection of the anticoagulant heparin to prevent the formation of blood clots. When the procedure is over, protamine is injected into a blood vessel to "turn off" the heparin. This can cause severe allergic reactions, even death, in a small percentage of people who have previously been treated with insulin containing protamine. Thus, even if an insulin is marketed as a "human" insulin, its effects upon antibody production may be significant if it contains the animal protein protamine.

As you may guess, I strongly oppose the frivolous use of insulins containing protamine. In the United States, the only insulin containing protamine is NPH (called isophane overseas). NPH or mixtures of NPH and other insulins are widely available and should be avoided. People who require very small doses of insulin, such as children, may be best treated with diluted insulin (see page 287) for accurate dose measurement. Unfortunately, there is no diluting fluid made for either of our two remaining long-acting insulins.* I therefore am now obliged to prescribe three or more daily doses of diluted NPH for small children. I also use small amounts of NPH mixed with regular before meals for some patients with gastroparesis (see Chapter 22).

A list of the insulins that I consider possibly suitable appears on page 284.

STRENGTHS OF INSULINS

The biological activity of insulin is measured in units. At small doses, 2 units of insulin should lower blood sugar exactly twice as much as 1 unit. An insulin syringe is therefore graduated in units, and the one shown in Figure 16-4 is also calibrated in half-units. The lines are far enough apart so that even ¼ unit can be reasonably estimated if you

---

* My favorite long- and intermediate-acting insulins, ultralente and lente, were taken off the market in 2006 because they were less profitable to the manufacturers. Diluting fluids were available for these insulins. Although the American Diabetes Association made no protest when these discontinuations were announced, there has been an uproar over this intrusion upon patient care in the U.K.

have good eyesight or use a magnifier. The syringe we recommend is designed for a concentration of 100 units per cc, and can dispense up to ³⁄₁₀ cc, or 30 units. The insulin's strength is designated U-100, meaning "100 units per cc." In the United States and Canada, this is the only insulin concentration sold, so you need not specify the strength when you purchase insulin. Other strengths, such as U-40 and U-80, are sold in other countries, and the scales on the syringes in these countries are designed for those strengths. A special strength for regular insulin, U-500, is available to physicians in the United States, upon request from the manufacturers, for special applications. The syringes for U-40 and U-80 strengths are not sold in the United States.

If you travel overseas and happen to lose or misplace your insulin, you may be unable to secure the U-100 strength locally. You can make the best of this by purchasing U-40 or U-80 insulin, together with U-40 or U-80 syringes. You should draw your usual doses in units into the new syringes with the new insulin.

CARING FOR YOUR INSULIN

Insulin is stable until the expiration date printed on the label, if refrigerated. A slight loss of potency may occur if insulin is stored at room temperature longer than 30–60 days. This is especially true of Lantus (glargine) insulin, which may lose a significant amount of potency 30 days after you remove the first dose, even if it's stored in the refrigerator.* Levemir (detemir) insulin also has a limited shelf life, about twice that of Lantus. Regular, NPH, Humalog, and Novolog insulins can usually be safely stored at room temperature for up to a year. I'm not sure about Apidra insulin.

Insulin can become partially deactivated with or without a change in its appearance, leading to unexpectedly elevated blood sugars. When I receive a distress call from a patient who has had higher than usual blood sugars for several days, I ask a number of questions in order to determine the source of the blood sugar elevation. Have there been dietary indiscretions? Is there a possible infection? Or might the insulin be somewhat deactivated, perhaps by reuse of syringes (see

---

* For this reason and because studies have found it to be associated with increased cancer incidence, I do not recommend Lantus.

page 272)? Even slight cloudiness of a clear insulin is a certain sign of deactivation. So is the appearance of visible clumps within, or a gray precipitate on the wall of, a vial of NPH insulin (normally cloudy) that will not disappear when it's shaken. Deactivation of insulin, however, may not be possible to distinguish simply by looking. If diet or infection seems unlikely to be the source of the blood sugar elevation, I advise my patient to discard all insulin currently in use and to utilize fresh vials, even if the insulin looks okay.

Here are some simple rules for routine care of your insulin:

- Keep unused insulin in the refrigerator until you are ready to use it for the first time. Vials in current use may be kept at room temperature for convenience, but Lantus, Levemir, and Apidra (glulisine) are best stored in the refrigerator.
- Never allow insulin to freeze. Even after it thaws out, it may no longer possess its full strength. If you suspect it may have frozen, discard it.
- If your home reaches temperatures above 85°F (29°C), refrigerate all your insulin when not in use. If your insulin has been exposed to temperatures in excess of 99°F (37°C) for more than 1 day, discard it.
- Do not reuse your insulin syringes unless you follow the procedure beginning on page 272.
- Do not put insulin in prolonged sunlight or in closed, unattended motor vehicles, glove compartments, or car trunks. These areas can become overheated on a sunny day, even in winter. If you inadvertently leave insulin in a hot vehicle, discard it. This rule also applies to blood sugar test strips and to meters if the screen darkens.
- Do not routinely keep insulin close to your body, as in shirt pockets.
- When you invert your insulin vial to fill your syringe, observe the level of insulin. When the level drops below the lower edge of the label on the inverted vial, discard the vial. This is especially necessary with normally cloudy insulin (NPH) because the concentration of active particles may change as you use it up.
- If you plan to travel to an area with a warm climate where you may not be able to refrigerate your insulin, consider a product called Frio, mentioned on page 77. This is a small fabric wallet with pellets sewn into the lining. It's available in five sizes in the United Kingdom and two in the United States. When the wallet is

soaked in water for 20 minutes, the pellets will form a gel. As the water in the gel slowly evaporates through the pores of the wallet, it will keep insulin at a safe temperature without recharging for at least 48 hours at a surrounding air temperature of 100°F (38°C).

HOW INSULIN AFFECTS YOUR BLOOD SUGARS OVER TIME

It's important for you to know when your insulin will begin to affect your blood sugar and when it will finish working. This information is printed on the insert in the insulin package. The published information, however, may be inaccurate for patients on our regimen. The reason for this is that we use very small doses of insulin, while most published data are based upon much larger doses. As a rule, larger nonphysiologic doses tend to start working sooner and finish working later than smaller doses. Furthermore, the action time of an insulin will vary somewhat from one person to another and from smaller to larger doses. Nevertheless, Table 17-1 is a reasonable guide to the approximate starting and finishing times of the insulins we recommend when used in physiologic (as opposed to the usual industrial) doses. *Your response may not follow a typical pattern,* but at least this table can serve as a starting point.

Insulin action will be speeded considerably if you exercise the region of your body into which you inject. As a consequence, it may be, for example, unwise to inject long-acting insulin into your arm on a day that you lift weights or into your abdomen on a day that you do sit-ups.

A NOTE ABOUT MIXING INSULINS

In a word, don't.

Two different insulins should never be mixed — with the single exception of the specific situation discussed on pages 397–398. Other than that, mixing of insulins has no useful purpose, even though it is advocated by the ADA and even though you can purchase mixtures that are marketed by pharmaceutical companies. Mixing a long-acting insulin with a rapid-acting one results in an insulin that no longer has either the long- or rapid-acting properties.

TABLE 17-1

APPROXIMATE ACTION TIMES OF PREFERRED INSULINS*

U.S. brand name	Abbreviation	Generic name of insulin	Speed of action	Action time after injection†	
				Action starts	Action ends
Humalog‡	H	Lispro	Most rapid	10 minutes	6–8 hours (but assume 5 hours)
Novolog	NO	Aspart	Second most rapid	15 minutes	6–8 hours (but assume 5 hours)
Apidra	AP	Glulisine	Second most rapid	15 minutes	6–8 hours (but assume 5 hours)
regular insulin Novolin R‡	R	Regular (crystalline outside U.S.)	Rapid	40–45 minutes	8–10 hours or more (but assume 5 hours)
regular insulin Novolin N‡**	N	NPH (isophane outside U.S.) (?) (cloudy)	Inter-mediate	1½–3 hours	12 hours if injected in the morning; 4–6 hours if injected at bedtime (apparent)
Levemir	L	Detemir	Long	Slowly over 4 hours	18 hours if injected in the morning; 6 hours if injected at bedtime (apparent)

* These times will vary from one person to another and even from one time of day to another.

† Doses exceeding 7 units will usually start sooner, last longer, and act less predictably than smaller doses. See page 321.

‡ Can be diluted for use by children (see page 287).

** Doses of NPH that exceed 7 units may have a peak of action at about 8 hours after injection.

ABBREVIATED DESIGNATIONS FOR THE VARIOUS INSULINS

When you're filling in the information on your GLUCOGRAF data sheets, it will be more convenient for you and your doctor if you use the abbreviated designations shown in the "Abbreviation" column of Table 17-1—NO, H, AP, R, N, or L—instead of the full names. Since it's implied, you also needn't write out the word "units" when noting insulin doses. Seven units of regular insulin would abbreviate as "7 R," and so on. If you forget these abbreviations, make up your own.

ARE THE PREFERRED INSULINS EQUALLY POTENT?

If we ignore the differences in timing, 1 unit of each of these insulins will have the same effect upon blood sugar as 1 unit of any of the others, with the striking exception of Humalog (H), Novolog (NO), and Apidra (AP). NO and AP insulins are about 50 percent more potent than regular (R), the only remaining rapid-acting, true human insulin. Humalog is about two and a half times as potent as regular. This information is extremely important, but has not been disclosed by the reigning powers.

DO YOU NEED A PRESCRIPTION FOR INSULIN?

Yes and no. In the United States, Humalog, Novolog, and Levemir require a prescription from your doctor. NPH and regular may be purchased without a prescription in most states. Local regulations are subject to change. For insurance coverage, you will need a prescription for all insulins.

WHY DO WE USE THE LONGER-ACTING INSULINS?

Levemir, our preferred longer-acting insulin, serves a purpose different from that of the rapid-acting insulins. Indeed, for our regimens it has but one principal task—to keep blood sugar from rising while fasting (see the discussions of gluconeogenesis and the dawn phenomenon on page 96). It is our basal insulin. It is not intended to prevent the blood sugar rise after eating. Furthermore, it is not used to lower a blood sugar that is too high—it works too slowly for that. A secondary purpose of longer-acting insulins in mild type 2 diabetes is to help delay or prevent beta cell burnout. As you'll see later, we may use a rapid-acting insulin to cover meals, whether or not the longer-acting insulin is used to cover the fasting state. Which insulin to use, and when, depends upon blood sugar profiles.

WHY I NO LONGER USE LANTUS INSULIN

The package insert for Lantus insulin warns that it may lose potency 30 days after the stopper of the vial has been punctured, even if it is stored in the refrigerator. One would have to inject at least 30 units of this insulin daily in order for this to make sense economically, if we consider that there is another long-acting insulin, Levemir, that lasts twice as long.

Some years ago, an internationally renowned diabetologist, Dr. Ernst Chantelau, pointed out the scientific likelihood that Lantus could cause a higher incidence of cancer than other insulins. The evidence lay in the high affinity of Lantus for the growth hormone (IGF-1) receptors on the surface of cancer cells. Several diabetologists were interviewed by the media, but I was the only one who supported Chantelau's theory. After receiving a confirmatory scientific study from Germany, the European Association for the Study of Diabetes contracted with investigators in Sweden, Scotland, and the U.K. to review the excellent records of insulin use and cancer occurrence kept by these nations. All but the U.K. study supported the German results.

Why use an insulin that has even a very small risk of promoting cancer when an equally good and less costly one already exists?

WHEN DO WE USE RAPID-ACTING INSULIN?

If you're a type 1 diabetic—or a type 2 diabetic who is following our diet and using oral medication and still experiencing blood sugar increases after one or more meals—injecting regular (R), Humalog

(H), Apidra (AP), or Novolog (NO) insulin prior to these meals is indicated. By sheer coincidence, the 5-hour (assumed) action time of regular corresponds approximately to the time most of us require to digest fully a mixed meal of protein and carbohydrate, and to experience the final effect of the meal upon blood sugars. Regular insulin should usually be injected 45 minutes before a meal, so that it starts to work just as we start to eat. This timing may vary from one meal to another or for different individuals.

The beta cells of some type 2s, however, may enjoy enough of a rest from one or two small doses of Levemir that they can produce sufficient insulin to cover meals. Since everyone is different, your insulin regimen must be custom-tailored to normalize your personal glucose profile. All this takes more effort on the part of your physician than just the prescription of one or two daily shots of a long-acting insulin.

Because of their very rapid action, Humalog, Novolog, and Apidra are also the insulins that we frequently use to lower high blood sugars. Since elevated blood sugars are the cause of the long-term complications of diabetes, we naturally want to see them come down to normal as fast as possible. In Chapter 19, "Intensive Insulin Regimens," we will teach you how to rapidly get high blood sugars down to your target, using one of the rapid-acting insulins. If your doctor finds that your blood sugars are rarely elevated or appear to rapidly drop down on their own, then it may not be necessary to use additional insulin for this purpose.

DILUTING INSULIN

Many type 2 diabetics, mild type 1 diabetics, and small children with type 1 diabetes require such small doses of injected insulin that dosage cannot be measured accurately enough with any of the syringes currently on the market. For such people, 1 unit might lower blood sugar by more than 300 mg/dl (versus only 10 mg/dl for a very obese type 1 or a very obese insulin-requiring type 2 adult). A measurement error of ¼ unit would therefore be equivalent to more than 75 mg/dl for a small child. To solve this problem we dilute the insulin. This is very easy. Your physician or pharmacist can secure, at no charge, empty sterile insulin vials from some insulin makers (e.g., Eli Lilly and Company and Novo Nordisk). The manufacturers will also provide, at no cost, the appropriate diluting fluids for some of the insulins you use. As of this writing, there is no diluting fluid for Apidra. This can be circumvented by switching to the equipotent Novolog (NO), for which a diluent is readily available. Since there is no diluent for Levemir, the best we can do is to dilute NPH. Because NPH is only intermediate-acting (not long-acting), some small children may have to get up to six shots per day.

If your pharmacist is unwilling to perform the dilution for you, either find a pharmacy with a compounding chemist or do it yourself as follows:

1. Have clear instructions from your physician as to how much insulin and how much diluting fluid should be put into a vial. If your doctor writes "dilute 2:1" (say "two to one"), this means 2 parts of diluent, or diluting fluid, for every 1 of insulin, and so on. He may want to give you a few sterile 3 cc syringes* for this purpose. They will contain about ten times as much as the 25- or 30-unit syringe you use for injections. Using the larger syringe will speed up the preparation of your vials.

2. Each vial can hold only 10 cc of fluid. You should write down how many cc of diluting fluid and insulin you will need, remembering that the sum of the two cannot exceed 10 cc. Thus, if your doctor tells you to dilute your insulin 3:1, you might use 6 cc of diluent and 2 cc of insulin.

3. All diluting fluids should be crystal clear, like water. Make sure that the label of the diluting fluid you are using specifies that it is for the insulin you want to dilute.† There is no diluting fluid for Levemir.

4. Pierce the empty vial with the needle of your 3 cc syringe. Draw out air to the dose of diluent you wish to transfer (1, 2, or 3 cc, et cetera).

5. Move the needle and syringe to the diluting fluid vial and inject the air. Invert the syringe and vial and hold vertically while you slowly withdraw the predetermined amount of fluid. Keep the tip of the needle near the stopper of the vial to avoid drawing in air. Be sure to expel any bubbles in the syringe.

---

* They should be supplied with relatively wide-bore (21–23 gauge) needles.
† Eli Lilly and Company provides diluting fluid for Humalog, regular, and NPH insulins, but Novo Nordisk supplies diluents only for Novolog insulin.

6. Inject the diluent into the empty vial from which you took the air, and withdraw more air if you will be delivering more fluid.

7. Repeat steps 4, 5, and 6 until the amount of diluent that you had written down is in the originally empty vial.

8. Draw another 1, 2, or 3 cc of air (depending upon how much insulin you will be transferring) from the vial you've been filling with diluent, but this time inject the air into the insulin vial. Invert the syringe and vial and, holding vertically, draw out the predetermined amount of insulin. Keep the tip of the needle near the stopper of the vial to avoid drawing in air. (If you're working with NPH [cloudy] insulin, remember to shake the insulin vial vigorously 6–10 times immediately before withdrawing the insulin; see Figure 16-6, page 271.)

9. Inject the insulin into the vial to which the diluent had been added.

10. Repeat steps 8 and 9 until the designated amount of insulin has been added to the diluent.

11. Using a permanent-ink felt-tip marker, label the newly diluted insulin vial with the expiration date that appears on the insulin vial, the type of insulin (use the designation ND, HD, LD, NOD, or RD to indicate that the insulin has been diluted), and the ratio of diluent to insulin used (2:1, 3:2, 4:1, or whatever it happens to be). Cover your writing with clear tape to prevent it from rubbing off.

12. Put the vial of diluted insulin in the refrigerator for storage until its first use.

I've seen many people, including doctors, nurses, and pharmacists, become confused about how much diluted insulin to inject. With that in mind, we will run through a couple of examples to show you how simply this can be computed.

Example 1. Your doctor wants you to inject 2¼ units of insulin, but yours has been diluted 1:1. For every 2 parts of liquid in the syringe, only 1 part, or half, is insulin. To get 2¼ real units of insulin, you will have to inject twice as many diluted units ($2 \times 2\frac{1}{4} = 4\frac{1}{2}$) as they're measured on the scale of the syringe—which is easier to estimate, especially with the new syringes that are calibrated every ½ unit.

Example 2. Your doctor wants you to inject 1¼ units of insulin, but yours has been diluted 4:1. This time, for every 5 parts of liquid only

1 part is insulin, so we must multiply real units by 5 to set our dose: $5 \times 1\frac{1}{4} = 5\frac{5}{4} = 6\frac{1}{4}$ units on the syringe.

I don't really expect my patients to compute the diluted units they must take. In the case of the second example, I would ask you to take 6¼ diluted units. If this were Humalog insulin, I'd write "6⁺ HD" on your data sheets in the usual doses box at the top of the form.*

HUMALOG, NOVOLOG, AND APIDRA: NEW MOST-RAPID-ACTING INSULINS

These three insulins were developed by three different manufacturers to overcome regular insulin's inability to rapidly cover fast-acting dietary carbohydrates. They cannot, however, circumvent the Laws of Small Numbers relating to large amounts of dietary carbohydrate. Since fast-acting carbohydrate foods (bread, pasta, fruit, and so on) usually contain large amounts of carbohydrate, the hazards of using such foods and covering them with large amounts of insulin will still exist. Furthermore, these foods will still raise blood sugar faster than the new insulins can lower it for people with normal digestion.

There are some applications of these insulins that the manufacturers may not have considered. For instance, if it is inconvenient to take regular insulin 40–45 minutes before a meal, you can take one of the above insulins 15–20 minutes before the meal. They should be fast enough to cover small amounts of slow-acting carbohydrate without the 40–45 minute delay. This can be very valuable when you eat out, as you will learn in Chapter 19. Also, insulin users who previously used regular insulin to lower an elevated blood sugar will benefit by using a most-rapid-acting insulin. They will get blood sugar down more rapidly. This, too, will be discussed in Chapter 19. *Note that studies show Humalog to act somewhat more rapidly than Novolog or Apidra.*

The use of the most-rapid-acting insulins is complicated further by the fact that for most of us, they are more potent than regular insulin. For example, 1 unit of Humalog will lower my blood sugar

---

* Note that we use the symbols ⁺ and ⁻ to indicate that a dose is just above or just below the nearest whole unit on a syringe scale. So 1⁻ means ¾ unit and 3⁺ means 3¼ units.

2½ times as much as 1 unit of regular; 1 unit of Novolog or Apidra will lower it 1½ times much as regular.

NONINJECTABLE INSULINS

Although several insulins that do not require injection may come on the market, none are of use for the precise control of blood sugars that we seek.

I will personally answer questions from readers for one hour every month. This free service is available by visiting www.askdrbernstein.net.

18

Simple Insulin Regimens

This chapter and the next describe a number of specific insulin regimens. As you read, please refer back to Table 17-1 (page 284) for descriptions of the various insulins and their speed of action—for instance, our long-acting insulin will be Levemir.

The particular regimen that suits you will depend to a considerable degree upon your blood sugar profiles. Your physician must decide whether you need long-acting insulin to cover the fasting state, short-acting insulin to cover meals, or both. In either event, she will require blood sugar profiles and related data, covering as many days as she designates, prior to every office visit or telephone call for fine-tuning of doses. Remember that "related data" includes the times of meals, whether you overate or underate, the times of exercise (including seemingly inconsequential activity such as shopping), the times and doses of blood sugar medications, infections or illnesses you may have had, when and how many glucose tablets you took to correct a low blood sugar—in short, anything that might have affected your blood sugar. Bedtime blood sugar readings are especially important information, because an increase or decrease overnight should most certainly affect the determination of your bedtime dosage of longer-acting insulin.

To give you some examples of how we might use insulin to bring your blood sugar levels into target range, let's consider the following blood sugar profile scenarios.

SCENARIO ONE: FASTING BLOOD SUGARS ARE HIGHER THAN BEDTIME BLOOD SUGARS

Let's say you're taking the highest useful dosage of an insulin-sensitizing agent (ISA) at bedtime. Your fasting (i.e., before-breakfast, empty-stomach) blood sugars are still consistently higher than your bedtime blood sugars. Because of this, you probably require long-acting insulin at bedtime. Before we'd start you on insulin, however, we'd examine your data sheet carefully in order to make certain that you finished your last meal of each day *at least* 5 hours prior to your bedtime blood sugar measurement. No one should be given a long-acting insulin to cover an overnight blood sugar increase *caused by a meal* unless delayed stomach-emptying (see Chapter 22) is present.

For people who customarily sleep 8 hours or longer, we usually start with long-acting Levemir at bedtime. Because of the dawn phenomenon (see page 97), a result of rapid removal of insulin from the bloodstream by the liver near the time of arising in the morning, it's wise to take this dose no more than 8½ hours before the morning dose. The bedtime insulin will usually appear to have lost much of its action 9 hours after the injection but will start working again after about 3 hours—when the dawn phenomenon ceases.

For type 1 diabetics and for some type 2s, Levemir does not usually last the entire night, despite claims to that effect by the manufacturer. This is also true of Lantus, the "long-acting" insulin that I don't recommend. If a bedtime injection of Levemir lasts the entire night, it may be because the dose you injected is so large that blood sugar drops too low in the middle of the night. It is therefore wise to set an alarm for 4 hours after the bedtime dose to make sure your blood sugar is not more than 10 mg/dl below your target. If it is, you will have to split your bedtime dose into two doses, each slightly less than half the initial dose, one taken at bedtime and the other 4 hours later. This inconvenience was not necessary with the old ultralente insulin that was discontinued by Eli Lilly and Company because it was considered to be unprofitable. This is just another reason why I believe diabetes is generally treated as an orphan disease, where profit is more important than the patient.

294   *Treatment*

Estimating the Dose

Your physician may want to use this simple method for estimating your starting bedtime insulin dose. Generally, 1 unit of regular, NPH, or long-acting insulin* lowers blood sugar 40 mg/dl for a 140-pound, nonpregnant adult whose pancreas produces no insulin. Since your beta cells may still be producing some insulin, we'd abide by the Laws of Small Numbers and cautiously assume initially that 1 unit of regular, NPH, or Levemir would, over a period of hours, lower your blood sugar 80 mg/dl, just so we wouldn't bring it dangerously low and risk hypoglycemia.

We would then proceed as follows.

First, we'd look at your blood sugar profiles. The first number we want is the minimum overnight blood sugar increase over the past week. For each night, we'd subtract your bedtime blood sugar from your fasting blood sugar for the following day, then use the difference for the night with the lowest rise. For this calculation, bedtime must be *at least* 5 hours after finishing supper. For small children, we accomplish this by asking parents to get a painless "tushy stick" while the child is sleeping.

The second number we'd want is the maximum amount that we'd expect 1 unit of long- or intermediate-acting insulin to lower your overnight blood sugar. To get this number, we'd take the maximum anticipated blood sugar drop from 1 unit. Since our initial conservative rule of thumb is that 1 unit of Levemir or NPH will lower a 140-pound type 2's blood sugar by 80 mg/dl, we would divide 140 by your weight in pounds and then multiply the result by 80 mg/dl. If your weight is 200 pounds, the equation would look like this: $(140 \div 200) \times 80 = 56$. So your initial estimated blood sugar drop will be 56 mg/dl from 1 unit.

Let us assume, for example, that your lowest overnight blood sugar rise in the past week was 73 mg/dl. We'd take 73 mg/dl and divide it by the number you derived from the above equation, or 56. Your trial

---

* Novolog and Apidra are about 1½ times as potent as the other insulins. Humalog is about 2½ times as potent. For the three other insulins I recommend (regular, Levemir, and NPH), as noted in the previous chapter, except for the speed with which each insulin acts, 1 unit of one insulin is equivalent to 1 unit of any of the others.

bedtime dose of Levemir would be 73 ÷ 56 = 1.3 units. This is your starting bedtime dose. Rounding off the dose to the nearest ¼ unit gives you 1¼ units, which you can abbreviate on your data sheet as 1⁺ L, or just over 1 unit.

Fine-Tuning the Dose

That was pretty easy, but it was only a starting point. Most probably this dose won't be perfect—likely too low or possibly even a little too high. To fine-tune the bedtime insulin, you merely record bedtime and fasting blood sugars for the first few days after starting the insulin. If the minimum overnight blood sugar rise was less than 10 mg/dl, you've likely hit the proper dose on the first try. If the rise was greater, your physician may want you to increase the bedtime dose by as little as ¼ unit every third night, until the minimum overnight rise is less than 10 mg/dl.*

Even one overnight hypoglycemic episode can be quite frightening, especially if you live alone. Such an event can easily turn you off to insulin therapy, so it's wise to take some simple precautions to ensure it doesn't happen. On the night that you take your first shot (and on the first night of any increase in dosage), set your alarm clock to ring 6 hours after your bedtime injection. When the alarm sounds, measure your blood sugar, and correct it to your target value if it's too low (see Chapter 20, "How to Prevent and Correct Low Blood Sugars"). Even one low blood sugar event suggests that the bedtime dose should be reduced.

With the possible exception of growing teenagers, people with infections or delayed stomach-emptying, and the obese, most of us usually require less than 8 units of Levemir at bedtime.

Levemir in doses greater than 7 units, in addition to creating a lower blood sugar, tends to last longer. This may be responsible for blood sugars that are too low in the late morning, or even in the afternoon. There are at least two ways to prevent this. First, you can split the insulin into two or more approximately equal doses. These should be injected at bedtime, but into different sites. If your required dose is 9 units, you might inject 4 units into your arm and the other 5 into your abdomen. You may recall that large doses are not absorbed with consistent timing or total action, so two or more smaller injections

_____

* I have some patients whose blood sugars are so easy to control that we shoot for zero blood sugar change throughout the day.

have the advantage of making the absorption of both doses more pre-dictable. The same syringe can be used for the second, third, and so on.

The most effective way to generate level blood sugars throughout the night was suggested by Pat Gian, the woman who runs my office: split the bedtime Levemir into two approximately equal shots, one taken at bedtime and the other taken 4 hours later.

SCENARIO TWO: BLOOD SUGAR RISES DURING THE DAY, EVEN IF MEALS ARE SKIPPED

If your blood sugar rises during the day even though you're taking the maximum dose of one or more ISAs to cover meals, it's time for you and your physician to perform another experiment.

This time you want to determine whether meals have caused your increase or whether blood sugar has increased independently. It's very unusual, by the way, for fasting blood sugars to rise during the day if you don't require insulin at bedtime, usually to compensate for the dawn phenomenon (which, as we've said, is the tendency in many dia-betics for blood sugars to go up overnight, and perhaps for up to 3 hours after arising). In order to determine when and how much your blood sugar is rising during the day:

- Start your day with a blood sugar measurement.
- If you're taking an ISA in the morning, continue with your present dose.
- Check blood sugar again 1 hour after arising.
- Do not eat breakfast or lunch, but plan on supper — at least 12 hours after this second morning blood sugar measurement.
- During the day, continue to check blood sugars approximately every 4 hours, and certainly 12 hours after the second morning test.
- If, even with a maximum dose of your ISA, your blood sugar rises more than 10 mg/dl during the 12-hour period — without any drops along the way — you probably should be taking a long-acting (that is, basal) insulin when you arise in the morning.*

---

* See page 300 for our introduction to the concepts of basal and bolus insulin dosing.

This dose of basal insulin is calculated the same way we calculated the bedtime dose in the first scenario. Because fasting twice in one week is unpleasant, we may try to wait another week before performing this experiment again to see if our basal dose is adequate. Further experiments in subsequent weeks may be necessary for fine-tuning of this insulin dose.

MONITORING YOUR INSULIN REGIMEN

Once you take insulin, it is essential that you and your family be familiar with the prevention of hypoglycemia (low blood sugar). To this end, you and those who live or work with you should read Chapter 20, "How to Prevent and Correct Low Blood Sugars."

If you are taking only longer-acting insulin as described in this chapter and are strictly following our dietary guidelines, it might not be necessary to measure blood sugar every day for life. Nevertheless, it's wise to assign one day every week or two for measuring blood sugar on arising, right before and 2 hours after meals, and at bedtime, just to make sure that your insulin requirements are not increasing or decreasing. If any of your blood sugars are consistently 10 mg/dl above or below your target, advise your physician.*

It's essential that you also measure blood sugar before and after exercising. If, in your experience, your blood sugar continues to drop one or more hours after finishing your exercise, you should check your blood sugar hourly until it levels off.†

As you shall read in Chapter 21, "How to Cope with Dehydration, Dehydrating Illness, and Infection," it is important whenever you suffer such an illness to secure daily blood sugar profiles and report them to your physician.

Many patients and physicians routinely increase the basal morning dose if before-breakfast blood sugars are repeatedly elevated. This is the wrong dose to change. It's the bedtime dose that controls fasting blood sugar, and therefore that dose should be adjusted accordingly.

---

* See page 316 if you've forgotten how we arrive at a blood sugar target.
† Insulin users must always check blood sugar before they drive and hourly while driving. Ditto for operating potentially dangerous machines. Scuba divers should probably check blood sugars after every 20 minutes of diving.

After fine-tuning of bedtime and, if necessary, morning doses of long-acting insulin, your pancreatic beta cells may recover enough function eventually to prevent a blood sugar rise after meals. This frequently turns out to be the case for mild type 2 diabetics. If, however, you still routinely experience a blood sugar rise of more than 10 mg/dl at any time after any meal, you'll probably require premeal injections of a rapid-acting insulin, as described in the next chapter.

OTHER CONSIDERATIONS

Weather-Related Changes in Insulin Requirements

Some people experience a sudden decline in their insulin requirements when a long period of cool weather (e.g., winter) is abruptly interrupted by significantly warmer weather. This phenomenon can be recognized by blood sugar well below target when the weather suddenly becomes warmer. In such individuals, insulin requirements will rise in the winter and drop in the summer.* The reason for this effect is speculative, but may relate to the increased dilation of peripheral blood vessels during warm weather and the resultant increased delivery of blood, glucose, and insulin to peripheral tissues. Whatever the cause, keep careful track of your blood sugar whenever the weather warms suddenly, since potentially severe hypoglycemia can result if insulin dosages are not adjusted.

Air Travel Across Time Zones

Long-distance travel that requires you to shift your clock by 2 hours or less shouldn't have a major effect upon your dosing of ISAs or basal insulins covering the fasting state. It should certainly have no effect upon the use of rapid-acting insulin or insulin-sensitizing agents intended to cover meals. A problem does arise when travel shifts the time frame by 3 or more hours and you're taking different doses of long-acting medication in the morning and at bedtime. The situation becomes particularly complex if you travel halfway around the world, so that day and night are reversed.

---

* Some diabetics who also have the disease lupus erythematosus may experience just the opposite — lower insulin requirements in cold weather and higher requirements in warm weather.

When the time shift amounts to 2 hours or less, you need only take your morning medication upon arising in the morning and your bed-time medication at bedtime. One solution to handling larger time shifts is to effect a gradual transition, using 3-hour intervals over a period of days. To do this, you must keep track of the time "back home." If, for example, you're traveling east, so that the time back home is earlier, on your first day away you would take both of your basal doses 3 hours later on the "back home" clock. On the second day, you would take them 6 hours later, and so on. Thus, if your new location to the east of home is in a time zone 6 hours later than it was at home, it would take you 2 days to achieve a full transition. You would do just the opposite when traveling west. This procedure can be inconvenient because it requires that you set an alarm clock for absurd hours just to take an insulin shot or a pill—and then, you hope, go back to sleep.

Several of my patients routinely save themselves this kind of annoy-ance when they travel. At their destinations, they continue to take their morning dose when they arise in the morning and their bedtime dose when they go to bed. They check their blood sugars every 2 hours while awake and lower them, if too high, using the method described in Chap-ter 19, "Intensive Insulin Regimens." If their blood sugars drop too low, they raise them using the method described in Chapter 20. Frankly, this is the approach I use myself. Neither I nor my patients have gotten into trouble this way. This carefree approach can cause problems if the bed-time dose is considerably different from the morning dose. If this is the case, the gradual transition of 3 hours per day is certainly safer.

Splitting Larger Doses of Insulin

My patients and I have observed that as larger doses of insulin are injected, the effects upon blood sugar become less predictable. This is due in part to day-to-day variations in absorption of large injections. After some trial and error, I arrived at a cutoff point of 7 units as the largest single injection I would want an adult to take (smaller for chil-dren). Therefore, if an insulin-resistant patient requires 20 units of Levemir at bedtime, I ask him to take 3 separate injections in 3 sepa-rate sites of 7 units, 7 units, and 6 units, all using the same syringe.

I will personally answer questions from readers for one hour every month. This free service is available by visiting www.askdrbernstein.net.

19

Intensive Insulin Regimens

A ll type 1 diabetics but the mildest should be treated with rapid-acting insulin before meals as well as long-acting insulin in the morning and at bedtime to cover the fasting state. This roughly mimics the way that a nondiabetic's body releases insulin to maintain normal blood sugars. Generally, the nondiabetic body when fasting has a constant, relatively low level of insulin in the bloodstream. This is the baseline, or *basal*, insulin level to prevent gluconeogenesis, the conversion of protein stores (muscles, vital organs) into glucose. Without it, they would "melt into sugar water," as the ancients observed when diabetes was first described in writing.

During the fasting state (sleeping, between meals), the pancreas stores the insulin it creates in preparation for the next time the body is exposed to food, while maintaining the low basal release rate. Upon eating and for the first 5 or so hours thereafter, the body receives what's known as a *bolus* of insulin—a greater rate of release—until the glucose derived from meals is stored in the tissues (see Figure 1-2, page 47). As you may recall from Chapter 6, "Strange Biology," the body has counterregulatory hormones that keep blood sugar from dropping too low so that one doesn't become hypoglycemic. So for those of us who make little or no insulin, essentially what we're trying to do with long- and rapid-acting insulins is to create a rough approximation of a steady basal rate and an appropriate bolus rate.

If you are a type 2 diabetic and preprandial (before-meal) use of ISAs does not prevent your blood sugars from routinely increasing by more than 10 mg/dl at any time prior to the next meal, it's probably time for you to use a rapid-acting insulin—Humalog, Novolog, Apidra, or regular—before meals.

Much of this chapter consists of guidelines for computing insulin timing and doses in various situations. They are essentially pretty simple calculations, and your physician or health care provider can and indeed should make them for you. I have included them here for several reasons. First, you should understand the information that goes into customizing a dose of insulin, so that you know there's no mystery involved. Second, if you understand how these calculations work, you can also more clearly see what incorrect insulin doses look like, and, we hope, avoid them. Finally, despite the dramatic findings of the Diabetes Control and Complication Trial, many physicians and health care professionals are still under the false impression that normalized blood sugars are dangerous or impractical or impossible. My hope is that by including these calculations, I can help you help your health care provider take better care of you.

If you're not the "math type," you can certainly skip the calculations, but do not skip the entire chapter. Herein lies important information about adjusting your insulin dosages or timing to accommodate common variations in your daily routine, such as eating out, and how to adjust your insulin if you skip a meal or have a snack. (Later in this chapter, you will learn why I rarely advocate snacking.)

DO YOU REQUIRE RAPID-ACTING INSULIN BEFORE EVERY MEAL?

The use of rapid-acting insulin prior to every meal or snack may help to preserve the function of any beta cells that you may still have. Nevertheless, you might not feel terribly enthusiastic about multiple daily injections. It's possible, however, that you may only require insulin before some meals and not others. Several of my patients, for example, maintain normal blood sugars by injecting a rapid-acting insulin before breakfast and supper and taking an ISA several hours before lunch. One patient injects before breakfast and supper, and has no medication before the small lunch she eats prior to her workout at the gym. The ultimate determinant of when you require preprandial rapid-acting insulin is your glucose profile. If blood sugar remains constant before and after every meal except supper, then you need a rapid-acting insulin only before supper.

You may recall, from our discussion of the dawn phenomenon on page 97, that both your own and injected insulins appear to be less effective when you wake up in the morning. This is why virtually all the people I've seen who require any premeal bolus insulin must at least have a dose before breakfast.

THE MOST-RAPID-ACTING INSULINS: HUMALOG, NOVOLOG, AND APIDRA VERSUS REGULAR FOR COVERING MEALS

Please reread Table 17-1 on page 284.

Clearly, when compared to regular insulin, Humalog has both advantages and disadvantages. Figure 19-1 illustrates the reason for a minor dilemma. As you can see, Humalog has a high early peak level in the blood, and then after 2 hours its level drops below that of regular (R). Attempting to match this peak with the action of carbohydrate upon blood sugar is very difficult for several reasons. I won't go into them all, but consider the following:

• The timing and shape of the peak will vary from one injection to the next.
• They will also vary with the size of the dose.

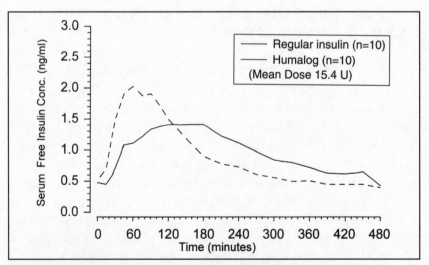

*Baseline insulin concentration was maintained by infusion of 0.2 mU/min/kg human insulin.

Fig. 19-1. *Serum insulin levels and action times of rapid-acting insulins: regular insulin versus Humalog (lispro). Note that the "industrial-sized" mean dose, 15.4 units, is far larger than the physiologic doses recommended in this text.*

- The appearance of carbohydrate in the blood will vary over time and from meal to meal.
- The flatter peak of regular insulin is easier to match with slow-acting carbohydrate than is the sharp peak of Humalog, Novolog, or Apidra with either slow- or fast-acting carbohydrate.

On the other hand, for most of us, regular must be injected about 40–45 minutes prior to a meal in order to start working as the meal starts to raise blood sugar. Humalog will start working about 15 minutes after injection. This short time interval makes for great convenience if you don't know precisely when your meal will be served, as when dining out (see later in the chapter). With this in mind, I usually recommend that patients cover meals with regular when time permits, but take Humalog when time is tight. I will usually, therefore, refer to regular as the premeal bolus insulin. This does not rule out the use of the other rapid-acting insulins for situations to be discussed later in the chapter.

There are yet additional complexities to using the three analog insulins.* First of all, their effect upon blood sugar is not as consistent, at least for me and my patients, as that of regular. Second, as mentioned earlier, these are, in our experience, 1½ to 2½ times more potent than regular, so that their doses must be only four-tenths (for Humalog) to two-thirds (for Novolog and Apidra) the dose of regular for the same net effect upon blood sugar.

From here on, for the sake of brevity, I will refer only to Humalog when discussing the most-rapid-acting insulins.

HOW MANY MINUTES BEFORE A MEAL SHOULD REGULAR INSULIN BE INJECTED?

Our goal is to minimize or totally prevent any blood sugar increase during or after meals. To achieve this, you must take your shot far enough in advance so that the insulin begins to lower blood sugar as your food starts to increase blood sugar. Yet you should not take it so

---

* Only two of the insulins we discuss (regular and NPH) have the same molecular structure as human insulin. All the others have slightly different structures and are therefore called "analog" insulins, not "human" insulins.

far ahead of the meal that blood sugar drops faster than digestion can keep up with it. The best time to inject regular, for most of us, is about 40–45 minutes before eating. The most common exception would occur if you have gastroparesis, or delayed stomach-emptying. Our approaches to the diagnosis of this condition and to appropriate timing of preprandial insulin if you have it are described in Chapter 22.

There are, however, a few people who absorb all of the rapid-acting insulins very slowly and must inject regular insulin, say, 1½ hours before a meal. Since this can be very inconvenient, we might use Humalog at a lower dose and inject it perhaps 1 hour before the meal.

Determining When to Inject

The following experiment should be useful in determining how long before a meal you should inject your regular insulin. This test can be conclusive only if your starting blood sugar is near normal—perhaps below 140 mg/dl and level for at least the prior 3 hours.

First, inject regular insulin 45 minutes before your planned mealtime. Now, measure blood sugars 25, 30, 35, 40, 45, et cetera minutes after the shot.

The point in time when your blood sugar has dropped 5 mg/dl determines when you should start eating. If this point occurs at 25 minutes, don't even bother to measure further just start to eat. If no drop is seen at 45 minutes, then delay the meal and continue checking blood sugar every 5 minutes until you see at least a 5 mg/dl drop. Then begin your meal. It shouldn't be necessary to repeat this experiment unless your preprandial dose of regular is changed by 50 percent or more at some future date.

If your starting blood sugar is higher than 140 mg/dl when you perform this experiment, the lack of precision in blood sugar measurement and insulin sensitivity may be greater than the 5 mg/dl drop that we're looking for. Just put off the experiment until your blood sugar is nearer to normal. In the meantime, assume the 45-minute guideline.

Is There Room for Error?

Suppose after performing the above experiment you find that your regular insulin should be injected 40 minutes before eating—which is the case for many of us. How far off can you be without getting into trouble?

Eating 5 minutes early or late makes no significant difference. If you eat 10 minutes too soon, your blood sugar may rise during the meal, but it probably will return to its starting point by the time we assume the regular finishes acting, about 5 hours after injecting. This is not serious, especially if it occurs only occasionally. If blood sugars go up significantly with every meal over many years, you would probably be at risk for long-term complications of diabetes. If you eat 15 or 20 minutes too soon, your blood sugar may go so high (say 180 mg/dl) that you become slightly resistant to the injected insulin. If this occurs, your blood sugar will not drop all the way to the premeal level when the regular finishes its action. If it happens often, your risk for developing the long-term complications of diabetes will increase.

What if you delay your meal by 10 or 15 minutes beyond the proper time after your shot? Now you're asking for trouble! Regular starts to work slowly, but its effect on blood sugar accelerates over the first 2 hours or so. Even a delay of 10 minutes can send your blood sugar dropping more rapidly than a low-carbohydrate meal can raise it. This, of course, can be hazardous.

USING A MOST-RAPID-ACTING INSULIN WHEN DINING OUT

Part of the pleasure of eating out is having someone else serve you something you can't make at home, but the difficulty for the insulin-taking diabetic is that you're served on their schedule, not yours. Hostesses, restaurants, and airlines—as well intentioned as they may be—rarely serve you at the time they promise. For nondiabetics, waiting may be annoying. For those of us who are diabetic, annoyance is compounded with danger. When planning your premeal bolus insulin shot, you cannot afford to rely on the word of your hostess, waiter, or airline staff. I've been taking premeal bolus regular insulin for more than forty years and have been "burned" more times than I care to count. Now that we have the most-rapid-acting insulins, I inject a dose when I see the waiter approaching my table with the first course. If I suspect that the main course will be delayed, I split my dose in half and take the second half when the waiter arrives with the main course. You should do the same. A transient blood sugar elevation is a small price to pay for the assurance that you will not experience severe hypoglycemia because the meal was delayed. If you eat a low-carbohydrate meal very slowly, even a transient blood sugar increase can be avoided.

As these newer insulins are more potent than regular insulin, the dose should be reduced as explained on page 287.

Nowadays, most airlines serve meals only on overseas flights. Unless you are traveling first class, or possibly business class, you will probably have no choice as to meal content. It is therefore wise to bring along your own food — or at least the protein portion, such as canned fish or meat or even some cheese. Usually you will be served a slow-acting carbohydrate in the form of a salad or vegetables. Again, this is a time for using a most-rapid-acting insulin, perhaps Novolog, 20 minutes before you begin to eat.

By the way, never order "diabetic" meals when traveling by air. As of this writing, airlines are still serving as "diabetic" meals a high-carbohydrate diet loaded with simple sugars. The salads in these meals may even contain fruit. My trick is to preorder "seafood" or even a kosher meal when I reserve my flight. This ensures that I get reasonable portions of protein. Unfortunately, many airlines do not serve seafood for breakfast. On airlines that serve nothing but drinks and a bag of peanuts, you may actually be better off. You can pack your own brown-bag breakfast or lunch, stick to your diet, and time exactly when you're going to take your shot and eat your food.

One warning: If you have gastroparesis, *never* inject an insulin for a meal that is more rapid than regular, as it will work faster than your stomach can empty the food. Use regular insulin.

OTHER MEALTIME CONSIDERATIONS

Must Meals Be Eaten at the Same Time Every Day?

Ever since the introduction of long-acting insulin in the late 1930s, diabetics have been advised that they must have meals and snacks at the same times every day. This very inconvenient rule still appears in current literature describing the treatment of diabetes. Prior to our use of low doses of long-acting insulins to cover the fasting state, physicians prescribed 1 or 2 large daily doses of long-acting insulin to cover both the fasting state and meals. (Most still do.) Such regimens never succeed in controlling blood sugars, and hypoglycemia is an ever-present threat. Patients are told to eat meals and several snacks at exactly the right times, to offset the continuous blood sugar drop caused by the long-acting insulin.

But if, as outlined in this chapter, we now cover our meals with rapid-acting insulin, we're free to eat whenever we want, provided we take our shot beforehand. We can also skip a meal if we skip the shot. When I was in medical training and worked 36-hour shifts, I sometimes skipped breakfast and ate lunch at 3 A.M. On some days I did not eat at all. This worked out fine because I followed the flexible insulin regimen described here.

What If You Forget to Take Your Regular 45 Minutes Before Eating?

If it's now less than 15 minutes before a predetermined mealtime (e.g., your lunch break at work), take a smaller dose of Humalog instead of regular.

If you ate your meal after forgetting your regular insulin, take Humalog instead—immediately—but don't forget that the amount of Humalog should be only four-tenths your usual dose of regular. If you were to use Novolog or Apidra, the dose would be half that of regular.

HOW TO ESTIMATE PREPRANDIAL DOSES OF REGULAR INSULIN

We know that for type 1 diabetics who make no insulin at all, 1 unit of regular insulin usually lowers blood sugar 40 mg/dl in a slim 140-pound adult. We also know that 1 gram of carbohydrate raises blood sugar 5 mg/dl. Thus 1 unit of regular usually covers 8 grams of carbohydrate. We also know that 1 unit of regular insulin covers *approximately* 2 ounces of protein.

There are variables, however. These figures apply only to people who produce none of their own insulin and who are not insulin-resistant. Doses must be tailored to the individual, so if you're obese, pregnant, or a growing child, you may require more insulin than these guidelines suggest. On the other hand, if your beta cells are still producing some insulin, you may need considerably less insulin than indicated here. I have adult patients who require only one-tenth as much insulin as I do.

Another variable in figuring a proper dose of regular is our old friend the dawn phenomenon. The regular insulin you inject before eating will be perhaps 20 percent less effective at breakfast than at other meals, even though it comes from the same vial.

The biggest factor is, of course, what you eat. Since we cannot know exactly how regular insulin will affect you until you begin to use it, your initial trial doses before meals must be based upon your precisely formulated meal plan. With that, we can make a reasonably safe initial estimate of how much insulin you're likely to need.

It's not easy for your physician to balance out all these variables and come up with just the right doses of regular insulin on the first attempt. Because of this, we try, for safety's sake, to underestimate your insulin needs initially, and then gradually to increase your preprandial doses after checking subsequent blood sugar profiles. This is yet another example of the Laws of Small Numbers in action. Because of the complexity of this task, let us examine how your physician might proceed with two very different scenarios.

Scenario One

You're a type 1 diabetic and are switching to our regimen from an outdated regimen of 1 or 2 large daily doses of intermediate- or long-acting insulin. Remember that many type 2 diabetics eventually lose nearly all beta cell function and then, in effect, have type 1 diabetes. So this scenario would apply to these people too.

Assume that the meal plan you negotiated with your physician is the following:

Breakfast: 6 grams carbohydrate, 3 ounces protein
Lunch: 12 grams carbohydrate, 4½ ounces protein
Supper: 12 grams carbohydrate, 6 ounces protein

Because we want to play it safe and stay with the lowest possible insulin doses, we will for the moment ignore any effect of the dawn phenomenon upon your breakfast dose, as well as the possibility of insulin resistance due to obesity. Our approximate calculations, based on the numbers mentioned above for a 140-pound adult, are as follows:

To cover carbohydrate: number of grams ÷ 8 = units of regular insulin

To cover protein: number of ounces ÷ 2 = units of regular insulin

Breakfast

- 6 grams of carbohydrate ÷ 8 = ¾ unit of regular insulin (which you'd note on your data sheet as 1⁻ – R)*
- 3 ounces of protein ÷ 2 = 1.5 unit of regular (1 R)
- Total trial dose for breakfast will be 2¼ units of regular (2⁺ R)

Lunch

- 12 grams of carbohydrate ÷ 8 = 1½ units of regular (1.5 R)
- 4½ ounces of protein ÷ 2 = 2¼ units of regular (2⁺ R)
- Total trial dose = 3¾ units of regular (4⁻ R)

Supper

- 12 grams of carbohydrate ÷ 8 = 1½ units of regular (1.5 R)
- 6 ounces protein ÷ 2 = 3 units of regular (3 R)
- Total trial dose = 4½ units of regular (4.5 R)

Your physician will probably want to lower these doses if your pancreas is making any insulin (as shown either by his or her educated guess or by the C-peptide test; see page 57).

It's virtually certain that your trial doses will be a bit too high or too low. In other words, your blood sugars may either rise or drop after some or all of these meals. It is most likely, however, that your postprandial blood sugars will not be dangerously low, unless you have gastroparesis. If you're insulin-resistant, you may need much more insulin on the second try.

Both you and your physician will want to get your blood sugars into line as rapidly as possible. So you'll probably be asked to fax, phone, or bring in your blood sugar profiles during the second day (and perhaps subsequent days) of this intensive insulin regimen for fine-tuning of doses. Remember that the important blood sugar measurements for fine-tuning your doses of premeal insulin are at least 5 hours after each dose of regular, Novolog, Apidra, or Humalog, as we assume this is the time it takes for the insulin to finish working. Let's assume that on the first day your blood sugar profile looked like this:

---

* Remember from Chapter 17 that 1⁻ means ¾ unit and 1⁺ means 1¼ units.

5 hours after breakfast: increased 70 mg/dl
5 hours after lunch: decreased 20 mg/dl
5 hours after supper: increased 25 mg/dl

Clearly, our initial insulin doses were a bit off and require adjustment to prevent further increases or decreases of more than 10 mg/dl. These changes are easy, if you remember that for most 140-pound adults who make no insulin (type 1 diabetics), 1 unit of regular lowers blood sugar by 40 mg/dl. If you weigh 100 pounds, 1 unit of regular will lower you about 56 mg/dl, or (140 ÷ 100) × 40 mg/dl. If you weigh 180 pounds, 1 unit of regular will lower you about 30 mg/dl, or (140 ÷ 180) × 40 mg/dl. We will assume, for this exercise, that your weight is close enough to 140 pounds to use the 40 mg/dl drop from 1 unit of regular. Type 2 diabetics might do better by using Table 19-1 (page 319).

Now let's look again at the hypothetical blood sugar profiles and work out the changes in preprandial regular that will be necessary:

Meal	Blood sugar change	Change ÷ 40 mg/dl	Change in dose rounded off to nearest ¼ unit
Breakfast	+70 mg/dl	+1.75	+2⁻ R
Lunch	−20 mg/dl	−0.5	−0.5 R
Supper	+25 mg/dl	+0.625	+0.5 R

We now fine-tune our premeal bolus of regular insulin by making the above changes to the original trial doses.

Meal	Trial dose	Change	New dose
Breakfast	2⁺ R	+2⁻	3.5 R
Lunch	4⁻ R	−0.5	3⁺ R
Supper	4.5 R	+0.5	5 R

That was pretty easy. Remember, however, that the content of your meals, in terms of grams of carbohydrate and ounces of protein, must be kept constant from one day to the next, because your insulin doses will not be changing every day. If you're consistently hungry after a particular meal, you can increase the amount of protein at that meal, but you must then have the extra protein every day. When you raise the protein portion of your meal, you look at your blood sugar profiles (or your physician does) to see how much your blood sugar goes up, and increase your dose of regular insulin for that meal accordingly. Do not increase your carbohydrates beyond 6 grams for breakfast, 12 grams for lunch, and 12 grams for supper—the Laws of Small Numbers dictate that the resultant rise and requirement for excess insulin will cause real problems with your blood sugar normalization attempts.

Scenario Two

You have type 2 diabetes and are following our diet. You've been taking an ISA in the morning and/or at bedtime. Your blood sugars are fine when you skip meals, but they go up after meals, even with the maximum doses of your ISA.

Since you're not a type 1 diabetic and are making some insulin of your own, we cannot use the simple rules that apply to those who make essentially no insulin. We have to assume that your beta cells still make a portion of the insulin needed to cover your meals, yet we do not know the magnitude of that portion. Furthermore, we don't know how much your insulin resistance will affect your injected insulin requirements. So we see how much a meal will raise your blood sugars without premeal bolus regular insulin. We then use this blood sugar increase as a guide for the doses you will be needing. We do not use this method with type 1s because their blood sugars might go so high without insulin as to cause the dangerous condition known as ketoacidosis.

Further fine-tuning of preprandial regular insulin might be performed by reviewing your blood sugar profiles over a week. If you've been taking a premeal ISA, as assumed in this scenario, you probably have already collected blood sugar profiles that show how much your blood sugar increases after each meal. If these profiles cover only 1 day, okay. If they cover a week, better. We want to start you with the lowest reasonable insulin doses, so we pick the smallest blood sugar increases that we can find for each meal, and then adjust your preprandial insulin accordingly. To find the increase before you begin taking regular insulin, subtract the preprandial blood sugar from the 3-hour postprandial blood sugar measurement (we wait 3 hours to allow the effect of the meal to be near its highest level).

On pages 294–295, we showed you how to compute a starting dose of long-acting insulin to cover overnight blood sugar rises. We can use the same simple formula to calculate initial doses of regular insulin to cover meals. But for safety's sake, and to obey the Laws of Small Numbers, we're deliberately going to keep the trial doses on the low side. We'll use as a guide the blood sugar data you collected while you were taking your ISA, even though we might discontinue the ISA sometime after you start using premeal bolus regular insulin.

To finish this example, let us assume that your 3-hour postprandial increases in blood sugar over the past week can be summarized as follows:

Smallest increase after breakfast: 105 mg/dl
Smallest increase after lunch: 17 mg/dl
Smallest increase after supper: 85 mg/dl

Now we must estimate the premeal bolus doses of regular insulin that would approximately offset these increases. You may remember that our preliminary formula in approximating trial doses of Levemir or NPH insulin (see pages 293–296) was that 1 unit of insulin will lower a 140-pound, insulin-requiring type 2 diabetic's blood sugar by 80 mg/dl. Your physician may want to be even more conservative and assume that 1 unit will lower your blood sugar by 90 mg/dl. We now only need to divide the above postprandial blood sugar increases by 90 to get the trial doses of premeal bolus regular insulin, as in the following table:

Meal	Blood sugar increase	Increase ÷ 90 mg/dl	Rounded off to nearest ¼ unit for trial dose of R
Breakfast	105 mg/dl	1.17	1⁺ R
Lunch	17 mg/dl	0.19	0.25 R
Supper	85 mg/dl	0.94	1 R

The above trial dose of R should be taken 40 minutes before the meal. As in the previous scenario, you will need to take periodic blood sugar measurements to monitor the effect of the insulin. If after one day on the trial doses of premeal bolus regular insulin, your postprandial blood sugars still go up by more than 10 mg/dl at 5 hours, your physician may ask you to increase the appropriate preprandial doses by

¼ unit or more. (Note that we now look at 5-hour blood sugars instead of 3-hour values, because we assume injected regular insulin requires 5 hours to finish working.) If your postprandial blood sugar elevations hardly respond to the ¼-unit increase, your physician may choose 1-unit increases. We rarely increase an initial preprandial dose in steps greater than 1 unit because of the danger of hypoglycemia, but in a very heavy person we may need 2-unit increases.

The above trial-and-error procedure should be repeated until your 5-hour postprandial blood sugars do not consistently change from the preprandial values by more than 10 mg/dl up or down. This all assumes that the carbohydrate and protein contents of your meals remain constant.

If, on this regimen, it turns out that your blood sugars are very stable, we'd eventually adjust your insulin so that changes after meals are less than 5 mg/dl.

WHAT ABOUT SNACKS?

If you've ever been on one of the conventional regimens that utilizes 1 or 2 large daily doses of longer-acting insulin, you're probably familiar with mandatory snacks. These are required, usually midway between meals and at bedtime, in the hopes of offsetting the continuous blood sugar–lowering effect of large amounts of insulin, hopefully preventing multiple daily episodes of hypoglycemia.

Our regimen, as you know, uses such low doses of Levemir insulin that blood sugars tend to remain level during the fasting state. With our regimen, there is no need for mandatory snacks. This does not mean that you must wait until the next meal before eating if you're hungry. Theoretically, you can eat a snack almost anytime, provided that you cover it with regular insulin, just as you would a meal. There are, however, some guidelines to remember.

Snacking Guidelines

Try to avoid snacks during the initial fine-tuning stage of your insulin doses. This is especially true of bedtime snacks. Snacks and their doses of regular insulin can confuse the issue of what caused what change in blood sugar. If, for example, you wake up with a high or low fasting blood sugar, did the problem originate in your bedtime dose of long-acting insulin, or in the dose of regular that you took for the snack?

Anytime you snack, try to wait until your prior meal has been fully digested, and the dose of regular insulin for that meal has run its course, at least 5 hours after the preprandial regular. Suppose you were to eat a snack 2 hours after a meal and then were to check your blood sugar 5 hours after the regular you took to cover the snack; you would have no way of telling whether it was the meal or the snack, and the respective doses of regular insulin, that were responsible for any increase or decrease in your blood sugar.

If you snack, don't eat "snack food." Try to snack on a food such as a single serving of sugar-free Jell-O brand gelatin (without maltodextrin) or three small sheets of toasted nori—that is, something that will not significantly affect your blood sugar and will not have to be covered with insulin. Most snacks other than these muddy the waters when you're trying to analyze data. If you really make no insulin you shouldn't snack, because your blood sugar depends almost entirely on what you eat and inject. Snacking interferes with meticulous blood sugar control. Full type 1s who do snack will have to refrain from correcting high blood sugars until 5 hours after the bolus injection of regular or Humalog for the snack. If you make some insulin and your routine injected doses have been fine-tuned, blood sugar corrections after a snack may not be needed, as you may be able to make enough insulin to prevent slightly elevated blood sugars (or "turn off" insulin production if blood sugars are heading too low). But if you make little or no insulin, you will still need to inject the correct dosage prior to the snack to cover it, and to check your blood sugar levels 5 hours later to make sure they do not differ from your target.

For these reasons, most of my patients do not snack on foods that will affect blood sugars. If you do snack, the same carbohydrate limit that applies to meals should also be applied to snacks. If you consume 12 grams of carbohydrate for lunch and for dinner, 12 grams of carbohydrate would be the upper limit for carbohydrate for any single snack. Lesser amounts of carbohydrate for a snack—as the Laws of Small Numbers would suggest—will naturally pose lesser problems.

If you're hungry several hours after a meal, check your blood sugar before snacking. Hunger may reflect hypoglycemia, reflecting in turn too much insulin, and should be treated with glucose tablets as indicated in Chapter 20, "How to Prevent and Correct Low Blood Sugars," and a possible reduction of your preprandial or basal insulin dosage the next day. ***An important rule for all diabetics: when hungry, check blood sugar.***

Estimating the Dose of Regular Insulin for a Snack

There are several different approaches to this problem.

The simplest is to decide in advance that you will eat for your snack exactly one-quarter the amount of carbohydrate and protein that you eat for lunch or supper. Remember that fat has no direct effect on blood sugar, so you need only consider the carbohydrate and protein. Cover the snack with exactly one-quarter the dose of regular that you take for the meal you selected. If your snack is one-third of your selected meal, then you'd naturally take one-third of your usual dose of regular for this meal—rounded off to the nearest ¼ unit. You should inject the regular insulin as far in advance of the snack as you would for a meal. In a pinch, you can take Novolog instead of regular and wait 20 minutes instead of, say, 45 minutes before snacking. But for this insulin, take only two-thirds of the dose that you would take for regular.

If you select a snack containing carbohydrate and/or protein that is not in the same proportion as one of your meals, use the computational method outlined on pages 308–309 for regular meals. To test the validity of your computations, skip lunch and lunch insulin and take the snack and snack insulin instead. Check your blood sugar before taking the snack insulin, and then check it again 2 and 5 hours after eating. This will help you determine the dosage correction to make when you next decide to do the same experiment (perhaps a few days later, as you may not wish to skip lunch two days in a row). You may want to try this several times to be sure of the dose. Thereafter, you won't have to skip lunch in order to have a snack.

If you've decided that your snacks will consist only of a small amount of protein (say, less than 3 ounces) and no carbohydrate, you can take your regular insulin 20 minutes before eating instead of 45 minutes before. This is because protein is converted to glucose much more slowly than is carbohydrate. Be sure to keep the protein and/or carbohydrate content of your snack(s) the same from one day to the next, as you probably won't want to do more experiments to determine doses of insulin.

Last but not least, *blood sugars will be easier for you to control if you don't snack at all,* or if you make your snack a small amount of sugar-free Jell-O (without maltodextrin) instead of real food. *It is important to remember that for covering a meal or snack, the dose of Novolog or Apidra should always be only half the equivalent dose of regular.*

A Final Warning About Snacks

Every new patient I see has read this book because I require it before I
will treat him or her. The great majority of new patients attempt to follow its teachings on their own and cannot understand why their blood
sugars are still on a roller coaster or their HgbA$_{1C}$ values are still elevated. I then ask if they snack and inevitably get responses such as these:

"Only on the right foods."
"Only a few times a week" (this usually means daily).
"Only some nuts" (usually a handful several times a day).

None of these people cover their snacks with insulin or eat consistent
amounts of food. These people are candidates for incretin mimetics (see
page 260) to control their cravings. (I do, however, have a few slim, very
active type 1 patients who actually require multiple small meals because
they cannot eat enough at one meal to last more than a few hours.)

WHAT SHOULD YOUR TARGET BLOOD SUGAR LEVEL BE?

In my experience, random blood sugars of nonobese, nonpregnant,
nondiabetic adults tend to cluster closely around 83 mg/dl (4.6 mmol/l).
Children tend to run slightly lower. About 1 hour after a high-
carbohydrate meal, many nondiabetics may have considerably higher
values. This, however, is not "natural," because for most of human history prior to the development of agriculture about ten thousand years
ago, high-carbohydrate meals were not usually available. Americans
now eat an average of about 156 pounds of added sugar per year, something that the average human would not have experienced in a lifetime
ten thousand years ago. Nowadays fast-acting carbohydrate accounts for
the largest part of energy consumption. So if we ignore elevated blood
sugars that may be encountered shortly after high-carbohydrate meals, a
"normal" value would be 83 mg/dl, perhaps even lower.

Several studies have demonstrated that risk for both cardiac and all
other causes of death increases as blood sugars or the equivalent values of HgbA$_{1C}$ exceed about 80 mg/dl.

With the above information in mind, for type 2 diabetics who use
no or very little injected insulin, I seek blood sugars of 80–85 mg/dl
(4.4–4.7 mmol/l). Since type 1s and type 2s who inject nontrivial

amounts of insulin cannot turn off injected insulin as their blood sugars drop, there always exists the possibility of going too low (hypoglycemia). I therefore throw in a small safety factor and ask such individuals *initially* to shoot for a target of 90 mg/dl (5 mmol/l). As you will learn in the next section, we try to correct blood sugars when they are above or below a target. Since we follow a low-carbohydrate diet, our target remains the same before, during, and after meals, as it probably was for our distant ancestors.

Under certain circumstances we will set a higher target:

- If someone's blood sugars prior to starting our regimen were very high, he or she will experience the unpleasant symptoms of hypoglycemia at blood sugars that are well above our 83 or 90 mg/dl. Thus if a new patient has had most blood sugars in the vicinity of 250 mg/dl, we might initially set a target of 140 mg/dl. We would then lower this target slowly over a period of weeks.

- Since the initial calculations of insulin doses may be too high, in spite of the precautions described earlier, it is wise to have a substantial safety factor. Thus one might set an initial target of 120 mg/dl and then slowly lower this over a period of weeks after it becomes apparent that no blood sugars less than 70 mg/dl have been encountered. This safety factor may also protect patients who at first make mistakes, because it is difficult to follow everything taught herein perfectly when starting out.

- Some insulin users, for whatever reason, are not meticulous in following what they have learned in this book or in my office — most commonly the dietary guidelines. These folks will inevitably experience roller-coaster blood sugars, although to a much lesser degree than in the past. Here again it is safer to use a target well above 90 mg/dl. A similar problem is encountered with people who experience unpredictable exercise, such as laborers and small children.

- Insulin pump users experience much greater uncertainty of insulin absorption than do those who inject. We therefore find it necessary to shoot for a higher than normal blood sugar, just to reduce the likelihood of severe hypoglycemia.

- Last but not least are those with gastroparesis (see Chapter 22). Here the unpredictable variations in blood sugars are great enough that a higher long-term target is frequently necessary in order to avoid very low values.

RAPID CORRECTION OF ELEVATED BLOOD SUGARS: CALCULATING THE DOSES OF RAPID-ACTING INSULINS

Sooner or later a dietary indiscretion, an infection, morning exercise, acute emotional stress, or even errors in estimating meal portions may cause your blood sugar to rise substantially over your target value. If your beta cells are still capable of producing moderate amounts of insulin, your blood sugar may drop back to target within a matter of hours. On the other hand, you may be like me and make little or no insulin, or you may be very resistant to your own insulin. If any of these is the case, your physician may want you to inject one of the most-rapid-acting insulins whenever your blood sugar goes too high.* (As you've probably noted, doses of insulin used to bring down elevated blood sugars are often referred to as "coverage.") Because these work faster than regular insulin, they are much preferred for this purpose. (If you are currently covering elevated blood sugars with regular insulin, use care when switching to one of the most-rapid-acting insulins; see "Some Final Considerations Regarding Humalog, Novolog, and Apidra Insulins," page 329.) To do this properly, you must first know how much ½ or 1 or 5 units of an insulin will lower your blood sugar; for Novolog and Apidra, it's usually 100 percent more than regular will.

This requires yet another experiment.

Wait until you have a blood sugar that is at least 20 mg/dl above your target (but this should not be an elevated measurement taken on arising—the dawn phenomenon can muddy the results of the experiment). To make sure that your prior mealtime bolus dose has finished working, this blood sugar should be measured at least 5 hours after your last dose. Be sure that you have taken your morning basal dose of Levemir. For this test, skip your next meal and the insulin bolus that covers it.

---

* For those who are not insulin-resistant, I avoid Humalog for this purpose because it is so powerful (½ unit will lower my blood sugar by 50 mg/dl). But many obese patients are so insulin-resistant that ½ unit may lower them by only 10 mg/dl. In such cases, Humalog is the ideal insulin because it works more rapidly than the others.

TABLE 19-1

SUGGESTED TRIAL EFFECT OF 1 UNIT OF
RAPID-ACTING INSULINS IN LOWERING
BLOOD SUGAR

Total daily basal dose of Levemir or undiluted NPH insulin*	1 unit NO or AP (full strength) might lower blood sugar		1 unit NO (3:1 dilution) or H (4:1 dilution)‡ might lower blood sugar		1 unit undiluted R might lower blood sugar	
2 units	320 mg/dl	17.7 mmol/l†	80 mg/dl	4.5 mmol/l	160 mg/dl	8.9 mmol/l
3	239	13.3	60	3.3	120	6.7
4	160	8.9	40	2.2	80	4.5
5	128	7.1	32	1.8	64	3.6
6	106	5.9	27	1.5	53	3
7	90	5	23	1.3	45	2.5
8	80	4.4	20	1.1	40	2.2
10	64	3.6	16	0.9	32	1.8
13	49	2.7	12	0.7	25	1.4
16	40	2.2	10	0.6	20	1.1
20	32	1.7	8	0.4	16	0.9
25	25	1.4	7	0.4	13	0.7

* If you have gastroparesis and must take more longer-acting insulin at bedtime in order to cover overnight emptying of your stomach, instead of using your bedtime dose to arrive at this number, substitute double your morning long-acting dose and don't add in the bedtime dose.
† Reminder: mmol/l, or millimoles per liter, is the standard international measure of blood glucose level (1 mmol/l = 18 mg/dl).
‡ We've diluted the Humalog 4:1 because it is so powerful that to lower my blood sugar by 15 mg/dl, I'd have to measure 0.15 unit, which is impossible. For people who are very insulin-resistant, dilution may not be necessary.

Now refer to Table 19-1, which suggests the amount that 1 unit of various rapid-acting insulins might lower your blood sugar, *for the purpose of this trial only*. The first column represents the sum of your daily doses of Levemir or NPH (children) that you are taking just to keep your *fasting* blood sugars level (your *basal* doses). The second column shows the amount that 1 unit of NO or AP will probably lower your blood sugar. The third column shows the amount that 1 unit, as read on a syringe, would likely lower blood sugar using a

3:1 dilution of NO or AP, or a 4:1 dilution of H. The last column shows the effect of 1 unit of R. (See page 288 for diluting instructions.) Again, *this table is only approximate.* Its only purpose is to suggest how much NO or AP you might try for this experiment. The column for diluted insulin is for those few individuals (children, for example) who find that a little goes a long way.

After recording your elevated blood sugar, determine the amount of your selected insulin suggested by the table to bring your blood sugar down to your current target. Let's assume that the sum of the doses of Levemir or NPH that will just keep your blood sugars level (if no meals) is 9 units. Then, by interpolating between lines in the table, 1 unit of NO will probably lower your blood sugar about 72 mg/dl. Let's further assume that your blood sugar at the time of this experiment is 175 mg/dl and that your target is 90 mg/dl. You therefore would like to lower your blood sugar 85 mg/dl. Dividing 85 by 72 yields 1.18 units of NO. Rounding down to the nearest quarter-unit, 1¼ units of NO should lower you about $1.25 \times 72 = 90$ mg/dl. This is certainly close enough, so you would inject 1¼ units.

Check and record your blood sugar again 4, 5, and 6 hours after the shot.* The lowest value will not only tell you how much your blood sugar dropped but also how long it took. For most of us, we assume that Humalog, Novolog, or Apidra finishes working in about 6 hours. If your lowest value occurs at or after 6 hours, you should in theory wait at least this long in the future before checking your blood sugars to see if the extra shot really brought you down to target. Let's say that the 1¼ units of NO in the above example brought your blood sugar from 175 mg/dl down to 81 mg/dl after 5 hours, and it did not drop further at 6 hours. Now you've learned that 1¼ units of NO will lower your blood sugar by 94 mg/dl (or 175 − 81). Divide 94 mg/dl by 1.25 units to find that 1 unit of NO will actually lower your blood sugar 75 mg/dl. Whatever this value turns out to be, write it down on your GLUCOGRAF data sheet in the box 1 UNIT ____ WILL LOWER BLOOD SUGAR. In this case, we have learned that our initial estimate that 1 unit would lower you 72 mg/dl was off by only

---

* Note that this experiment requires that you refrain from eating for 5 hours after your last shot of regular and then another 6 hours after the Novolog, for a total of 11 hours. With luck, you'll have to do this only once in your life.

4 percent. This can happen, and this is precisely why we do this experiment.

If at any point during this experiment your blood sugar drops 10 mg/dl or more below your target, immediately correct to target with glucose tablets, as detailed in the next chapter. This will offset the hazard of hypoglycemia. On your data sheet, record the number of glucose tablets that you used. After you have read the next chapter, you will understand how knowing the number of tablets will enable you to complete the above calculation without terminating or repeating the experiment.

As stated at the beginning of this chapter, it shouldn't be necessary for you to perform any of the above calculations on your own. This is the job of your health care professional, who can use our table and should have much more experience than you. He or she might want to try a simple option. For example, your doctor might instruct you to measure your 6-hour, post-lunch blood sugar and, if it's over 180 mg/dl, to inject 1 unit of NO and see how far your blood sugar drops in another 6 hours (without eating again). This will tell you approximately how much 1 unit will lower your blood sugar, without all the calculations.

WHEN TO COVER HIGH BLOOD SUGARS

Once you know how much 1 unit of one of the rapid-acting insulins will lower your blood sugar, you're in a position to bring down your blood sugar rapidly if it goes much above your target. All you need to do is to inject the proper dose. Within hours, your blood sugar will probably return to target. These extra doses are what is known as coverage. Once your insulin doses have been fine-tuned, it should rarely be necessary for you to cover with more than will lower you 60 mg/dl, unless you overeat, have an infection, or suffer from gastroparesis.

Never cover an elevated blood sugar if you have not waited for the last dose of regular or other rapid-acting insulin to finish working. After all, if two doses are working at the same time, your blood sugar can drop too low. This is one reason you should know how long it takes for a dose of any rapid-acting insulin to complete its action.

It is convenient to assume that the rapid-acting insulins continue their action for only 5 hours after injection, even though Table 17-1 (page 284) shows either 6–8 or 8–10 hours. The reason for our not-quite-correct assumption is that if we assumed even 6 hours for completion of action and you were to correct blood sugars at least 6 hours after each injection of the rapid-acting insulins (e.g., before meals and at bedtime), you would not only have inconveniently spaced meals and bedtime, but you also would have to remain awake at least 18 hours daily, leaving you only 6 hours of sleep. We therefore assume a 5-hour action time for convenience, on the reasonable assumption that blood sugar drop thereafter will be minimal. Thus we arrive at a prime guideline for correcting elevated blood sugars: *Wait at least 5 hours from your last shot of a rapid-acting insulin before correcting elevated blood sugars.*

Suppose target blood sugar is 90 mg/dl and you wake up in the morning and find that your fasting blood sugar is 110, an elevation of 20 mg/dl. If 1 unit of NO lowers you 40, you'd immediately inject ½ unit as coverage. If you plan on having breakfast in 40 minutes, just take this ½ unit as a separate shot, in addition to your usual breakfast dose of regular.

Another time you may find that 5 hours after your lunchtime regular was injected, your blood sugar is 60 mg/dl above your target. If 1 unit of H lowers you 80 mg/dl, take 1⁻ units of H right away.

A major variation from the 5-hour rule applies to *children* and to anyone who sleeps more than 9 hours overnight and has meals spaced less than 5 hours apart. These people should correct elevated blood sugars only upon arising in the morning, unless an alarm is set to ring during the night for a 5–7 hour postdinner correction. This alarm could also signal the time for the nightly dose of longer-acting insulin so that less than 9 hours elapse between the night dose and the morning dose, as dictated by the dawn phenomenon (see the next section).

After you cover with one of the rapid-acting insulins, you should check your blood sugar when the insulin has finished working, to make sure that the numbers from your original experiment were correct.

USING HUMALOG, REGULAR, NOVOLOG, OR APIDRA TO COVER THE DAWN PHENOMENON

Many of us find that blood sugar increases during the short interval between arising in the morning and eating breakfast. This is why, during the first few weeks on our regimen, it is necessary to check blood sugar not only upon arising but also when you sit down for breakfast. If such an increase occurs regularly, you should cover it before it occurs—on arising—with the appropriate dose of the fastest-acting insulin that you can easily measure. This will prevent the dawn phenomenon increase. I find it necessary to take ½ unit of R every morning upon arising, in addition to any coverage I might need for a slightly elevated fasting blood sugar. If I were to use NO or AP for this purpose, I would have to estimate ¼ unit, which would be imprecise.

IF RESULTS DON'T MATCH EXPECTATIONS

Under certain circumstances, one of these insulins will not lower your blood sugar as much as you would expect based upon your calibration. Let's take a look at some factors that can cause this.

Your insulin is cloudy. If your blood sugar does not drop as much as you expect, hold the insulin vial to the light to make sure that it's not cloudy. Compare it with a fresh vial to be sure. All insulin except NPH should be crystal clear; if it is even the slightest bit cloudy it has been deactivated and should be discarded. Also discard the vial if it has been frozen, kept in a hot place, or kept out of the refrigerator for more than three months, since temperature extremes will affect its potency. According to the manufacturers, Levemir and Lantus are more likely to deactivate at elevated temperatures than NO, H, and R. I'm not certain about AP.

Your fasting blood sugar was high on arising in the morning and you can't get it down. The dawn phenomenon causes more insulin resistance in the morning for some people than for others. If you start the day with an elevated blood sugar, you may require more coverage to bring down the elevation at that time than you would 3 or more hours later in the day. If you find that early-morning coverage is not very effective, review your blood sugar profiles with your physician. You'll probably be told that you should increase your coverage by one-third, one-half, or some other proportion during the first few hours after you wake up. More than 3 hours after arising, this increase in coverage should no longer be necessary.

To prevent overnight blood sugar increases, be sure to wait at least 5 hours (preferably 6) between your supper premeal bolus and your bedtime basal insulin and correct accordingly. You may do better by reducing your protein at supper, and certainly you should not eat bedtime snacks. Be sure to take your bedtime basal (Levemir) insulin less than 9 hours before your morning basal dose.

Your blood sugar was higher than 200 or 300 mg/dl. At such high blood sugars we become more resistant to the effects of injected insulin. This increased resistance may become very significant as blood sugar rises above 250 mg/dl. But the point at which resistance becomes significant is not precise, and its magnitude is difficult to determine. We rarely encounter such high blood sugars once insulin doses and diet are appropriate. If you do measure a very high blood sugar, cover it with your usual calibration and wait the usual 5 hours or so. Then check your blood sugar again. If it has not come all the way down to your target, take another coverage dose based on the new less elevated blood sugar. This time the coverage will probably be fully effective.

Infections. If your coverage or any other insulin dose is less effective than usual, you may have an infection. We once discovered that a patient had an intestinal inflammation called diverticulitis only because he was wise enough to telephone me when his blood sugars were a little less responsive to insulin than usual. *It's important that you notify your physician whenever you find that your insulin appears to be losing its efficacy.* See Chapter 21, "How to Cope with Dehydration, Dehydrating Illness, and Infection."

INTRAMUSCULAR SHOTS WILL GET YOUR BLOOD SUGAR DOWN FASTER

Intramuscular shots of a rapid-acting insulin can be quite useful for bringing down elevated blood sugar more rapidly than our usual subcutaneous shots. You should not ordinarily use them for your usual premeal doses of regular insulin, and you should never inject Levemir, Lantus, or NPH into a muscle—it makes no sense to speed up the action of a long-acting insulin.

Typically, an intramuscular shot of any rapid-acting insulin will begin to lower an elevated blood sugar within about 10 minutes. It will finish acting at least 1 hour sooner than your usual subcutaneous injection, and it will have your blood sugar close to your target within about 2–3 hours. Because I have trouble estimating very small doses of AP, NO, or H for a 10 mg/dl reduction, I would estimate ¼ unit of R and inject it intramuscularly.

Problems to Consider
With intramuscular shots, you may experience several problems that you do not encounter with subcutaneous shots, unless you want to try your outer thighs. Because of this, I give my patients the option of using or not using this method of self-injection, and fully appreciate the feelings of those few who turn it down. Here are some obstacles you may confront.

Fat arms. If you have fat arms, don't even try intramuscular shots. If you have a lot of fat over the deltoid muscle on your upper arm (see Figure 19-2), the needle on any insulin syringe will be too short to penetrate the underlying muscle.

Missing the muscle. Even moderately slim people sometimes "miss" the muscle because even the longer (½-inch) needle sometimes may not penetrate deeply enough. Since we cannot always tell whether or

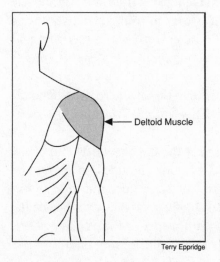

Deltoid Muscle

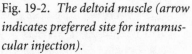

Fig. 19-2. *The deltoid muscle (arrow indicates preferred site for intramuscular injection).*

not the needle hit the muscle, we sometimes must wait as long before rechecking our blood sugars as we would for a subcutaneous shot.

Hitting a blood vessel. You are much more likely to hit a blood vessel than with subcutaneous injections. This can be briefly painful. You can also get blood on your shirt if you shoot right through the sleeve as I do. I estimate that I hit a blood vessel once in every thirty intramuscular injections. (See page 276 for instruction on using hydrogen peroxide to remove bloodstains from clothing.)

Pain. If for whatever reason you're unable to throw the needle in rapidly like a dart, all your intramuscular shots may be briefly painful. If so, do not even bother to attempt them.

Intramuscular Injection Technique

Please refer to Figure 19-2 as you read the following step-by-step instructions. Do not use a syringe with the new short needles. I keep on hand a supply of syringes with ½-inch (12.7 mm) needles just for intramuscular shots.

1. Locate your deltoid muscle, illustrated in Figure 19-2. It begins at the shoulder and ends about one-third of the way down your upper arm. It's wide at the shoulder and tapers to a V shape farther down. You may be able to feel the V with your fingers if you lift your arm to the side until it is parallel to the floor. This will tighten the muscle and make it feel harder. We usually use the deltoid muscle because it is easy to find, is relatively large and thick, and is less likely to be covered with a deep fat pad than most other muscles (except, for most of us, the outer thighs).

2. Now, allow your nondominant arm (left if you're right-handed) to dangle loosely at your side. This will relax the muscle, so that the needle can penetrate easily.

3. The site for injection will be near the upper (wider) end of the deltoid, about 1½ inches below your shoulder (at about the position of the arrow in Figure 19-2). We use the wide end of the muscle because you are less likely to miss it with the needle, and because you would not want to pierce the axillary nerve, which is located near the tip of the V, at the lower end.

4. As your nondominant, target arm dangles loosely at your side, pick up the syringe with your dominant hand and "throw" the needle straight into the injection site as you would a dart—but, of course, don't let go of the syringe. Do not grab any flesh, as you do for subcutaneous shots. Do not inject at an angle, but go in perpendicular to the skin. Be fast, as a slow intramuscular shot can hurt. Push in the plunger rapidly to inject your insulin. Now pull out the needle. Touch the injection site with your finger to make sure you have not bled.

5. If the shot hurts, you probably hit a small blood vessel, so be prepared for some blood. In such a case, press the injection site firmly with a finger. Hold it there for about a minute. This will prevent or stop any bleeding. If you do not press, you will develop a slightly painful lump where the blood accumulates under the skin. The lump will turn yellow or black-and-blue after a number of hours. If you inject through your shirt or blouse and get it bloody, apply hydrogen peroxide, as described on page 276.

Once you have given a number of intramuscular shots using your dominant hand, try switching hands and arms. This may seem cumbersome at first, but with practice you will be able to inject into either arm.

"MIXED" THERAPY — INSULIN PLUS ISAs

As indicated previously, if you are still making some insulin and are insulin-resistant, you may be able to take the rapid-acting version of Glucophage (metformin) instead of regular insulin before certain meals. This will depend upon your postprandial blood sugar profile. There may be no therapeutic advantage to such a substitution, but it might be more convenient. Remember, however, that you will probably have to wait at least 60 minutes before starting your meal. It is usually more convenient to take a shot of regular insulin, since the waiting time after injecting is generally only 40–45 minutes, even less for some people.

A more important use for an ISA in combination with insulin occurs if you are overweight or have polycystic ovarian syndrome

(PCOS; see Appendix E) and your bedtime dose of long-acting insulin is more than 8–10 units. This suggests that you may have insulin resistance, which may partly respond to one of the ISAs. Recall that ISAs increase your sensitivity to insulin. Large doses of insulin help build fat, of course, and can also cause further down-regulation, or desensitization, of insulin receptors. If you're obese, the less insulin you have in your system storing away fat, the better. So there may be some advantage to reducing your bedtime insulin dose.

If your physician decides to add Glucophage XR or Actos to your bedtime regimen, he or she will want you to build up the dose gradually while simultaneously reducing your dose of basal insulin. We use the extended-release (XR) version of Glucophage because it will keep working all night and is not likely to cause the digestive discomfort sometimes found with the more-rapid-acting version. If your bedtime insulin requirements are not reduced while taking the maximum recommended dose of Glucophage XR or Actos before sleeping, then the bedtime oral agent is serving no purpose and should be discontinued. The FDA warns against using Avandia or Actos if you are taking insulin, as there is a small risk of congestive heart failure (due to fluid retention) in susceptible individuals who take insulin plus these medications.* This restriction does not apply to Glucophage or to the insulin-mimetic agents.

IS IT NECESSARY TO RECORD DAILY BLOOD GLUCOSE PROFILES AFTER INSULIN DOSES HAVE BEEN FINE-TUNED?

Type 1 diabetics, and those type 2s whose beta cells are producing little or no insulin, tend to show significant blood sugar changes following relatively small changes in what they eat, their activity level, and so on. If your blood sugars commonly show changes of more than

---

* Insulin in large doses causes fluid retention. Avandia and Actos can also cause fluid retention. It is likely that the people reported to have developed heart failure while taking both Avandia or Actos and insulin were taking large doses of insulin to cover the usual high-carbohydrate diabetes diet currently advocated by the ADA.

10 mg/dl in the course of a day, you probably should measure your blood sugar profiles daily for the rest of your life. Such frequent monitoring is necessary so that you can correct high blood sugars with insulin or low blood sugars with glucose tablets (see Chapter 20, "How to Prevent and Correct Low Blood Sugars").

I've seen many individuals on our regimen whose blood sugars are quite stable even though they require the 5 daily shots typical of intensive insulin therapy. These people usually require small doses of insulin—typically for adults, under 8 units daily for all doses combined. If you fit into this category, your beta cells are probably still producing some insulin. This enables your system automatically to smooth out the peaks and valleys that your blood glucose profile would otherwise show. With such stable blood sugars (varying less than 10 mg/dl daily), there's no reason to bother taking daily blood sugar profiles. You would, instead, prepare a full blood glucose profile (seven tests) for 1 day every two weeks. If you spotted a change in your blood sugar ranges, you'd check the next few days to see if it continued. If it did, you would contact your physician, who might want to explore the possible reasons for such changes. If you become ill, or if, say, you have a school-age child who brings home a cold, you might want to check your blood sugar profiles every day. If your physician has prescribed oral or injected steroids for other disorders such as asthma or bursitis, you should be checking and recording your blood sugars, as they will certainly increase.

SOME FINAL CONSIDERATIONS REGARDING HUMALOG, NOVOLOG, AND APIDRA INSULINS

Perhaps as a result of reading one of my prior books, you may already be covering elevated blood sugars with regular insulin. If this is the case, be very careful when switching to Humalog, Novolog, or Apidra for this purpose. I and many of my patients have found them to be more effective than regular—that is, a given dose is likely to lower blood sugar more than the same dose of regular. For example, I find that while 1 unit of regular will lower my blood sugar 40 mg/dl, 1 unit of Humalog will lower it 100 mg/dl and 1 unit of Novolog or Apidra will lower it 80 mg/dl. I advise, therefore, that you initially take half as much Novolog or Apidra or 40 percent as much Humalog as your prior regular for this purpose. Based upon the initial effect on your blood sugar, you can then adjust subsequent doses of these analog insulins. The same consideration applies if you eat out and use an analog insulin to cover a meal.

We have also observed that when Humalog is used to cover meals, blood sugars are less predictable than with regular. This result was not mentioned in reports of clinical trials of Humalog, probably because the trial population followed a high-carbohydrate diet and had such wide blood sugar fluctuations that this effect was not apparent.

It's certainly worth mentioning that the rapid-acting insulins are usually available in small (3 cc) cartridges. These can be carried in a jacket pocket or small purse without creating an unsightly bulge. When using cartridges, insert a needle and pull back on the plunger of the syringe very slowly. Do not inject air into the cartridge. If you draw out too much insulin, do not inject it back into the cartridge. Squirt the excess into a plant or wastebasket.

INSULIN PUMPS

Much effort and expense are being devoted to promote and market insulin pumps. These devices were designed to make multiple daily injections easier. They also do away with the need for long-acting insulins.

The instruments consist of two basic elements:

- A pump unit about the size of a small pocket calculator, which you can hang from a belt, keep in a pocket, attach to your arm, or pin to your clothing.
- Large-bore plastic tubing that stays in your skin, typically just above your waist. The plastic tubing, which is inserted into the skin through a large, retractable needle, usually should be changed every 2–3 days.

The pump unit can be loaded with a supply of any rapid insulin that lasts a number of days before refilling is necessary. It delivers a tiny basal flow of insulin all day long, giving an effect similar to that of 3 daily injections of long-acting insulin. This basal rate can be pre-set by the user on a remote control and can even be set to change automatically at various times of the day. Premeal bolus or corrective doses are readily produced by setting the dose and then pushing a button.

Insulin pumps offer the following advantages over multiple daily injections:

- There is no need to carry a number of insulin syringes when away from home, but catheters and other supplies must accompany you.
- Corrective injections are elegantly simple.
- Pumps can be set to automatically increase the basal delivery rate shortly before arising in the morning, thereby circumventing problems associated with the dawn phenomenon. They thus render it unnecessary for you to arise early on weekends to take your long-acting insulin.

On the other hand, insulin pumps can pose some problems:

- The initial cost of the pump is considerable.
- The cost of disposable supplies is much greater than that of insulin syringes.
- Pump failure, tubing coming out of the skin, insulin coagulation, tubing blockage, or kinking can occur in spite of sophisticated alarms and safeguards. As a result, ketoacidosis has occurred overnight in many type 1 users.
- There is a moderate incidence of infections at injection sites. Many of these have formed abscesses requiring surgical drainage.
- Severe hypoglycemia is more common among pump users, possibly because of mechanical problems.
- Insulin pumps cannot be used to give intramuscular injections for more rapid lowering of elevated blood sugars.
- All of the long-term (seven-plus years) pump users that I have seen had fibrosis (scar tissue formation) at their injection sites. This had impaired their insulin absorption so much that even high doses failed to control their blood sugars. In addition, blood sugar effects of pump boluses appeared to be inconsistent in these individuals.
- Until recently, pump delivery rates could not be set for less than 0.1 unit per hour. This makes it necessary for basal dosing to be in multiples of 2.4 units per day, thereby preventing fine adjustments of basal insulin. For example, consider someone who requires 6 units of basal insulin daily. With a pump she would

have to take either too little, 4.8 units (2×2.4), or too much, 7.2 units (3×2.4). Some pump manufacturers now make their products adjustable to 0.025 unit per hour, which solves this problem for most adults, but not for small children.

- Many people are turned off by the idea of constantly having large-bore tubing sticking in their abdomens.
- Users experience at least some inconvenience with the four S's—sleep, showers, swimming, and sex.
- Over the past five years, the FDA has received reports linking 7,170 deaths to infusion pump problems. This probably reflects gross underreporting of actual events. FDA officials believe that software and design problems underlie this situation.
- Raising or lowering an insulin pump above or below the injection site can cause siphoning that will speed up or slow down the delivery rate by up to 123 percent if above the site, or 73 percent if below the site. This effect was much smaller with the Omni-Pod, which uses no tubing. The above variations in delivery rate can render blood sugar control impossible.

In our experience, insulin pumps do not provide better blood sugar control than multiple injections. Contrary to a common misconception, they do not measure what your blood sugar is and correct it automatically. Furthermore, most pumps are programmed to produce meal boluses that are computed to cover varying amounts of carbohydrate, totally ignoring both dietary protein and the Laws of Small Numbers.

The OmniPod uses both a slimmer needle (28 gauge) and a short length of very fine tubing. The pain is virtually eliminated, and the long-term problems caused by a large foreign body (i.e., the tubing) under the skin are considerably reduced. The basal infusion rate, however, is still a bit too great (0.05 units per hour) for most people taking physiologic doses of basal insulin. This may be improved in the future.

INHALABLE INSULIN

In 2006, Pfizer introduced an inhalable insulin. I reviewed it in the previous edition of this book and recommended against it. The FDA eventually agreed with my appraisal and banned its use. It is likely that other inhalable insulins will become available in the future. They will all have at least one inherent problem—uncertain absorption from one dose to the next—in other words, unpredictable effects upon blood sugar. Since insulin injections, if done our way (see Chapter 16), should be painless, and their effects are quite precise when given in physiologic doses, there is no likely benefit of inhalable insulin.

> I will personally answer questions from readers for
> one hour every month. This free service is available by
> visiting www.askdrbernstein.net.

20

How to Prevent and Correct Low Blood Sugars

U se of medications such as insulin or the obsolete sulfonylurea-type and newer, similar oral hypoglycemic agents (OHAs) that provoke increased insulin production exposes you to the ever-present possibility that your blood sugars may drop far below your target value.* Because your brain requires glucose in order to function properly, a deficit of glucose — or hypoglycemia — can lead to some occasionally bizarre mental symptoms. In extreme cases, it can result in death. Although severe hypoglycemia can be dangerous, it is preventable and treatable. I encourage you to have your family, close friends, or workmates read this chapter so they will be able to assist you in the event you have a hypoglycemic episode and cannot correct it alone. I mention OHAs repeatedly in this chapter because of the hazard of hypoglycemia they pose. Please remember that for oral medications I recommend insulin-sensitizing agents (ISAs) and insulin mimetics, while I oppose the use of OHAs.

HYPOGLYCEMIA: THE BASICS

For our purposes in this chapter, we will use the term "hypoglycemia" to designate any blood sugar that's more than 10 mg/dl below target.

---

* It has been claimed that the insulin-sensitizing agents (ISAs) cannot cause abnormally low blood sugars. This is not so. As we discussed in Chapter 15, I've seen it happen — in a very mild diabetic who was using it to facilitate weight loss. Nevertheless, this is a rare occurrence.

"Mild" hypoglycemia is any blood sugar that's 10–20 mg/dl below target. As it drops lower, it's progressively more "severe," and can, if left uncorrected, become the condition known as neuroglycopenia, which means "too little glucose in the brain."

Glucose diffuses in and out of your brain slowly, whereas blood sugar in the rest of your body can rapidly drop to zero in an hour from an intramuscular overdose of rapid-acting insulin. Many diabetics develop physical symptoms or signals that enable them to recognize a hypoglycemic episode and think clearly enough to measure blood sugar and correct it.

When blood sugar drops slowly, neuroglycopenia can occur at about the same time that physical symptoms appear. You may not be aware of them, however, because your brain, severely deprived of glucose, is less capable of comprehending these things. "Hypoglycemia unawareness" (reduced or absent ability to experience early signs of hypoglycemia) is also common in individuals who have recently had frequent hypoglycemic episodes, because of a phenomenon called down-regulation of adrenergic receptors (see page 358). It can also in theory be caused by a class of cardiac drugs (beta blockers) that slow the heart and lower blood pressure. In reality, however, this may not be true. If you do not notice physical symptoms, you may not be able to think clearly enough to realize that your blood sugar is too low, and your cognitive state may deteriorate.

Progression of Symptoms of Neuroglycopenia
Following is a partial list of the signs and symptoms of hypoglycemia as they progress, ranging from mild (early) to severe (late), which together make up neuroglycopenia.

- Delayed reaction time—e.g., failure to slow down fast enough when driving a car.
- Irritable, stubborn behavior and lack of awareness of the physical symptoms of hypoglycemia (see the box on page 340).
- Confusion, clumsiness, difficulty speaking, weakness.*
- Somnolence (sleepiness) or unresponsiveness.

---

* One study has shown these symptoms to occur when blood sugar drops to 45–65 mg/dl. Furthermore, symptoms were found to continue for 45 minutes after blood sugars were normalized.

- Loss of consciousness (very rare if you do not take insulin).
- Convulsions (extremely rare if you do not take insulin).
- Death (extremely rare if you do not take insulin).

Some Common Causes of Hypoglycemia

In various chapters, particularly those covering insulin, we've discussed a number of different potential causes of low blood sugar. Following is a list of some common causes.

- Not waiting at least 5 hours after a prior dose of rapid-acting insulin before correcting an elevated blood sugar. This is especially dangerous at bedtime.
- Too much delay before eating a meal after taking a rapid-acting insulin or classic OHAs, such as the old sulfonylureas and similar newer agents.
- Delayed stomach-emptying after a meal (see Chapter 22).
- Reduced activity of counterregulatory hormones during certain phases of the menstrual cycle.
- Sudden termination of insulin resistance after abatement of illness or stress that required higher than usual doses of classic OHAs or insulin.
- Injecting from a fresh vial of insulin after having used progressively higher doses of insulin that has slowly lost its activity over a period of months.
- Switching from an insulin pump to manually injected insulin without lowering the dose.
- Incorrectly assuming that the most-rapid insulins are equivalent in potency to regular insulin (see page 329).
- Eating less than the planned amount of carbohydrate or protein for a meal or snack.
- Taking too much insulin or OHA.
- Engaging in unplanned physical activity or failing to cover physical activity with appropriate carbohydrates.
- Drinking too much alcohol, especially prior to or during a meal.
- Failure to shake vials of NPH insulin vigorously before using.
- Inadvertently injecting long-acting or premeal bolus insulin into a muscle.
- Injecting near a muscle that will be strenuously exercised.
- Long-term treatment with intravenous gamma globulin, causing random intermittent recovery of beta cells in type 1 diabetics.

- Using insulin that contains protamine (NPH; see page 279).
- Taking aspirin in large doses, or anticoagulants, barbiturates, antihistamines, or certain other pharmaceuticals that may lower blood sugar or inhibit glucose production by the liver (see Appendix C).
- A sudden change from cool weather to warm weather.

Common Signs and Symptoms of Hypoglycemia

Hunger. This is the most common early symptom. A truly well-controlled, well-nourished diabetic should not be unduly hungry—unless he's hypoglycemic. This symptom, although frequently ignored, should not be. On the other hand, hunger is also very often a sign of tension or anxiety. One cannot assume that it automatically signals hypoglycemia. Perhaps half of so-called insulin reactions may merely reflect hunger pangs provoked by mealtime, emotional factors, or even high blood sugars. When blood sugars are high, the cells of the body are actually being deprived of glucose, and you may feel hungry. Thus, hunger is very common in poorly controlled diabetics. *If you feel hungry, measure your blood sugar!*

Impaired visual acuity. Even mild hypoglycemia can make for difficulty in reading street signs or fine print. More severe hypoglycemia can cause double vision.

Elevated pulse rate. Always carry a watch with a sweep second hand. Know your maximum resting pulse rate. When possible symptoms of hypoglycemia appear and you have no handy means of testing your blood sugar (a sign of gross negligence), measure your resting pulse. Many people find it more convenient to measure the temporal pulse (at the temple, on the side of the head between the eyebrow and hairline) or the carotid pulse (on the side of the neck just below the lower edge of the jaw and about 1–3 inches forward of the ear) than the radial, or wrist, pulse. If your resting pulse exceeds your *maximum* resting value by more than one-third, assume hypoglycemia. This measurement may be normally elevated if you've been walking about during the prior 10 minutes. Your health care professional can help you learn how to measure your pulse. This exercise should never be necessary since, of course, you have your blood sugar meter with you at all times.

Nystagmus. This symptom may be demonstrated by slowly moving your eyes from side to side while keeping your head immobile. If another person is asked to watch your eyes, she will notice—when your blood sugar is low—that they may jerk briefly in the reverse direction, or "ratchet," instead of moving smoothly. You can observe the effect of this by looking at the sweep second hand of your watch. If it seems occasionally to jump ahead, you are experiencing nystagmus (actually, as your eyes jumped to the side for brief instants, you missed seeing bits of motion of the second hand).

Absence of erections. For a man, a fairly reliable sign of early-morning hypoglycemia is awakening without an erection, assuming that he ordinarily experiences morning erections. Failure to experience an erection when sexually stimulated likewise suggests hypoglycemia if this is not a usual problem.

Denial. As hypoglycemia becomes more severe, or if blood sugar has been dropping slowly, many patients will be certain that their blood sugars are fine. An observer suspecting hypoglycemia should insist on a blood sugar measurement before accepting the diabetic's denial.

TREATING MILD TO MODERATE HYPOGLYCEMIA, WITHOUT BLOOD SUGAR OVERSHOOT

Historically, the advice for correction of low blood sugar has been to consume moderately sweet foods or fluids, such as candy bars, fruits, cookies, hard candies, peanut butter crackers, orange juice, milk, and soda pop. Such treatment has never worked properly, for reasons you can probably guess, knowing what you now know about various foods and how they affect your blood sugar.

These moderately sweet foods contain mixtures of slow- and rapid-acting carbohydrates. If, for example, you eat or drink enough that the rapid-acting carbohydrate in these foods raises your blood sugar from 40 mg/dl up to your target of 83 mg/dl over the course of half an hour, you may have simultaneously consumed so much slow-acting carbohydrate that your blood sugar will go up by 300 mg/dl several hours later.

In the old days, before I learned to maintain my blood sugar in normal ranges, my physicians insisted that very high blood sugars after hypoglycemic episodes were due to an "inevitable" hypothetical effect they called rebound, or the Somogyi phenomenon.* Once I learned to avoid the usual foods for treating low blood sugar, I never experienced blood sugar rebound. Nevertheless, the scientific literature does describe occasional *mild* insulin resistance that lasts up to 8 hours following an episode of very low blood sugar. This is not the dramatic rebound caused by eating the wrong thing to bring up blood sugar.

Hypoglycemia can be hazardous, as the list of its progression on page 335 demonstrates. We therefore want to correct it as rapidly as possible. Complex carbohydrate, fructose, lactose (in milk), and even sucrose, which is used in most candies—all must be digested or processed by the liver before they will fully affect blood sugar. This delay makes these types of carbohydrate poor choices for treating hypoglycemia. Furthermore, you need to know exactly how much your blood sugar will rise after eating or drinking something to raise it. With most of the traditional treatments you must continually check your blood sugar many hours later to gauge the unpredictable effect.

Raising Blood Sugars Predictably

What, then, can we use to raise blood sugars rapidly with a predictable outcome? The answer, of course, is glucose.

Glucose, the sugar of blood sugar, does not have to be digested or converted by the liver into anything else. Unlike other sweets, it's absorbed into the blood directly through the mucous membranes of the stomach and gut. Furthermore, as we discussed in Chapter 14, "Using Exercise to Enhance Insulin Sensitivity and Slow Aging," we can compute precisely how much a fixed amount of glucose will raise blood sugar. If you have type 2 diabetes and weigh about 140 pounds, 1 gram of pure glucose will likely raise your blood sugar about 5 mg/dl— provided that your blood sugar is below the point at which your pancreas starts to make insulin to bring it down. If you weigh 140 pounds and have type 1 diabetes, 1 gram of glucose will raise your blood sugar about 5 mg/dl no matter what your blood sugar may be, because you

---

* If your physician still believes what he learned in medical school about this fictional phenomenon, ask him to read "The Somogyi Phenomenon—Sacred Cow or Bull?," *Archives of Internal Medicine* 1984; 144:781–787.

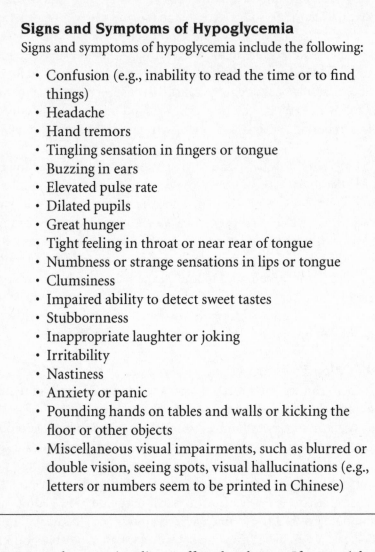

Signs and Symptoms of Hypoglycemia

Signs and symptoms of hypoglycemia include the following:

- Confusion (e.g., inability to read the time or to find things)
- Headache
- Hand tremors
- Tingling sensation in fingers or tongue
- Buzzing in ears
- Elevated pulse rate
- Dilated pupils
- Great hunger
- Tight feeling in throat or near rear of tongue
- Numbness or strange sensations in lips or tongue
- Clumsiness
- Impaired ability to detect sweet tastes
- Stubbornness
- Inappropriate laughter or joking
- Irritability
- Nastiness
- Anxiety or panic
- Pounding hands on tables and walls or kicking the floor or other objects
- Miscellaneous visual impairments, such as blurred or double vision, seeing spots, visual hallucinations (e.g., letters or numbers seem to be printed in Chinese)

cannot produce any insulin to offset the glucose. If you weigh twice that, or 280 pounds, 1 gram will raise your blood sugar only half as much. A 70-pound diabetic child, on the other hand, will experience double the blood sugar increase, or 10 mg/dl per gram of glucose consumed. Thus, the effect of ingested glucose on blood sugar is inversely related to your weight. Table 20-1 gives you the approximate effect of 1 gram glucose upon low blood sugar for various body weights.

If you have handled glucose tablets, be sure to wash your hands before rechecking your blood sugar. If a source of water is not available, lick the finger you intend to prick to remove any residual

- Uncontrolled extension, stretching, or movement of the arms or legs
- Poor physical coordination (e.g., bumping into walls and dropping things)
- Tiredness
- Convulsions
- Weakness
- Sudden awakening from sleep
- Shouting while asleep (or awake)
- Rapid shallow breathing
- Nervousness
- Light-headedness
- Faintness
- Hot feeling
- Cold or clammy skin, especially on the neck
- Restlessness
- Insomnia
- Nightmares
- Pale complexion
- Nausea
- Slurred speech
- Nystagmus (see page 338)

Several of these symptoms may occur at the same time. One symptom alone may be the only indicator. In some cases, there may be no clearly apparent early signs or symptoms at all.

glucose. You can dry the finger by wiping it on your clothing or a handkerchief.

Do not keep glucose tablets near your blood sugar meter or test strips!

Many countries have available as candies or confections products that contain virtually all of their nutritive ingredients as glucose. These glucose tablets are usually sold in pharmacies. Some countries even have glucose tablets marketed specifically for the treatment of hypoglycemia in diabetics. Table 20-2 lists a few of the products with which we are familiar.

TABLE 20-1

EFFECT OF 1 GRAM GLUCOSE UPON
LOW BLOOD SUGAR

Body weight		1 gram glucose will raise low blood sugar	
35 pounds	16 kilograms	20 mg/dl	1.11 mmol/l
70	32	10	0.56
105	48	7	0.39
140	64	5	0.28
175	80	4	0.22
210	95	3.3	0.18
245	111	3	0.17
280	128	2.5	0.14
315	143	2.2	0.12

Of the glucose tablets listed, I personally prefer Dex4 bits because they're very easy to chew, raise blood sugar quite rapidly, taste good, are conveniently packaged, and are inexpensive. They are also small enough that they usually need not be broken in halves or quarters to make small blood sugar adjustments (except for small children). Dex4 products are available at most pharmacies in the United States, Canada, and possibly the U.K. The bits come in jars of 60. Larger Dex4 tablets contain 4 grams of glucose and are packaged in vials of 10 and jars of 50. These are appropriate for people who weigh more than 220 pounds (100 kg). For smaller children I prefer Smarties or Winkies* because of their tiny size. Most glucose tablets begin to raise blood sugar in about 3 minutes and finish after about 45 minutes, if you don't have gastroparesis. (If you do, see Chapter 22.)

With this background in mind, how should you proceed when you encounter a low blood sugar?

---

* Both are available at kosher stores. Winkies are available at Rosedale Pharmacy, (888) 796-3348; Smarties are available at www.smartiesstore.com.

TABLE 20-2

GLUCOSE TABLETS USED FOR TREATMENT OF HYPOGLYCEMIA BY DIABETICS

Country of manufacture	Name of product	Grams of glucose per tablet	1 tablet will raise blood sugar of 140-pound person with low blood sugar approximately	
USA, Canada	Dex4 bits	1	5 mg/dl	0.28 mmol/l
USA	SweeTARTS or Wacky Wafers	2*	10	0.56
USA, Canada	Smarties or Winkies†	0.4	2	0.11
USA, Canada	Dex4	4	20	1.10
U.K., Canada	Dextro Energy	3	15	0.83
USA, Germany	Dextro Energen	4	20	1.10

* Tablet size may vary.
† Ideally suited for children because of their small size.

USING GLUCOSE TABLETS

If you experience any of the symptoms of hypoglycemia detailed earlier—especially hunger—measure blood sugar. If blood sugar is 5 mg/dl or more below target, chew enough glucose tablets to bring blood sugar back to your target. If you have no symptoms but discover a low blood sugar upon routine testing, again take enough glucose tablets to bring blood sugar back to your target. Having no symptoms is *not* a valid reason for not taking tablets. A low blood sugar without symptoms carries more risk than one with symptoms. If you weigh about 140 pounds and your blood sugar is 60 mg/dl but your target is 83 mg/dl, then you might eat 5 Dex4 bits. This would raise your blood sugar, according to Table 20-2, by 25 mg/dl, bringing you to 85 mg/dl. If you are using Dextro Energen, you'd take 1 tablet. Simple.

If your low blood sugar resulted from taking too much insulin or OHA, it may continue to drop after taking glucose if the insulin or OHA hasn't finished working. You should therefore recheck your blood sugar about 45 minutes after taking the tablets, to rule out this possibility and to see if you're back where you belong. If blood sugar is still low, take additional tablets and keep testing every 45 minutes—

sooner if it is dropping rapidly. If you have delayed stomach-emptying, you may have to wait as much as 2 or more hours for the full effect.*

What if you're out of your home or workplace and don't have your blood sugar meter? (A major crime, as noted earlier.) If you think you're hypoglycemic, play it safe and take enough tablets to raise your blood sugar about 40 mg/dl (2 Dex4 tablets, for example). You may worry that this will bring you too high. If you take insulin, this poses no problem. Simply check your blood sugar when you get back to your meter. If it's above your target, take enough corrective insulin to bring you back to target, but be sure to wait 5 hours after your last dose of rapid-acting insulin. If you don't take insulin, your blood sugar should eventually come back on its own, because your pancreas is still making some insulin. It may take several hours, or even a day, depending upon how rapidly you can produce insulin. In any event, you may have saved yourself from an embarrassing or even disastrous situation.

WHAT IF BLOOD SUGAR IS LOW JUST BEFORE A MEAL?

Take your glucose tablets anyway. If you don't, you may become very hungry, overeat, and be too high hours later. The medication you take for a meal is intended to keep your blood sugar level. So if it was too low before a meal, it will be too low after if you don't take your glucose but eat properly.

WHAT IF YOUR SYMPTOMS PERSIST AFTER YOU HAVE CORRECTED THE HYPOGLYCEMIA?

Many of the symptoms of hypoglycemia are actually effects of the hormone epinephrine (which you may know as adrenaline). If you do not have the problems listed in the section "Hypoglycemia Unawareness" later in this chapter, your adrenal glands will respond to hypoglycemia by producing epinephrine. Epinephrine, like glucagon,

---

* This time frame can be greatly reduced by drinking a glucose solution (see page 396).

signals the liver to convert stored glycogen to glucose. It is epinephrine that brings about such symptoms as rapid heart rate, tremors, pallor, and so on. (Beta blocker medications may interfere with the ability of epinephrine to cause these symptoms.) Epinephrine has a half-life in the blood of about 1 hour. This means that an hour after your blood sugar comes back to target, about half the epinephrine you made may still be in your bloodstream. This can cause a persistence of symptoms, even if your blood sugar is normal. Thus, if you took some glucose tablets an hour ago and still feel symptomatic, check your blood sugar again. If it's on target, try to control the temptation to eat more. If your blood sugar is still low, more tablets are warranted.

COPING WITH THE SEVERE HUNGER OFTEN CAUSED BY HYPOGLYCEMIA

Mild to moderate hypoglycemia can cause severe hunger and an associated panic. The drive to eat or drink large amounts of sweet foods can be almost uncontrollable. New patients, before starting our regimen, have told me stories of eating an entire pie, a jar of peanut butter, or a quart of ice cream, or drinking a quart of orange juice in response to hypoglycemia. Before I stumbled onto blood sugar self-monitoring and learned how to use glucose tablets, I did much the same. The eventual outcome, of course, was extremely high blood sugar several hours later.

Since the effects of glucose tablets are so predictable, the panic element has vanished for me and for most of my patients.

Unfortunately, rapid correction of blood sugar does not always correct the hunger. This may be somehow related to the long half-life of epinephrine and the persistence of symptoms even after restoration of normal blood sugars. My patients and I have successfully coped with this problem in a very simple fashion. You can try the same trick we use.

First, consume the appropriate number of glucose tablets.

If overwhelming hunger persists, consider what might satisfy it. Typical options include a full meal (such as another lunch or supper), half a meal, or a quarter of a meal. A full meal means exactly the amounts of carbohydrate and protein that you would ordinarily eat at that meal. Half a meal means exactly half the protein and half the carbohydrate.

Even if your blood sugar has not yet come back to target, since you know you have consumed the proper amount of glucose to eventually bring it back, you can confidently inject the amount of insulin or swallow the dose of the OHA that you normally use to cover that meal. For half a meal, take half the dose; for a quarter of a meal, take one-quarter the dose.

Don't frustrate yourself by waiting the usual 40–45 minutes or so after injecting regular insulin, or the 20 minutes after injecting a most-rapid insulin, or the 60–120 minutes after taking an OHA. Just inject and eat. An extra meal now and then won't make you fatter or cause harm. Since you're eating within the controlled boundaries of your meal plan and not gorging on sugars or unlimited amounts of food, you're still abiding by the Laws of Small Numbers.

If you know how much insulin or OHA you usually take to cover a certain snack, you might have the snack instead of the meal.

HOW FAMILY AND FRIENDS CAN HELP YOU CATCH A HYPOGLYCEMIC EPISODE WITHOUT MUTUAL ANTAGONISM

Two of the most common effects of hypoglycemia can make the job of helping you difficult and unpleasant. These effects are irritability, nasty behavior and failure to recognize your own symptoms. At my first interview with many new patients and their families, instances of violence during hypoglycemic episodes are commonly reported. The most common scenario I hear goes like this: "Whenever I see that he's low, I hand him a glass of orange juice and tell him to drink it, but he throws the juice at me. Sometimes he throws the glass too." Such stories come as no surprise to me because as a teenager I used to throw the orange juice at my mother, and when I was first married, I did the same to my wife. Why does this happen, and how can we prevent such situations?

First, it's important to try to understand what's going on in the minds of you and the family member or partner during a bout with hypoglycemia. The cognitive difficulties that accompany severe hypoglycemia can make the slightest frustration or irritation overwhelming. Your low blood sugar may cause you to act bizarrely, as if intoxicated — and in a sense, you are intoxicated. Because your thinking is impaired, you may be totally unaware that your blood sugar is low. The similarity to drunkenness is not a coincidence, since the higher cognitive centers of the brain, which control rational behavior, are impaired in both cases.

You probably have learned that high blood sugars are to be avoided, and at some level, you remember this, perhaps even cling to it, despite your hypoglycemia. If someone tries to cajole you into eating something sweet, you may decide that it's the *other* person who's irrational. This is especially true if the other person has done the same thing in the past, when blood sugars were actually normal or even high. In "self-protection" against the supposed irrational attempt to get you to eat something sweet, you instinctively may become violent. Most commonly, this occurs if an attempt is made to put food or drink in your mouth. You might view this as an "attack." In less rational moments, you may even decide, since you know that high blood sugars are harmful, that your spouse or relative is trying to kill you.

The helping relative, usually a spouse or parent, may be terrified to see such strange behavior. If your loved one has been through many such encounters, he or she may, for self-protection, keep candies or other sweets around the house in the hope that you will eat them and thus avoid such situations. The fear can be exacerbated if your loved one has seen you unconscious from hypoglycemia, or is merely aware that hypoglycemia can cause dire consequences. On other occasions, when your blood sugar wasn't really low, your loved one may have erroneously asked you to eat something sweet. Such erroneous diagnoses are especially common during family squabbles. The spouse or parent may feel that "his blood sugar is low, and that's why he's yelling at me." Your loved one would rather play it safe and give you something sweet, even if your blood sugar isn't low.

There is a solution to this apparent dilemma. First of all, both parties must recognize that, as a rule, about half of the time that the relative suspects hypoglycemia, you do not have low blood sugar; the other half of the time, blood sugar is indeed low.

No one has ever contradicted me when I've made this point.

Encouraging a diabetic to eat sweets when hypoglycemia is suspected, despite conventional teaching, does as much harm as it does good. A better approach would be for the loved one to say, "I'm worried that your blood sugar may be low. Please check it and let me know the result so that I'll feel less anxious." As a patient, you should realize that living with a diabetic can often be as much or more of a strain than having diabetes. You, the diabetic, owe some consideration to the needs of your loved ones. Try to look upon the request to check your blood sugar not as an intrusion but as your obligation to relieve someone else's fear. With this obligation in mind, you should automatically check your blood sugar if asked, just to make the other person feel better. It doesn't matter whether your blood sugar is low or normal. If your blood sugar is low, you can correct it and find out why. If it's normal, then you probably will have defused the situation, and now you'll be able to get back to whatever you were doing, unworried that blood sugar is off target. When you look at blood sugar as something like a clock that you can set—and reset—you take some of the mystery out of it, and can diminish the emotion involved.

If you're without your meter, take enough glucose tablets to raise your blood sugar about 40 mg/dl—again to make the other person feel better. This is the least you can do for someone who may worry about you every day.

Believe it or not, this simple approach has worked for me and for many of my patients. As I've said previously, I went through this with my parents and have gone through it with my wife. Spouses report that it relieves them of a great burden. Some wives have even cried when expressing their gratitude.

HOW FAMILY AND FRIENDS CAN HELP WHEN YOU ARE CONSCIOUS BUT UNABLE TO HELP YOURSELF

This more serious hypoglycemic state is often characterized by extreme tiredness and inability to communicate. You may be sitting and banging your hand on a table, walking around in a daze, or merely failing to respond to questions. It's important that those who live or work with you learn that this is a fairly severe stage of hypoglycemia. The likelihood that it's hypoglycemia is so great that valuable time may be wasted if treatment is delayed while someone fumbles about trying to measure your blood sugar. It's quite possible that if you're given glucose tablets you will not chew them, and may even spit them out.

The treatment at this stage is glucose gel by mouth.

Glucose prepared as a syrupy gel is sold in the United States under several brand names. At least one of these products is not pure glucose (dextrose) but contains a mixture of long- and short-acting sugars, and therefore will not exert its full effect as rapidly as we'd like. At present, I ask my patients to purchase Dex4 gel. It is packaged in a plastic tube (like toothpaste) with a replaceable screw cap. Each tube contains 15 grams of glucose. From Table 20-1 (page 342), we see that this amount will raise the blood sugar of a 140-pound person by 75 mg/dl (15 × 5). An appropriate dose for most adults in this condition would be about 1 full tube.

Some of the tubes of decorative icing used to write on birthday cakes contain almost pure glucose (dextrose), so you might save money by purchasing those. Look in the baking section of most supermarkets, but make sure of the contents and weight. To convert ounces to grams, multiply by 30. Make sure that the major ingredient is glucose, as some brands are mostly sucrose, which works too slowly.

We recommend that 2 tubes of a glucose gel, secured together with a rubber band, be placed at strategic locations about your house and place of work, as well as in luggage when you travel with a companion. It should not be refrigerated, as it may harden when cold. To administer, someone should insert the tip of an open tube into the corner of your mouth, in between your lower gum and your cheek, and slowly squeeze out a *small amount.* You will probably swallow this small amount. After you swallow, a bit more of the gel should be gently squeezed from the tube. Within 5 minutes of ingesting an entire tube, you should be able to answer questions.

When you have fully recovered, check and correct your blood sugar to your target. Since you may have wiped the sticky gel off your mouth with your hands, you should wash them before sticking your finger.

Although glucose gels may not be available in many countries, they are available on the Internet. Most industrialized nations have pharmacies and surgical dealers that sell flavored glucose drinks to physicians for performing oral glucose tolerance tests. These are usually bottled in 10-ounce (296 ml) screw-top bottles that contain 100 grams of glucose. A dose of 2 fluid ounces (60 ml) will provide about 20 grams of glucose, enough to raise the blood sugar of a 140-pound person by 100 mg/dl. *Tiny amounts* can be administered with the help of a plastic squeeze bottle. Whoever feeds you the liquid or gel must exercise caution, as the possibility exists that you could inhale some of it, causing you to choke. Using a liquid is potentially much more hazardous than using a gel in this respect, so administer only a tiny amount (about 1/4 tsp.) for each swallow.

TREATING HYPOGLYCEMIA IF YOU ARE UNCONSCIOUS

Hypoglycemia is not the only cause of loss of consciousness. Stroke, heart attack, a sudden drop in blood pressure, and even a bump on the head can render you unconscious. In fact, very high blood sugar (above 400 mg/dl) over several days, especially in a dehydrated individual, can also cause loss of consciousness. We will assume, however, that if you are carefully observing the treatment guidelines of this book, you will not allow such prolonged blood sugar elevation to occur.

If you're found unconscious by someone who knows how to rapidly check your blood sugar, a measurement may be made. Treatment should not be delayed, however, while people are scampering about trying to find your testing supplies.

The treatment under these conditions is injection of glucagon, a hormone that rapidly raises blood sugar by causing the liver and muscles to convert stored glycogen to glucose. It is imperative, therefore, that those who live with you know how to give an injection. If you use insulin, you can give them some practice by teaching them how to give you insulin injections. Glucagon is sold in pharmacies in many countries as the Glucagon Emergency Kit. This consists of a small plastic box containing a syringe filled with an inert waterlike solution and a little vial of white powder (glucagon). The kit also contains an illustrated instruction sheet that your family should read before an emergency develops. The user injects the water into the vial, withdraws the needle, shakes the vial to dissolve the powder in the water, and draws the solution back into the syringe. The tip of the long needle must be submerged in the liquid. For adults, the entire contents of the syringe should be injected, either intramuscularly or subcutaneously; lesser amounts should be used for small children. Any of the sites shown in Figure 16-1 (page 265) can be used, as can the deltoid muscle (see Figure 19-2, page 325), the outer thigh, or even the calf muscle. Your potential benefactors should be warned that if they choose the buttocks, injection should go into the upper outer quadrant, so as not to injure the sciatic nerve. An injection may be given through clothing, provided it is not too thick (for example, through a shirtsleeve or trouser leg, but not through a coat, a jacket, or a trouser pocket).

Under no circumstances should anything be administered by mouth while you are unconscious. Since you will not be able to swallow, oral glucose could asphyxiate you. If your glucagon cannot be found, your companions should dial 911 (in the United States) for the emergency medical service, or take you to the emergency room of a hospital.

When an individual has lost consciousness from hypoglycemia, he may experience convulsions. Signs of this include salivation, tooth-grinding, and tongue-biting. Although the last can cause permanent damage in the mouth, no attempt to intervene should be made. Your heroic savior will not be able to help you if you bite off her fingers. If possible, you should be turned to lie on your side with your head positioned so that your mouth is downward. This is to help drain excess saliva from your mouth so you won't breathe it in and choke.

You should begin to show signs of recovery within 5 minutes of a glucagon injection. You should fully regain consciousness and be able to talk sensibly within 20 minutes at most. If steady improvement is not apparent during the first 10 minutes, the only recourse is the emergency squad or hospital. The emergency squad should be asked to inject 40 cc of a 50 percent dextrose (glucose) solution into a vein. Individuals weighing under 100 pounds (45 kg) should receive proportionately smaller amounts (e.g., a 70-pound child would receive 20 cc of the dextrose solution).

Glucagon can cause retching or vomiting in some people. Your head should therefore be turned to the side so that if you do vomit, you won't inhale the vomitus. Keep a 4-ounce (120 ml) bottle of metoclopramide syrup on hand, attached with a rubber band to the Glucagon Emergency Kit. One gulp of metoclopramide, taken after you are sitting up and speaking, should almost immediately stop the feeling of nausea. Do not consume more than one gulp, as large doses can cause unpleasant side effects (see page 387). In the United States, metoclopramide is available only upon prescription by a physician.

One dose of glucagon can raise your blood sugar by as much as 300 mg/dl, depending upon how much glycogen was stored in your liver at the time of the injection and subsequently converted to glucose. After you've fully recovered your senses, you should check your blood sugar. If at least 5 hours have elapsed since your last dose of a rapid-acting insulin, take enough intramuscular (or subcutaneous) rapid-acting insulin to bring your blood sugar back down to your target. This is important, because if your blood sugar is kept normal for about 24 hours, your liver will rebuild its supply of glycogen. This glycogen reserve is of great value for protection from possible subsequent hypoglycemic events.

By the way, if we tried to give glucagon to someone twice in the same day, the second shot might not raise blood sugar. This is possible because liver glycogen reserves may have been totally depleted in response to the first injection. Thus, monitoring and correction of blood sugar every 5 hours for 1 full day is mandatory after the use of glucagon. Additional blood sugar measurements should be taken every 2½ hours to make sure that you're not again hypoglycemic, but do not correct for *high* blood sugars every 2½ hours; wait the full 5 hours since the last shot of rapid-acting insulin (see page 322).

Although reading about possible loss of consciousness may be frightening, remember that this is an extremely rare event, and usually results when a type 1 diabetic makes a major mistake, such as those included in the list on pages 336–337. I know of no case where a type 2 diabetic experienced severe hypoglycemia when using any oral medication that we recommend.

HOW TO DETECT HYPOGLYCEMIA WHILE YOU ARE SLEEPING

The signs of hypoglycemia during sleep include cold, clammy skin, especially on the neck, erratic breathing, and restlessness. It certainly helps to have a light sleeper sharing your bed. Parents should check diabetic children at night and should feel their necks.

KNOW WHY YOU WERE HYPOGLYCEMIC

Review your GLUCOGRAF data sheet after all hypoglycemic episodes, even mild ones. It's important that you reconstruct the events leading up to any episode of low blood sugar, even if it caused no notable symptoms. This is one of the reasons why we recommend (see page 80) that most insulin-taking diabetics keep faithful records of data pertinent to their blood sugar levels and why we go into so much detail in Chapter 5 teaching you how to record the information. Since severe hypoglycemia can lead to amnesia for events of the prior hour or so, habitual recording of relevant data can be most valuable for this scenario. It is certainly helpful to record times of insulin shots, glucose tablets, meals, and exercise, as well as to note if you overate or underate, and so on. Recording blood sugar data alone may not help you to figure out what caused a problem. If you experience a severe hypoglycemic episode or several mild episodes and cannot figure out how to prevent recurrences, read or show your GLUCOGRAF data sheet to your physician. Your doctor may be able to think of reasons that did not occur to you.

BE PREPARED

Hypoglycemia Supplies

Glucose tablets, glucose gel, and glucagon can each potentially save your life. They won't help if they're not around or are allowed to deteriorate. Here are some basic rules:

- Place supplies in convenient locations around your house and workplace.
- Show others where your supplies are kept.
- Keep glucose tablets in your car, pocket, or purse.
- When traveling, keep a full set of supplies in your hand luggage and also in your checked luggage—just in case a piece of luggage is lost or stolen.
- It may be wise to replace glucagon on or before the expiration date on the vial. In an emergency, however, it isn't necessary for your savior to worry about the expiration date. In the United States, glucagon is usually sold with very short dating. Many people are sold costly emergency kits marked with expiration dates only a few months later. Don't worry. Glucagon is sold as a freeze-dried powder that will probably remain effective for five years after the "expiration" date, unless of course it has been exposed to moisture or extreme heat (as in a closed car in the summertime). It retains its longevity especially if it is refrigerated. Once diluted, however, it is good for only 24 hours.
- Always replace supplies when some have been used. Never allow your stock to become depleted. Keep plenty of extra glucose tablets and blood sugar test strips on hand.
- Bacteria love to eat glucose. Once you have opened your bottle or package of glucose tablets, expect that within six months you

will see black spots on each tablet corresponding to bacterial colonies. Even unopened packages will present spotted tablets about one year after manufacture. These tablets will not kill you, but they may be unpleasant-tasting and too hard for easy chewing. Periodically take a look at your supply of glucose tablets.

Your Hypoglycemia Tool Kit

To make sure you are not caught unprepared by low blood sugars, you should always keep the following supplies on hand at both your home and your workplace.

If You Take OHAs or Even ISAs
- 1–3 bottles glucose tablets; always carry glucose tablets with you

If You Take Insulin and Do Not Live Alone, You Also Need
- One package of 3 tubes glucose gel
- Glucagon Emergency Kit
- 4-ounce bottle metoclopramide syrup

Emergency Identification Tags

If you use insulin or OHAs, you should wear an identification tag that displays a recognizable medical emblem, such as a red serpent encircling a red staff. The tag, which may be worn as a bracelet or necklace, should be engraved with a message that will advise emergency medical personnel of your diabetic status. If you take insulin, it might say "Diabetic—takes insulin." Since bracelets are more likely to be spotted by emergency personnel, I prefer them to the necklaces.

Most pharmacies and jewelers sell medical ID tags. Prices begin at $5 for stainless steel and go into hundreds of dollars for solid gold. The MedicAlert Foundation (2323 Colorado Avenue, Turlock, CA 95382) will keep a record of your medical history and will send you a stainless steel ID bracelet or necklace, with its emblem, for $40. Sterling silver or gold-plated IDs cost slightly more. MedicAlert will also engrave the tag for the same cost. All tags are stamped with your special ID number and with the foundation's "call collect" 24-hour telephone number. By phoning this number, a hospital or paramedic can secure your name and address, contact information for your next of kin and physician, a list of all your medical conditions, and the doses of medications that you take. You can obtain an application form by writing to the above address, by phoning (888) 633-4298, or by going to www.medicalert.org.

Diabetics who do not take medications that can cause hypoglycemia would also be wise to wear a MedicAlert bracelet, if only to discourage the automatic use of intravenous glucose infusions—a common practice of emergency personnel on victims of motor vehicle accidents, heart attacks, and so on.

Emergency Alarm Service

If you live alone, you may want to consider using an emergency alarm system. These can automatically phone a friend, relative, or emergency squad when you push a button on a necklace. The system can also be activated if you do not "check in" at predetermined time intervals. The least expensive system that I have encountered is supplied by the MedicAlert Foundation. Their "failure to check in" alert unfortunately can only be activated at 24-hour intervals, so you could be unconscious for 24 hours before someone is notified.

The Continuous Glucose Monitor (CGM)

Most of us have jobs that bring us into contact with other people during the day and family with whom we have contact after work. These contacts offer considerable protection from severe hypoglycemia, as colleagues and relatives will intervene if you start walking into walls or talking silly. A sleeping partner can frequently pick up on the labored breathing and cold, clammy skin or damp nightclothes that accompany hypoglycemia and then awaken you and ask you to check your blood sugar.

If you live or sleep alone, or if your sleeping partner is an extremely deep sleeper, however, you don't have this protection at night.* A backup is available.

Several companies are now marketing continuous glucose monitors.† A CGM works via a tiny sensor implanted beneath the skin,

---

* Many insulin users will awaken automatically when blood sugar gets too low during sleep, so these people have built-in protection.
† Search the Web for "continuous glucose monitor" to compare different models.

using a technique similar to that used for insulin pump tubing. The sensor constantly measures glucose concentration in the tissue fluid present at its subcutaneous location. A combined power supply and radio transmitter attaches to your skin or clothing. The transmitter sends up to several hundred glucose readings daily to a small portable receiver that you can keep in a pocket. The number displayed is approximately equal to the blood sugar about 20 minutes prior to the reading. So if you had taken a reading with your conventional method 20 minutes ago, this would be roughly the same as the reading from the sensor right now.

Also displayed is an up or down arrow to indicate whether blood sugar is increasing or decreasing. What's most valuable is an audible alarm that can be set to sound at any selected blood sugar value and also to signal rapid drops in blood sugar.

There are some potential problems associated with these devices, so they're not for everyone.

- One of the CGM manufacturers has disclosed reports of sensors breaking off in the skin, requiring surgical removal.
- The sensor remains under the skin for 3 days. During this time, there is always the possibility for inflammation or infection (probably a low risk).
- Fibrosis, or scar tissue, can potentially build up at the sensor site over time (although how long this would take is as yet unclear) and eventually make measurements less accurate.
- Measurements are inherently less accurate than ordinary blood sugar monitoring, so the devices need to be calibrated against finger-stick blood sugars about twice daily. For now, at least, I would recommend that any blood sugar correction be made based on finger-stick measurements.
- Both the equipment and the disposable sensors with associated supplies are quite costly and may not be covered by insurance.
- Advertising for these products may falsely imply (but not state outright) that a sensor–insulin pump combination will automatically monitor and inject insulin to keep blood sugars on target around the clock.
- The sensor is typically implanted in the abdomen but may have a bulky exterior.
- The sensor will typically work for only 3 days, because the enzyme used is then depleted.

- The setup requires training to use, usually provided by a salesperson.

While CGMs have at best limited usefulness at the moment, it is entirely feasible — just from an engineering perspective — that they will vastly improve over time and even be able to act as an artificial pancreas. That said, I'm not holding my breath — this technology has been around for decades, and manufacturers have made plenty of money by employing it shoddily. One can still hope, however, that some brilliant entrepreneur will develop a highly accurate and timely monitor that can provide constant, accurate blood sugar readings. One manufacturer has already applied to the FDA for approval in the United States. I suspect, however, that it will pose the same problems as are found with insulin pumps and will not give the same accuracy and precision that we get with injection and an accurate blood sugar meter.

If I were living alone, I'd use a CGM to protect from nighttime hypoglycemic episodes and forget about using an insulin pump.

"HYPOGLYCEMIA UNAWARENESS"

Some diabetics have absent or diminished ability to experience the warning signs of hypoglycemia. This occurs under six circumstances that have been documented in the scientific literature:

- Impaired delivery of glucose to the brain.
- Severe autonomic neuropathy (injury, by chronically high blood sugars, to the nerves that control involuntary bodily functions).
- Adrenal medullary fibrosis (destruction, by chronically high blood sugars, of the cells in the adrenal glands that produce epinephrine). This is especially common in long-standing poorly controlled diabetes.
- Blood sugars that are chronically too low.
- The use of beta-blocking medication for treatment of hypertension or cardiac chest pain. A recent study disproves this, but I'm not certain of its universal validity.
- The use of large (nonphysiologic) doses of insulin, as is common for individuals on high-carbohydrate diets.

All of these situations result in lowered production of, or sensitivity to, epinephrine, the hormone that produces tremor, pallor, rapid pulse, and other signs that we identify with hypoglycemia. It is ironic that epinephrine production or sensitivity is most commonly diminished in those whose blood sugars have been chronically either very high or very low.

Injury to the autonomic nervous system by elevated blood sugar is discussed on pages 65–66. Individuals whose heart rate variation on the R-R interval study is severely diminished may be especially susceptible to this problem.

People who have frequent episodes of hypoglycemia or chronically low blood sugar tend to adapt to this condition. They appear to be less sensitive to the effects of epinephrine, which, when repeatedly released in large amounts, down-regulates its own receptors. This condition cannot be predicted by R-R studies. It is, however, readily detectable if you measure your own blood sugar frequently. If caused by chronically low blood sugar, this condition can be reversed by taking measures to ensure that blood sugar is maintained at normal levels.

Hypoglycemia unawareness can deprive one of potentially lifesaving warning signals. To compensate for this disability, blood sugar should be checked more frequently. For some rare insulin users, it may be necessary, for example, to measure blood sugar every hour for 5 hours after meals, instead of only once or twice after each meal. Fortunately, we have the tools to circumvent this problem; we need only to use them diligently.

I frequently encounter patients who do not take glucose tablets for low blood sugar measurements because they "feel fine" or are "about to eat anyway." These are just the people who are most likely to lose consciousness or find themselves in an automobile accident.

Whether or not you have hypoglycemia, it is essential that you check your blood sugar before driving a car and—after finding a place where you can safely stop your vehicle—every hour while driving.

POSTURAL HYPOTENSION — THE GREAT DECEIVER

Syncope, or fainting, is fairly common as people get older. It is especially common among diabetics. Even more common is near-syncope. This is merely the feeling that you will pass out unless you lie down right away. Simultaneously, your surroundings may look gray or your vision may fade. There are many causes of syncope and near-syncope. These include cardiac and neurological problems, certain medications, and dehydration. These causes are not nearly as common in diabetics as are sudden drops in blood pressure caused by autonomic neuropathy or by inappropriate use of antihypertensive medications—especially diuretics ("water pills") and alpha-1 adrenergic antagonists, such as prazosin and terazosin.

When most of us stand from a seated, supine, or squatting position, the brain sends a message to the blood vessels in our legs to constrict reflexively and instantly. This prevents blood from pooling in the legs, which would deprive the brain of blood and oxygen. If you've had high blood sugars for many years, the nerves that signal the vessels in the legs may conduct the message poorly (a sign of autonomic neuropathy). A drop in blood pressure upon standing, called postural, or orthostatic, hypotension, occurs when this pooling in the legs occurs. For some, the heart may bring blood pressure back up by increasing its rate and amount of contraction. Unfortunately, this does not occur for many diabetics with autonomic neuropathy.

Alternatively, if you eat a big meal, blood may concentrate in your digestive system, also depriving the brain. The normal mechanisms that protect the brain from this shunting of blood may be deficient if you have autonomic neuropathy. It is in part to gauge the potential for these reactions that I measure supine and standing blood pressures, and perform R-R interval studies on all my diabetic patients. A study of medical (mostly nondiabetic) outpatients in the United States suggests that 20 percent of individuals over age 65 and 30 percent of those over age 70 have documentable postural hypotension. For diabetics the incidence is probably much greater.

A common scenario for syncope or near-syncope involves the diabetic who gets up in the middle of the night to urinate and keels over on the way to the bathroom. A simple way to avoid this is to sit on the edge of the bed with your feet dangling for a few minutes before standing.

Another syncope scenario involves the person who goes to the toilet and passes out while trying to produce a bowel movement or urinate. Again, the reflexes that prevent the shunting of blood away from the brain are blunted by autonomic neuropathy.

If syncope is caused by transient low cerebral blood pressure as a result of autonomic neuropathy, one should lay the victim out flat and elevate his feet high above his head. He should return to consciousness almost immediately.

The symptoms of syncope are similar to those of moderate to severe hypoglycemia. In both cases, the brain is being deprived of a basic nutrient—oxygen in the case of syncope, glucose in the case of hypoglycemia. Furthermore, postural hypotension can also occur as a result of hypoglycemia. Some symptoms of near-syncope include faintness, visual changes, and disorientation.

Whatever the cause of fainting or near-syncope, blood sugar must be checked to rule out hypoglycemia. If blood sugar is normal, no amount of glucose will cure the problem. People with recurrent postural hypotension will usually find relief by wearing surgical stockings of 30–40 mm compression. If these are inadequate, waist-high surgical panty hose should be used.

SOME NEW INFORMATION

In 2011 we published in the *Journal of Allergy and Immunology* my discovery that at least 20 percent of diabetics (types 1 and 2) have an inherited disorder called common variable immunodeficiency (CVID). This involves inadequate blood levels of immunoglobulins (antibodies). About one-tenth of these individuals are so severely affected that they develop nonhealing infections or malignancies. The treatment for CVID is intravenous gamma globulin—usually several times per month. All of my insulin-using patients who get gamma globulin experience frequent, unexpected dangerously low blood sugars or reductions in insulin requirements. This has been attributed to a partial but transient recovery of the beta cells that make insulin. These CVID patients must check their blood sugars every 1–2 hours, especially during the first week after an infusion. They must even set an alarm to awaken them once or twice during the night. Although this situation is rare, it can theoretically affect at least 2 percent of people with diabetes.

A FINAL NOTE

If you've heard horror stories about the frequency and severity of severe hypoglycemia in type 1 diabetes, the people you've been hearing about are probably taking industrial doses of insulin to cover large amounts of dietary carbohydrate. On our regimen, this hazard is virtually nil. Someone would have to make a major mistake, such as taking an insulin dose twice or not waiting the full 5 hours (or 6 hours before bedtime) before correcting an elevated blood sugar, for life-threatening episodes to occur. Many type 1 diabetics seek me out because of their frequent hypoglycemic episodes and not necessarily because of their high blood sugars. Our regimen takes care of both.

Please don't neglect to ask others to read this chapter. When you are most in need of help for treating hypoglycemia, you may be incapable of rendering it yourself. So show this chapter to your close relatives, friends, and coworkers and ask them to read it. It should increase their own confidence in coping with such situations, and the potential payoff to you may be considerable.

I will personally answer questions from readers for one hour every month. This free service is available by visiting www.askdrbernstein.net.

21

How to Cope with Dehydration, Dehydrating Illness, and Infection

When you experience vomiting, nausea, fever, diarrhea, or any form of infection, you should immediately contact your physician. I can't emphasize enough the importance of getting treatment and getting it fast. To drive home this point, I'll share the following experience.

Some years ago, I got a call from a woman at about four o'clock on a Sunday afternoon. She wasn't my patient, but her diabetologist was out of town for the weekend with no backup for emergencies. He had never taught her what I teach my patients — the contents of this chapter.

She found my Diabetes Center in the white pages of the phone book. She was alone with her toddler son and had been vomiting continuously since 9 A.M. She asked me what she could do. I told her that she must be so dehydrated that her only choice was to get to a hospital emergency room as fast as possible for intravenous fluid replacement. While she dropped off her son with her mother, I called her local hospital and told them to expect her. I got a call 5 hours later from an attending physician. He had admitted her to the hospital because the emergency room couldn't help her. Why not? Her kidneys had failed from dehydration. Fortunately, the hospital had a dialysis center, so they put her on dialysis and gave her intravenous saline (salt solution). Had dialysis not been available, she would likely have died. As it turned out, she spent 5 days in the hospital.

Clearly, a dehydrating illness is not something to take lightly, not a reason to assume your doctor is going to think you're a hypochondriac if you call every time you have one of the problems discussed in this chapter. This is something that could kill you, and you need prompt treatment.

Why is it, then, that diabetics have a more serious time with dehydrating illness than nondiabetics? Clearly it has something to do with blood sugars.

DEHYDRATION'S VICIOUS CIRCLE

If you are vomiting or have diarrhea, you've either been poisoned (unlikely) or have an infectious illness. If you have an infection, whether it's in your mouth, on your finger, or in your gastrointestinal tract, your blood sugar is most likely going to go up. So you're starting off with elevated blood sugars just by virtue of the infection. If you vomit or have diarrhea, you are losing fluid from a region in the body that normally contains fluid. That lost fluid is going to be replaced from the largest source of fluid in the body, the bloodstream. It's not that you're going to bleed into your stomach — your GI tract is full of blood vessels that are there in part for the exchange of fluids. That's how fluid is absorbed.

Your body naturally tries to maintain a balance, so when fluid disappears from one place, your body tries to replace it using water from your bloodstream. But as water diffuses out of your blood, glucose is left behind, and you end up with a higher blood sugar. In addition, blood vessels are a giant web throughout the body, but unlike a web, the vessels narrow as they travel out from the center, narrowing from inside the body to outside, from inside an organ to its surface, and so on. At any given time, much of the blood is in these narrow, peripheral vessels.

If your bloodstream has lost significant amounts of fluid, as you would in a dehydrating illness, the periphery is not going to be as well supplied as it would normally be. It's like having a whole new insulin resistance simply because insulin and glucose aren't adequately reaching the narrower vessels. Since less glucose will be delivered to the cells adjoining these vessels, your blood sugar concentration will continue to climb. Furthermore, the higher your blood sugars go, the more insulin resistance you will experience. The more insulin-resistant you are, the higher your blood sugars are going to be. A vicious circle.

To make the circle even more vicious, when you have high blood sugars, you urinate — and of course what happens then is that you get even more dehydrated and more insulin-resistant and your blood sugar goes even higher. Now your peripheral cells have a choice — either die from lack of glucose and insulin or metabolize fat. They'll choose the latter. But ketones are created by fat metabolism, causing you to urinate even more to rid yourself of the ketones, taking you to a whole new level of dehydration.

This sequence of events can happen in a matter of hours, as it did with the woman just described. So the name of the game is *prevention.*

How do you prevent illness from causing dehydration? Let's say you wake up in the middle of the night or in the morning and vomit or have a bout of diarrhea. What do you do? Call your physician and let him or her know — even if it's two o'clock in the morning, call your doctor. Even if it turns out to be just something you ate and it's a transient episode, call your doctor or the emergency medical service.

We all get sick from time to time, but if you're on our diet and treatment plan, and if you're reasonably healthy, you shouldn't get sick any more frequently than the average person (unless you have CVID; see page 360) — and probably less frequently than the average diabetic. For diabetics, however, such illness can pose special problems.

As you know, sickness or infection can cause your blood sugar to increase, and injected insulin — even if you don't normally take insulin — can help preserve beta cell function during illness (as well as help keep your blood sugar under control and thereby reduce dehydration). One of the most pressing concerns for diabetics during illness is dehydration, which, as illustrated above, can lead to life-threatening consequences if not handled effectively and rapidly.

DIABETES AND DEHYDRATION: A DANGEROUS COMBINATION

Common causes of dehydration include multiple episodes of diarrhea or vomiting; fever with resulting perspiration; failure to drink adequate fluids, especially during hot weather or prolonged exercise; and very high blood sugars. You probably know that one of the hallmark symptoms of very high blood sugars is the combination of extreme thirst and frequent urination. From what you've already read in this chapter, you should understand the equation. Still, I think it's noteworthy enough to lay it out again for emphasis.

1. Dehydration causes transitory insulin resistance.*
2. During periods of dehydration, blood sugar will tend to rise.
3. High blood sugar, as you know, itself leads to insulin resistance and further blood sugar increase.
4. Blood sugar elevation from dehydration in addition to blood sugar elevation caused by the viral or bacterial infection that led to your vomiting, fever, or diarrhea causes further insulin resistance and blood sugar elevation.
5. High blood sugar causes further dehydration as your kidneys attempt to unload glucose and ketones by producing large amounts of urine.
6. Increased dehydration causes higher blood sugars, which in turn cause further dehydration. All of which brings us back to number 1.

The good news is, however, that simple interventions can halt this spiraling of blood sugars and fluid loss. It's the purpose of this chapter to give you the knowledge to prevent the sort of grave consequences experienced by the lady who called me on that Sunday afternoon—or worse, death.

KETOACIDOSIS AND HYPEROSMOLAR COMA

There are two acute conditions that can develop from the combination of high blood sugars and dehydration. The first is called diabetic ketoacidosis, or DKA. It occurs in people who make virtually no insulin on their own (either type 1 diabetics or type 2 diabetics who have lost nearly all beta cell activity). Very low serum insulin levels, combined with the insulin resistance caused by high blood sugars and dehydration, result in the virtual absence of insulin-mediated glucose transport to the tissues of the body. In the absence of adequate insulin,

---

* It is absolutely important when experiencing dehydrating illness not to do anything that would hasten dehydration—and that includes the use of certain medications, such as ACE inhibitors and diuretics. Never discontinue a medication without discussing it with your doctor, so ask your physician as soon as you experience such an illness about ceasing use of these and similar medications. If you're unsure, most pharmacists can tell you if a particular drug can facilitate dehydration.

the body metabolizes stored fats to produce the energy that tissues require to remain alive. A by-product of fat metabolism is the production of substances called ketones and ketoacids. One of the ketones, acetone, is familiar as the major component of nail polish remover. Ketones may be detected in the urine by using a dipstick such as Keto-stix (see Chapter 3, "Your Diabetic Tool Kit"). Ketones may also be detected on the breath as the aroma of an organic solvent, which is why unconscious diabetics are often mistaken for passed-out drunks.

Ketones and ketoacids are toxic in very large amounts. More important, your kidneys will try to eliminate them with even more urine, thereby causing further dehydration. Some of the hallmarks of severe ketoacidosis are large amounts of ketones in the urine, extreme thirst, dry mouth, nausea, frequent urination, deep labored breathing, and high blood sugar (usually over 350 mg/dl).

The other acute complication of high blood sugar and dehydration, hyperosmolar coma, is a potentially more severe condition, and occurs in people whose beta cells still make some insulin. ("Hyperosmolar" refers to high concentrations of glucose, sodium, and chloride in the blood due to inadequate water to dilute them.) Diabetics who develop this condition usually have some residual beta cell activity, making enough insulin to suppress the metabolism of fats, but not enough to prevent very high blood sugars. As a result, ketones may not appear in the urine or on the breath. Because this condition most commonly occurs in elderly people, who do not become very thirsty when dehydrated, the degree of dehydration is usually greater than in ketoacidosis. Early symptoms of a hyperosmolar state include somnolence and confusion. Extremely high blood sugars (as great as 1,500 mg/dl) have been reported in cases of hyperosmolar coma. Fluid deficit may become so severe that the brain becomes dehydrated. Loss of consciousness and death can occur in both the hyperosmolar state and in severe DKA.

The treatment for DKA and hyperosmolar coma includes fluid replacement and insulin. Fluid replacement alone can have a great effect upon blood sugar because it both dilutes the glucose level in the blood and permits the kidneys to eliminate excess glucose. Fluid also helps the kidneys eliminate ketones in DKA. Our interest here, though, is not in *treating* these conditions — this must be done by a physician or in a hospital — but in *preventing* them.

VOMITING, NAUSEA, AND DIARRHEA

Vomiting, nausea, and diarrhea are most commonly caused by bacterial or viral infections sometimes associated with flulike illness. An essential part of treatment is to stop eating. Since you can certainly survive a few days without eating, this should pose no problem. But if you're not eating, it makes sense to ask what dose of insulin or ISA you should take.

Adjusting Your Diabetes Medication

If you're on one of the medication regimens described in this book, the answer is simple: you take the amount and type of medication that you'd normally take to cover the basal, or fasting, state and skip any doses that are intended to cover meals. If, for example, you ordinarily take Levemir, Lantus, or NPH as basal insulin upon arising and at bedtime, and a rapid-acting insulin before meals, you'd continue the basal insulin and skip the preprandial rapid-acting insulin for those meals you won't be eating. Similarly, if you take an ISA on arising and/or at bedtime for the fasting state, and again to cover meals, you skip the doses for those meals that you do not plan to eat.

In both of the above cases, *it's essential that the medications used for the fasting state continue at their full doses.* This is in direct contradiction to traditional "sick day" treatment, but it's a major reason why patients who carefully follow our regimens should not develop DKA or hyperosmolar coma when they are ill.

Of course, if you're vomiting, you won't be able to keep down oral medication and this poses yet another problem.

Remember, because infection and dehydration may each cause blood sugar to increase, you may need additional coverage for any blood sugar elevation. Such additional coverage should usually take the form of rapid-acting insulin. This is one of the reasons that we advocate the training of *all* diabetics in the techniques of insulin injection—even those who, when not sick, can be controlled by just diet and ISAs. Using insulin when you're sick may be especially important for you, because it helps to relieve the added burden on beta cells that leads to burnout. This is but one of the reasons it's mandatory that you contact your physician immediately when you feel ill. He or she should be able to tell you how much coverage with insulin will be necessary, and when to take it. The protocol for such coverage is discussed on pages 318–321, but because of its importance, it bears repeating here briefly:

1. Measure blood sugars on arising and every 5 hours thereafter.
2. Inject enough rapid-acting insulin at these times to bring your blood sugars down to your target value. Intramuscular shots are preferred (see pages 324–327) because of their more rapid effect, but subcutaneous injection is also acceptable. It is prudent to continue blood sugar measurements and insulin coverage, even during the night, for as long as blood sugars continue to rise.

If you're so ill that you cannot check your own blood sugars and inject your own insulin, someone else must do this for you, or you should be hospitalized. The potential consequences are so serious that you have no other options.

Medications to Be Discontinued

Certain medications that can accelerate dehydration or temporarily impair kidney function should be discontinued during a dehydrating illness. These include diuretics, ACE inhibitors, and certain arthritis medications such as NSAIDs (ibuprofen, Motrin, Advil) and COX-2 inhibitors. NSAIDs may, however, be used as a last resort to treat a fever only if other medications are ineffective. Discuss this with your physician before discontinuing any medication he has prescribed. If you can't reach him, then discontinue those listed here.

Controlling the Vomiting

The mainstay of treatment is fluid replacement, but if you've been vomiting, you'll probably be unable to hold anything down, including fluids. If symptoms disappear after vomiting once and you can keep things down, then there's likely no need for treatment to prevent further vomiting (*but still notify your physician*). Ordinary vomiting can usually be suppressed with Tigan (trimethobenzamide HCl) injections, administered every 3–5 hours if vomiting persists. Tigan should not be taken by mouth, as it will probably be vomited up before it can work. It is sold in the United States as a 100 mg/ml solution in 20 ml vials. For an adult, we usually inject a trial dose of 30 units with an insulin syringe. It is injected just like insulin. Small children can be started at 10 units. If vomiting persists 30 minutes after injection, the dose can be doubled. Because big injections leave large lumps under the skin, many users prefer to inject multiple 10-unit doses at different sites.

Tigan works for most people, but in about 20 percent of cases, it doesn't, which is all the more reason to contact your physician when you experience a potentially dehydrating illness. If vomiting or nausea continues for more than 3 hours, or if it cannot be halted by Tigan within 1 hour, he or she may want you to try a second or even a third dose or may prescribe a visit to a hospital emergency room to receive intravenous fluid (saline) and to have the cause established. Some surgical emergencies such as intestinal obstruction can lead to vomiting, as can poisoning, gastroparesis (see Chapter 22), DKA, and so on. Vomiting is a serious problem for people with diabetes, and should not be treated casually.

Large doses of Tigan can cause bizarre neurological side effects,* especially in children and in slim elderly people. The antidote to these effects would be one gulp of diphenhydramine elixir or sugar-free syrup (e.g., Benadryl), if you can hold it down. When vomiting has ceased, Tigan should probably not be administered more often than every 3 hours, or in doses greater than that prescribed by your physician. If Tigan doesn't work fully within 1 hour, take more and call your physician again.

Fluid Replacement

Once vomiting has been controlled, you should immediately begin to drink fluids. Two questions naturally arise at this point: What fluid? And how much? There are three factors that must be considered in preparing the fluid to be used.

First, it must be something you don't dislike. Second, it should contain no carbohydrate (therefore *no* Gatorade, Enfalyte, Oralyte, Glucerna, or sports drinks), but artificial sweeteners are okay. This guideline also contradicts conventional treatment, which usually calls for sweetened beverages to offset the excessive amounts of insulin that many diabetics use. Finally, the fluids should replace the electrolytes — sodium, potassium, and chloride — that are lost from the body when we lose fluids. Beverages commonly used by my patients include diet soda, diluted iced tea, seltzer, water, and carbohydrate-free bouillon or clear soup. To these fluids, we add electrolytes.

---

* Including tremors, lip-smacking, and neck-jerking.

To each quart of liquid, add:

Exactly but *no more than* 1 level teaspoon table salt (½ teaspoon if
it tastes too salty) (provides sodium and chloride)
Approximately but *no more than* ¼ teaspoon salt substitute (see
list, page 70) (provides potassium and chloride)

If the vomiting ceased after one episode without the need for Tigan,
it isn't necessary to add the salts to the fluid you consume.

In anticipation of these rare "sick days," you should always have on
hand several 2-quart bottles of diet soda or seltzer, or two empty
2-quart plastic iced tea pitchers. The pitchers can be used to store
whatever rehydration concoction you may prefer instead of diet soda.
When the need arises, one pitcher of fluid can be kept by your bed-
side, while the second is kept cool in the refrigerator.

The volume of fluid you will require each day when not eating
depends upon your size, since large people utilize more fluid than
small people. If your blood sugars are elevated or if your urine on dipstick is positive for more than moderate amounts of ketones, you will
need much more fluid than otherwise. The ongoing fluid requirement
for most adults without these problems comes to about 2.7 (women)
to 3.7 (men) quarts (or liters) daily while fasting.* In addition, within
the first 24 hours you should replace the estimated fluid loss caused by
vomiting, fever, or diarrhea. This may come to another few quarts, so
clearly you will have to do a lot of drinking. Your physician should be
consulted for instructions regarding your fluid intake while ill. Keep
an exact record of the volume of fluid consumed, as she may ask for it.
If for any reason you cannot consume or keep down the amount of
liquid that she or he recommends, you may have to be hospitalized to
receive intravenous fluids.

If you do have to be hospitalized for IV fluid replacement, you may
run into the difficulty of inexperienced or ignorant hospital personnel wanting to give you one or another standard IV solution that contains some sort of sugar — dextrose, glucose, lactose, lactated Ringer's
solution, fructose, and so on. Do not allow them to do so, and do not
assume they know more than you do about your situation. Insist upon

---

* Figure on 0.022 quarts per pound of body weight (0.048 liters per kilogram).
Thus, about 3 quarts (or 3 liters) for a person weighing 150 pounds (68 kilos).

a saline solution,* and if they balk, insist upon speaking with the hospital administrator and threaten malpractice and wrongful death lawsuits, if necessary, to persuade them of what you need. Although not usually effective outside the United States, such threats are usually effective here.

Diarrhea

First note that any diarrhea with bloody stools or fever requires the immediate attention of a physician or a visit to the emergency room. Here again we are faced with three basic problems: blood sugar control, control of the diarrhea to prevent further water and electrolyte loss, and fluid and electrolyte replacement.

The guidelines for blood sugar control are the same as if you have been vomiting (see above). Fluid and electrolyte replacement should be the same as for vomiting, except that 1 level teaspoon of sodium bicarbonate (baking soda) should be added to each quart of the electrolyte-replacement mixture. The primary treatment for diarrhea, as for vomiting, is to stop eating. Medications to relieve diarrhea, if any, should be specified by your physician. Some forms of diarrhea caused by bacteria, such as "traveler's diarrhea," may warrant the use of Pepto-Bismol (bismuth subsalicylate) and antibiotics such as ciprofloxacin or tetracycline.

In my experience, there is one antidiarrheal agent that has always worked, Lomotil (diphenoxylate HCl with atropine sulfate). This is a prescription drug that you should have your doctor prescribe (in advance of any illness) in both liquid form in a dropper bottle and as a tablet. The generic versions are much less expensive and just as effective. You should always have several bottles on hand. You will find dosing instructions on the package insert. If diarrhea continues, double the dose every hour until it ceases and continue the final dose every 3 hours until your physician advises you to discontinue. (Once the diarrhea ceases, it would be more convenient and cheaper for an adult to switch from the liquid to the tablet form of the drug. One 2.5 mg tablet is equivalent to 1 teaspoon or full dropper of the liquid.)

---

* Beware of D5 or D10 saline solutions. These contain dextrose (glucose) and will certainly raise your blood sugar and thereby cause further dehydration. For uncontrollable diarrhea, *half normal* saline should be used; otherwise, *normal* saline.

Overdosing will not only dry out your gut, which we are seeking, but also can dry out your larynx, mouth, nose, and eyes. Lomotil can also make you drowsy, but its effect on diarrhea is miraculous, in my opinion. If an equivalent to Lomotil is not available in your country, one 30 mg codeine tablet is equivalent to about 10 Lomotil tablets.

If diarrhea is accompanied by fever or bloody stools, *do not use Lomotil or codeine,* and see a physician immediately. This is because your gut may contain toxic agents that should not be retained.

FEVER

No doubt you've heard the advice "Drink plenty of fluids" for a fever. This is because a fever causes considerable fluid loss through the skin as perspiration. Your loss of fluid can be difficult to estimate, so your physician may want to assume that you'd require 1–2 more quarts of fluid daily than you'd normally need. Ordinarily, a mild fever helps to destroy the infectious agent (virus or bacteria) that is causing the fever. The tendency to sleep out a fever may also be beneficial. For a diabetic, however, the somnolence that you experience with a fever may discourage you from checking your blood sugar, covering with insulin, drinking adequate fluid, and calling your physician every few hours. If you don't have someone to awaken you every 20 minutes, you should use aspirin, acetaminophen (Tylenol), or ibuprofen (Advil or Motrin), in accordance with your doctor's instructions, to help fight the fever. Beware, however, that aspirin can cause false positive readings on tests for urinary ketones, so don't even test for ketones if you are using aspirin. *Never use aspirin or ibuprofen (or any of the NSAIDs) for a fever in children* because of the risk of Reye's syndrome. Excessive doses of aspirin or NSAIDs (naproxen, ibuprofen, and many others) can cause severe hypoglycemia. If at all possible, *try not to use NSAIDs, as the combination of these drugs with dehydration can cause kidney failure.* NSAIDs should **never** be used by people with kidney impairment. Acetaminophen can be highly toxic if used in doses greater than those indicated on the package label (3,250 mg/day for adults).

If you have a fever, the guidelines for blood sugar control and replacement of fluid are almost the same as indicated previously for vomiting. There is one difference, however. Since there is very little electrolyte loss in perspiration, it's not necessary to add salts to the fluid you consume if you're not vomiting or experiencing diarrhea. Certainly there is no reason not to eat if you feel hungry—but if you want to eat, cover your meals with your usual dose of insulin or ISA. If you're hungry for only a small meal, eat half or a quarter of your usual protein and carbohydrate, and cover it with only half or a quarter of your usual dose of insulin or ISA.

ADDITIONAL SUGGESTIONS FOR DEHYDRATING ILLNESS

Like hypoglycemia, dehydrating illness can be life-threatening to a diabetic. Encourage the people you live with to read this chapter carefully. The supplies mentioned should be kept in locations known to all. Phone your physician at the first sign of a fever, diarrhea, or vomiting. The chances are that he or she would much rather be contacted early, when dehydration and loss of blood sugar control can be prevented. Emergency situations make treatment more difficult, so you can make your life and your physician's a bit easier by phoning before major problems occur.

Your physician will probably ask you whether your urine shows ketones, so use the Ketostix whenever you urinate before you call. Also, let your doctor know if you have taken any aspirin in the prior 24 hours, as this can cause a false positive Ketostix reading. If you are not eating, your urine will certainly show "moderate" ketones. Your physician should therefore fear ketoacidosis only if it shows "high" ketones combined with high blood sugars (180 mg/dl or above). Always report your recent blood sugars when you phone your physician.

NONDEHYDRATING INFECTIONS

Most infections can cause elevation of blood sugars, from an infected toe to infected tonsils to infected heart valves. Most infections cause symptoms that are recognizable, such as burning upon urination if you have a urinary tract infection, coughing if you have bronchitis, and so on. So you'll get pretty prompt warning from your body that you should immediately contact your physician. If you have type 2 diabetes or early type 1, you certainly don't want your blood sugars to get so high that your remaining beta cells are destroyed. My friend Jay put off visiting a urologist until his blood sugars got so high that his type 2 diabetes became type 1 diabetes and he went from requiring no insulin to 5 daily insulin injections. Occult, or hidden, infections will not become readily apparent unless you notice that your blood sugars have become unreasonably high and you have the good judgment to contact your doctor.

By far the most common type of occult infection is that family of infections that affect dental structures. This includes infections that affect root canals, gums, and jawbones. A history of elevated blood sugars over a period of years predisposes diabetics to such infections; these infections, in turn, predispose diabetics to high blood sugars and severe insulin resistance.

If one of my patients calls our office and complains of recent-onset high blood sugars but no apparent accompanying infection (no coughing, for instance), we ask if she is reusing insulin syringes and contaminating insulin, making injections relatively ineffective (see page 272). If the answer is no, then we recommend a visit to the dentist immediately to search for an oral infection.

Among the things that your dentist should do are to examine your gums very carefully and to tap every tooth to see if one or more are tender. He or she should also touch each tooth with a chip of ice. Pain upon exposure to cold is the most common overt symptom of infection in the tooth or jawbone, in my experience. We have had patients with dentists who refused to do this and we've had to instruct the patients to find better dentists. This is one of those many cases of being a good, educated health care consumer in order to get proper treatment for your diabetes. In each case, when a new dentist performed these tests, a problem was found. If your dentist does find a problem, he or she will probably refer you to an endodontist or periodontist to treat the infection. Not only can dental infections cause blood sugar elevation, but there is now considerable evidence that combinations of dental bacteria in the bloodstream can actually play a role in heart attacks.

Even after such dental infections have been successfully treated, however, blood sugar elevations frequently continue for many months. If blood sugars don't return to your target immediately after treatment, an appropriate antibiotic should be prescribed and continued until blood sugars remain at their preinfection level. Many people require continuation of antibiotics for as long as a year after treatment to prevent further blood sugar increases. This is because the gum or tooth infection frequently spreads to the adjacent jawbone, causing osteomyelitis. When using oral antibiotics, always take a probiotic every day,* at least 2 hours before or after the antibiotic, to replace gastrointestinal bacteria killed by the antibiotic.

To help prevent dental infections, it is wise to arrange with your dentist for tartar and plaque to be removed from your teeth every three months. The best results are usually achieved by periodontists or their technicians. You should also brush your teeth at least twice daily and after meals floss from between your teeth any food that remains there. If your teeth are too tightly spaced for flossing, try Doctor's BrushPicks or GUM Soft-Picks, which are available at most pharmacies.

> I will personally answer questions from readers for one hour every month. This free service is available by visiting www.askdrbernstein.net.

---

* My current favorite probiotic is saccharomyces boulardii (brand name Florastor). It is available at most pharmacies.

22

Delayed Stomach-Emptying: Gastroparesis

A number of times throughout this book, you've come across the terms "delayed stomach-emptying" and "gastroparesis." As I explained in Chapter 2, elevated blood sugars for prolonged periods can impair the ability of nerves to function properly. It's very common that the nerves that stimulate the muscular activity, enzyme secretion, and acid production essential to digestion function poorly in long-standing diabetics. These changes affect the stomach, the gut, or both. Dr. Richard McCullum, a noted authority on digestion, has said that if a diabetic has any other form of neuropathy (dry feet, reduced feeling in the toes, diminished reflexes, et cetera), he or she will also experience delayed or erratic digestion.

Slowed digestion can be fraught with unpleasant symptoms (rarely), or it may only be detectable when we review blood sugar profiles (commonly) or perform certain diagnostic tests. The picture is different for each of us. For more than twenty-five years, I suffered from many unpleasant symptoms myself. I eventually saw them taper off and vanish after thirteen years of essentially normal blood sugars. Some of the physical complaints possible (usually after meals) include burning along the midline of the chest ("heartburn"), belching, feeling full after a small meal (early satiety), bloating, nausea, vomiting, constipation, constipation alternating with diarrhea, cramps a few inches above the belly button, and an acid taste in the mouth.

GASTROPARESIS: CAUSES AND EFFECTS

Most of these symptoms, as well as effects upon blood sugar, relate to delayed stomach-emptying. This condition is called gastroparesis diabeticorum, which translates from the Latin as "weak stomach of diabetics." It is believed that the major cause of this condition is neuropathy (nerve impairment) of the vagus nerve. This nerve mediates many of the autonomic or regulatory functions of the body, including heart rate and digestion. In men, neuropathy of the vagus nerve can also lead to difficulty in achieving penile erections. To understand the effects of gastroparesis, refer to Figure 22-1.

On the left is a representation of a normal stomach after a meal. The contents are emptying into the intestines, through the pylorus. The pyloric valve is wide open (relaxed). The lower esophageal sphincter (LES) is tightly closed, to prevent regurgitation of stomach contents. Not shown is the grinding and churning activity of the muscular walls of the normal stomach.

On the right is pictured a stomach with gastroparesis. The normal

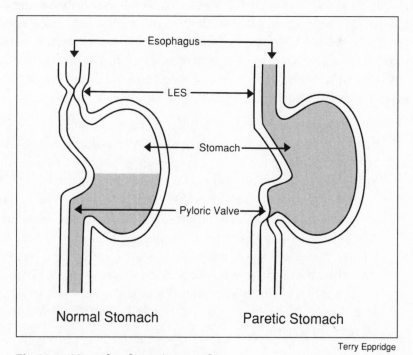

Terry Eppridge

Fig. 22-1. *Normal and paretic stomachs.*

rhythmic motions of the stomach walls are absent. The pyloric valve is tightly closed, preventing the unloading of stomach contents. A tiny opening about the size of a pencil point may permit a small amount of fluid to dribble out. When the pyloric valve is in tight spasm, some of us can sometimes feel a sharp cramp above the belly button. Since the lower esophageal sphincter is relaxed or open, acidic stomach contents can back up into the esophagus (the tube that connects the throat to the stomach). This can cause a burning sensation along the midline of the chest, especially while the person is lying down. I have seen patients whose teeth were actually eroded over time by regurgitated stomach acid.

Because the stomach does not empty readily, one may feel full even after a small meal. In extreme cases, several meals accumulate and cause severe bloating. More commonly, however, you may have gastroparesis and not be aware of it. In mild cases, emptying may be slowed somewhat, but not enough to make you feel any different. Nevertheless, this can cause problems with blood sugar control. Consuming certain substances, such as tricyclic antidepressants, caffeine, fat, and alcohol, can further slow stomach-emptying and other digestive processes.

Some years ago, I received a letter from my friend Bob Anderson. His diabetic wife, Trish, who was not my patient and has since passed away, had been experiencing frequent loss of consciousness from severe hypoglycemia, caused by delayed digestion. His description of an endoscopic exam, when he was allowed to look through a flexible tube into Trish's stomach and gut, paints a graphic picture.

> All this brings me to today's endoscopy exam. I watched through the scope and for the first time, I now understand what you have been saying about diabetic gastroparesis. Not until I viewed the inside of the duodenum did I understand the catastrophic effect of 33 years of diabetes upon the internal organs. There was almost no muscle action apparent to move food out of the stomach. It appeared as a very relaxed smooth-sided tube instead of having muscular ridges ringing the passage. I suppose a picture is worth a thousand words. Diabetic neuropathy is more than a manifestation of a tilting gait, blindness, and other easily observable presentations; it wrecks the whole system. This you well know. I am learning.

HOW DOES GASTROPARESIS AFFECT BLOOD SUGAR CONTROL?

Consider the individual who has very little phase I insulin release and takes rapid-acting insulin or one of the older-type (sulfonylurea) or newer pancreas-provoking OHAs before each meal. If he were to take his medication and then skip the meal, his blood sugar would plummet. When the stomach empties too slowly, it can have almost the same effect as skipping a meal. If we knew when the stomach would empty, we could delay the insulin shot or add some NPH insulin to the regular to slow down its action. The big problem with gastroparesis, however, is its *unpredictability*. We never know when, or how fast, the stomach will empty. If the pyloric valve is not in spasm, the stomach contents may empty partially within minutes and totally within 3 hours. On another occasion, when the valve is tightly closed, the stomach may remain loaded for days. Thus, blood sugar may plummet 1–2 hours after eating, and then rise very high, say 12 hours later, after emptying eventually occurs. It is this unpredictability that can make blood sugar control impossible if significant gastroparesis is ignored in people who take insulin (or the type of OHAs I don't recommend) before meals.

For most type 2 diabetics, fortunately, even symptomatic gastroparesis may not grossly impede blood sugar control, because they may still produce some phase I and phase II insulin. They therefore may not require significant amounts of injected insulin to cover their low-carbohydrate meals. Much of their insulin is produced in response to food in the intestines or to blood sugar elevation. Thus, if the stomach does not empty, only the low basal (fasting) levels of insulin are released, and hypoglycemia does not occur. Of course, the sulfonylurea and similar OHAs (which I don't recommend) can cause hypoglycemia under such circumstances. If the stomach empties continually but very slowly, the beta cells of most type 2s will produce insulin concurrently. Sometimes the stomach may empty suddenly, as the pyloric valve relaxes. This will produce a rapid blood sugar rise, caused by the sudden absorption of carbohydrate following the entrance of stomach contents into the small intestine. Most beta cells of type 2 patients then cannot counter rapidly enough. Eventually, however, insulin release catches up and blood sugar drops to normal, if a reasonable regimen is followed. If your supper doesn't fully leave your stomach before you sleep, you may awaken with a high morning blood sugar due to emptying overnight, even though your bedtime blood sugar was low or normal.

In any event, if you do not require insulin or use a sulfonylurea-type OHA before meals, there is no hazard of hypoglycemia due to delayed stomach-emptying. This assumes that any long-acting insulin or sulfonylurea is administered in doses that cover only the fasting state, as discussed in prior chapters. The traditional use of large doses of these medications, meant to cover both the fasting and fed states, brings with it the hazard of postprandial hypoglycemia when gastroparesis is present.

DIAGNOSING GASTROPARESIS

When I treat new patients who require premeal rapid-acting insulin, I always test them for gastroparesis before I negotiate a new meal plan. If your physician does not know how to do an R-R interval study (see page 65) and you have symptoms or blood sugar profiles like the ones described in this chapter, he should assume you have gastroparesis. If your R-R study at the initial physical exam is grossly abnormal, he can be quite certain of gastroparesis. Remember that this study checks the ability of the vagus nerve to regulate heart rate. If the nerve fibers going to the heart are impaired, the branches that activate the stomach are probably also inevitably impaired. In my experience, the correlation of grossly abnormal R-R studies with demonstrable gastroparesis is very real.*

Diagnostic Tests
Given the physical symptoms or the abnormal R-R study, your physician may want to consider further tests to evaluate your condition. The most sophisticated of these studies is the gamma-ray technetium scan. This test is performed at many medical centers, and is quite costly. It works this way: You eat some scrambled eggs to which a

---

* If, during an R-R study, your heart rate varies only 28 percent between inhaling and exhaling, then you will likely have mild gastroparesis. If the variation is about 20 percent, gastroparesis will probably be what I call moderate, and if less than 15 percent, I would call it severe.

minute amount of radioactive technetium has been added. A gamma-ray scanner trained on your abdomen measures (from outside your body) the low levels of radiation the technetium emits as the eggs pass from your stomach into your small intestine. If the gamma radiation drops off rapidly, the study is considered normal.

A less precise study can be performed at a much lower cost by any radiologist. This is called the barium hamburger test. In this test, you eat a quarter-pound hamburger and then drink a liquid that contains the heavy element barium. Every half hour or so, an X-ray photo is taken of your stomach. Since the barium shows up in these photos, the radiologist can estimate what percentage of the barium remains in your stomach at the end of each time period. Total emptying within 3 hours or less is usually considered normal.

Despite their theoretical usefulness, neither of these studies is anywhere near 100 percent sensitive, because of the unpredictable nature of the paretic stomach. One day it may empty normally, another day it may be a bit slow, and on yet another day its emptying may be severely delayed. Because of this unpredictability factor, the study may have to be repeated a number of times before a diagnosis can be made. The possibility exists that you could have several normal studies but still have abnormal stomach-emptying. I therefore advise my patients against relying on either of these two tests. The R-R interval study is my gold standard (see page 65), because the status of the vagus nerve does not depend on how your stomach empties on a particular day.

Telltale Blood Sugar Patterns

Having medical tests is bad enough, but having to repeat them with conflicting results naturally proved quite annoying to my patients many years ago when I actually repeated them. Worse than annoyance, the studies are not cheap, and most insurance companies will not pay for repeats of the same study unless they're separated by many months. If you're regularly measuring your blood sugar levels and trying to keep them in the normal range, it's really not difficult to spot gastroparesis that's severe enough to affect blood sugars. For practical purposes, this is just the degree of gastroparesis that should concern us.

Following are some of the typical blood sugar patterns that I look for. To call these patterns, though, is slightly misleading. *The hallmark of gastroparesis is randomness, unpredictability from one meal to the next.* These "patterns" come and go in such a fashion that blood sugar profiles are rarely similar on 2 or 3 successive days. The first two patterns together are highly indicative of gastroparesis, while the third by itself is usually adequate for diagnosis.

- Low blood sugar occurring 1–3 hours after some (not necessarily all) meals.
- Elevated blood sugar occurring 5 or more hours after meals with no other apparent explanation.
- Significantly higher fasting blood sugars in the morning than at bedtime, especially if supper was finished at least 5 hours before retiring. If the bedtime long-acting insulin or ISA is gradually increased in an effort to lower the fasting blood sugars, we may find that the bedtime dose is much higher than the morning dose. On some days fasting blood sugar may still be high, but on other days it may be normal or even too low. We're thus giving extra bedtime medications to accommodate overnight stomach-emptying—but on some days the stomach doesn't empty overnight and fasting blood sugars drop too low.

Having seen such patterns of blood sugar, we can then perform a simple experiment to confirm that they really are caused by delayed emptying.

Skip supper and its premeal insulin or ISA one night. When you go to bed, be sure to take your basal (bedtime) insulin or ISA, then measure your blood sugar; measure your fasting blood sugar the next morning on arising. If, without supper, your blood sugar has dropped or remained unchanged overnight, gastroparesis is the most likely cause of the roller-coaster morning blood sugars.

Repeat this experiment several days later, and again a third time, after another few days. If each experiment results in the same effect, delayed stomach-emptying is virtually certain on one or more of the nights when you had eaten. When you had previously been eating suppers, at least *some* of the following mornings had shown an overnight rise in blood sugars. Since such rises occurred on nights when you had eaten supper, but *not* on the nights when you had *not* eaten, the rise must have been caused by food that did not leave your stomach until after you went to bed. Be very cautious when performing this experiment, as you may experience severe hypoglycemia upon arising or during the night. To play it safe, check your blood sugar midway through the night and correct it if it's below your target.

"False Gastroparesis"

I've seen a number of patients whose blood sugar profiles or physical symptoms could have been diagnostic of gastroparesis, yet their R-R interval studies were normal or only slightly impaired. These people had delayed stomach-emptying but well-functioning vagus nerves. The conflicting data obliged me to order upper gastrointestinal endoscopic studies for them. Endoscopy uses a thin, flexible, lighted fiber-optic cable to look directly into the stomach and duodenum.

The endoscopic tests demonstrated that they all had abnormalities unrelated to their diabetes. Such findings have included gastric or duodenal ulcers, erosive and atrophic gastritis, irritable gastrointestinal tract, hiatal hernia, celiac disease, and other gastrointestinal disorders such as tonic or spastic stomach. Each of these conditions required treatment distinct from treatment for diabetes. Only with hiatal hernias were we unable to at least partially alleviate the digestive problem. In such cases, however, surgical correction of the hiatal hernia is possible, but it may or may not normalize emptying. Blood tests for parietal cell antibodies, serum vitamin B-12, and ferritin might be performed to rule out autoimmune gastropathy as a cause of gastritis. Likewise, serum serotonin levels can be tested to rule out a carcinoid tumor.

The following suggestions for treating gastroparesis may or may not facilitate stomach-emptying for the above conditions but should certainly be tried. The loud and clear message from this is that the R-R interval study should be performed on every diabetic patient whose blood sugar profiles resemble those outlined above.

APPROACHES TO CONTROL OF GASTROPARESIS

It is worth noting that gastroparesis can be cured by extended periods of normal blood sugars. I've seen several relatively mild cases where special treatment was terminated after about one year, and blood sugar profiles remained flat thereafter. At the same time, R-R studies improved or normalized. Since my late teens, I experienced severe daily belching and burning in my chest. These symptoms gradually eased off, and eventually disappeared, but only after thirteen years of nearly normal blood sugars. My last R-R study was normal. The "sacrifices" in lifestyle required for treatment of gastroparesis may really pay off months or years later. The vagus nerve doesn't control only stomach-emptying — there are a number of other complications resulting from impaired vagus function that can be reversed by maintaining normal blood sugars. The regained ability to sustain a penile erection is an important one for many of my male patients.

Once gastroparesis has been confirmed as the major cause of high overnight blood sugars and wide random variations in blood sugar profiles, we can begin to attempt to control or minimize its effects. If your blood sugar profiles reflect significant gastroparesis, there is no way to get them under control only by juggling doses of insulin. There's just too much danger of either very high or very low blood sugars for such approaches to work. The only chance for effective treatment is to concentrate on improving stomach-emptying.

How do we do this?

We have four basic approaches. First is the use of medications. Second is special exercises or massage during and after meals. Third is meal plan modification utilizing ordinary foods, and fourth is meal plan modification utilizing semiliquid or liquid meals.

It's unusual for a single approach to normalize blood sugar profiles fully, so most often we try a combination of these four approaches, adapted to the preferences and needs of the individual. As these attempts start to smooth out blood sugars, we must modify our doses of insulin accordingly. The guidelines that we use to judge the efficacy of a given approach or combination of approaches are these:

- Reduction or elimination of physical complaints such as early satiety, nausea, regurgitation, bloating, heartburn, belching, and constipation
- Elimination of random postprandial hypoglycemia
- Elimination of random, unexpected high fasting blood sugars — probably the most common sign of gastroparesis that we encounter
- Flattening out of blood sugar profiles

Remember that the last three of these improvements may not be possible even without gastroparesis if you're following conventional dietary and medication regimens for "control" of your blood sugar. For example, I know of no way that will truly flatten out blood sugar profiles if you're on a high-carbohydrate diet and the associated large doses of insulin.

Medications That Facilitate Stomach-Emptying

There is no medication that will cure gastroparesis. The only "cure" is months or years of normal blood sugars. There are, however, some pharmaceutical preparations that may speed the emptying of your stomach after a meal if your gastroparesis is only mild or moderate in severity (see footnote on page 380). These will help smooth out your blood sugar profiles after that meal. Most diabetics with mild to moderate gastroparesis will require medication before every meal.

When gastroparesis is very mild, it may be possible to get away with medication only before supper. For some reason—perhaps because most people tend not to be as physically active after supper, and may have their largest meal of the day in the evening—digestion of supper appears to be more impaired than that of other meals. It is also likely that stomach-emptying is slower in the evening, even for nondiabetics.

Medications for gastroparesis may take the form of liquids or pills. The question immediately arises that if pills must dissolve in the stomach to become effective, just how effective are they going to be? My experience is that they're of questionable value unless chewed. The time required for a pill to dissolve in a paretic stomach is likely to be lengthy, and consequently the medication may take several hours to become effective. I prefer to prescribe only liquid medications or chewed tablets for stimulating gastric (stomach) emptying. All the medications described below are prescription-only, with the exception of Super Papaya Enzyme Plus and betaine hydrochloride with pepsin.

Cisapride suspension (Propulsid, Janssen Pharmaceutica) stimulates the vagus nerve to facilitate stomach-emptying. I usually prescribe 1 tablespoon (25 mg), 15–30 minutes before meals for adults. Many people will require 2 tablespoons for maximum effect. Larger doses appear to be of little added value. The manufacturer recommends doses only up to 20 mg (2 teaspoons) for the treatment of esophageal reflux disease. This condition is much more responsive to treatment than is diabetic gastroparesis, which as a rule requires the larger doses. The package insert also recommends a bedtime dose, which serves no purpose for gastroparesis. In many cases, cisapride alone will not bring about complete stomach-emptying. We may add other medications or methods if blood sugar profiles don't level off.

Cisapride can inhibit or compete for liver enzymes that clear certain medications from the bloodstream. Your physician should therefore review all your medications, especially antidepressants, antibiotics, statins, and antifungal agents, before prescribing cisapride.* Stimulating the vagus nerve will also slow the heart. Since diabetics with gastroparesis usually have an excessively rapid heart rate (more than 80 beats per minute) this is not often a problem. Some individuals, however, have a cardiac conduction defect that abnormally slows the heart. For such people, cisapride can stop the heart, resulting in death. Since, for many years, physicians have ignored this bold warning on the package insert, a number of deaths actually have occurred. The product has therefore been removed from the marketplace in many countries. It is still available in the United States at no charge as an "investigational drug" if prescribed by a gastroenterologist who has been cleared for its use by the investigational review board of his hospital. It is also available from pharmacies in New Zealand under the trade name Prepulsid (not a misspelling). It may be purchased via the Internet after searching for websites containing the words "pharmacy" and "New Zealand." Such a purchase will not be covered by your insurance (unless you happen to live in New Zealand), and with shipping charges, it can be expensive. Furthermore, many pharmacies in New Zealand refuse to ship to the United States. I've been told that some compounding pharmacies in the United States prepare cisapride. Since this agent works by stimulating the vagus nerve, it will not produce results if the nerve is almost dead — as with heart rate variability less than 13 percent on an R-R interval study.

Super Papaya Enzyme Plus has been praised by many of my patients for its rapid relief of some of the physical symptoms of gastroparesis — bloating and belching, for example. Some claim that it also helps to level off the blood sugar swings caused by gastroparesis. The product consists of pleasant-tasting chewable tablets that contain a variety of enzymes (papain, amylase, proteases, bromelain, lipase, and cellulase) that digest protein, fat, carbohydrate, and fiber while they are still in your stomach. You would normally chew 3–5 tablets spaced at the start of, during, and at the end of each meal. The tablets

---

* For a list of medications that should not be used with cisapride, go to www .propulsid-lap.com.

are available in most health food stores and are marketed by American Health, 2100 Smithtown Avenue, Ronkonkoma, NY 11779, (800) 445-7137, www.americanhealthus.com. They are also available from Rosedale Pharmacy, (888) 796-3348. Some of my kosher patients use a similar product called **Freeda Parvenzyme,** which is distributed by Freeda Vitamins, 47-25 Thirty-fourth Street, 3rd Floor, Long Island City, NY 11101, (800) 777-3737, www.freedavitamins.com. The small amount of sorbitol and similar sweeteners contained in these products should not have a significant effect on your blood sugar if consumption is limited to the above dose.

Domperidone (Motilium, Janssen Pharmaceutica) is not available in the United States. It can be purchased in Canada, the U.K., and perhaps some other countries. Pharmacies in Canada are no longer permitted to ship medications to the United States unless they are prescribed by a Canadian physician. It therefore may be necessary to purchase it via the Internet.* Since it is not available as a liquid, we ask patients to chew 2 tablets (10 mg each) 1 hour before meals and to swallow with 8 ounces of water or diet soda. I limit dosing to 2 tablets because larger doses can cause sexual dysfunction in men and absence of menses in women. These problems resolve when the drug is discontinued. Since it works by a mechanism different from those of the preceding products, its effects can be additive (that is, useful with other preparations). Janssen may market a liquid form of this product in the United States at some time in the future. In the meantime, some gastroenterologists are able to prescribe it, like Propulsid, as an investigational drug; it may also be available from some compounding chemists.

Metoclopramide syrup may be the most powerful stimulant of gastric emptying. It works in a fashion similar to domperidone, by inhibiting the effects of dopamine in the stomach. Because it can readily enter the brain, it can cause serious side effects, such as somnolence, depression, agitation, and neurologic problems that resemble parkinsonism. These side effects can appear immediately in some individuals or only after many months of continuous use in others. Because

---

* A number of Canadian pharmacies for an additional charge of $5 can secure prescriptions for distant foreign patients from Canadian physicians.

gastroparesis often requires doses high enough to cause side effects, I use this medication infrequently and limit dosing to no more than 2 teaspoons 30 minutes before meals.

If you use metoclopramide, you should keep on hand the antidote to its side effects—diphenhydramine elixir or sugar-free syrup (e.g., Benadryl). Two tablespoons usually work. *If side effects become serious enough to warrant use of the antidote, the metoclopramide should be immediately and permanently discontinued.*

Abrupt discontinuation of metoclopramide was reported to cause psychotic behavior in two patients after continuous use for more than three months. This information might suggest to your physician that it be gradually tapered off if it is to be discontinued after even two months of continuous use.

Erythromycin ethylsuccinate is an antibiotic that has been used to treat infections for many years. It has a chemical composition that resembles the hormone motolin, which stimulates muscular activity in the stomach. Apparently, when stimulation of the stomach by the vagus nerve is depressed, as with autonomic neuropathy, motolin secretion is diminished. Three papers delivered to the 1989 annual meeting of the American Gastroenterological Association demonstrated that this drug can stimulate gastric emptying in patients with gastroparesis. In people without gastroparesis, erythromycin can cause nausea unless taken after drinking fluids. I ask my patients to drink two glasses of water or other fluid before each dose. I prescribe erythromycin ethylsuccinate oral suspension just before meals. We start with 1 teaspoon of the 400 mg/tsp concentration, and increase to several teaspoons if necessary. As each teaspoon of this suspension contains 3.5 grams of sucrose (table sugar), it is necessary to increase slightly the doses of insulin covering meals to reduce blood sugar elevation while this medication is used. If the liquid is kept in a refrigerator, the taste begins to deteriorate after 35 days. At room temperature, the taste deteriorates after 14 days. I have seen no side effects from this medication. I insist that patients who use it chronically take 1 probiotic capsule (such as Florastor [saccharomyces boulardii]) once daily, at least 2 hours before or after each dose. This is to restore to the intestine natural bacteria that can be destroyed by this antibiotic. It is also wise to consume one 150 mg fluconazole tablet once a week to inhibit the growth of fungi in the GI tract or vagina. *I have not found erythromycin to be especially effective for treating gastroparesis, despite* *published studies.* However, mixing a few drops of **peppermint spirits** into a glass of water before eating has helped a few of my patients with mild gastroparesis.

Betaine hydrochloride with pepsin is a potent combination that can predigest food in the stomach by increasing acidity and adding a powerful digestive enzyme. It can be procured at most health food stores or at Rosedale Pharmacy, (888) 796-3348. Because of its acidity it should not be used by those with gastritis, esophagitis, or stomach or duodenal ulcers. Food that has been predigested will more likely pass through the narrowed pyloric valve of gastroparesis. We initially use 1 tablet or capsule midmeal. If no burning is perceived, we increase the dose to 2 and then eventually 3 or more tablets or capsules, spaced evenly throughout subsequent meals. *It should never be chewed or taken on an empty stomach.* Since betaine HCl with pepsin, unlike cisapride, does not attempt to stimulate the vagus nerve, it is frequently of value for even severe cases of gastroparesis.

Nitric oxide agonists are currently being used to relieve the effects of angina in patients with cardiac disease. My search for an agent that is effective for patients with more severe gastroparesis led to my investigation of this class of substances. Since they work by relaxing the smooth muscle in the walls of coronary arteries, I assumed that they could also relax the smooth muscle of the pyloric valve.

My initial trial was with a medication called isosorbide dinitrate. I had it prepared as a suspension in almond oil (with flavoring) so that it could coat the pylorus and work directly upon it. I had it compounded in a concentrate of 5 mg/tsp (1 mg/ml). I was pleased to see that my assumption proved correct—it was very effective for nearly all of my patients who used it. Thus far, it appears to be more successful than any of the agents described above. Nevertheless, it is only partially effective for more severe cases of gastroparesis.

This formulation can be prepared by any compounding chemist (see footnote on page 213). The only adverse effect I've observed has been headache in about 10 percent of the users. Although the headache usually resolves after several days of use, I try to prevent it by starting with very small doses that can then be gradually increased.

I recommend that initially ½ teaspoon be taken 30–60 minutes before dinner. After one week, we increase the dose to 1 teaspoon. If this fails to level off blood sugars at bedtime and the following morning, we continue 1 teaspoon for a week and then increase it to 2 teaspoons. If this is not fully effective, we then increase to 3 teaspoons. If this dose doesn't do the trick, I discontinue the treatment, as further increases are unlikely to be effective. Because multiple daily doses can cause the treatment to rapidly cease working, I do not recommend its use for meals other than dinner. It's been unusual for this formula to be totally ineffective. The liquid must be vigorously shaken before use.

If you have a cardiac condition, isosorbide dinitrate should not be used for gastroparesis unless approved by your cardiologist.

Unfortunately, isosorbide dinitrate usually stops working after a period of weeks to months. I therefore attempt to increase its effectiveness and lower blood sugar levels by applying a chemically similar product to the skin directly over the pylorus. What I prescribe is a nitroglycerine skin patch. These are available by prescription at any pharmacy in strengths of 0.1, 0.2, 0.4, and 0.8 mg. The patch is placed over the pylorus, which is located on the midline of the abdomen above the navel, about 1½ inches (37 mm) below the middle of the lowest rib where it forms an inverted V. The patch is applied on arising in the morning and removed at bedtime. We start with the 0.1 mg patch and, if necessary, increase the size each week if there are no adverse effects. As with isosorbide dinitrate, nitroglycerine should not be used for gastroparesis without your cardiologist's approval if you have a cardiac condition.

Another alternative is a clonidine adhesive skin patch. This product is sold as Catapres in all pharmacies to lower blood pressure and requires a prescription. It is a powerful smooth muscle relaxant. It can, however, cause somnolence (sleepiness) in some people. We therefore start at the smallest size (1 mg) for the first week and increase it to 2 mg for the second week, then 3 mg for the third week and thereafter. Although each patch will work for a week on most people, we remove it at bedtime and replace it the next morning. Since the patch's adhesiveness will be reduced after it's removed, you can use paper tape to keep it attached after the first day. If it causes tiredness, we lower the patch dosage or discontinue it.

Like the aforementioned nitric oxide agonists, it can stop working eventually. If it has been effective and stops working, we discontinue it and restart it after a couple of months. Some patients find that a patch will stop working after 3–4 days. For these people, we change to a new patch midweek.

The reason we remove the clonidine (or nitroglycerine) patch from the skin at bedtime is to slow down the development of tolerance to its action which eventually occurs. I also recommend continuously alternating daytime skin patches—one week on clonidine and one week on nitroglycerine.

Zofran (ondansetron) has been used for many years to prevent the nausea often caused by agents used for cancer chemotherapy. I have prescribed it for many patients and thus far have seen no adverse effects. It opposes nausea in part by helping food to go down instead of up. Zofran has been taken off the market in the United States for reasons that make no sense to me. Generic ondansetron is still available in capsules and oral disintegrating tablets from compounding chemists.* Although the original product was sold in 4 mg and 8 mg oral disintegrating tablets, strange laws in the United States limit copies to be made as 5 and 10 mg capsules, which is okay. I usually start patients at 5 mg about 30 minutes before a meal. I may then increase to 10 mg if necessary. The maximum daily dose is 25 mg. I would rate ondansetron as moderately effective, especially for mild to moderate gastroparesis, and certainly better than erythromycin and the smooth muscle relaxants.

Exercises That Facilitate Stomach-Emptying

The paretic stomach may be described as a flaccid bag, deprived of the rhythmic muscular squeezing present in a stomach that has a properly functioning vagus nerve. Any activity that rhythmically compresses the stomach can crudely replicate normal action. You may perhaps have observed how a brisk walk can relieve that bloated feeling. I therefore strongly recommend brisk walking for an hour immediately after meals—especially after supper.

A patient of mine learned a trick from her yoga instructor that eliminated the erratic blood sugar swings caused by her moderate gastroparesis. The trick is to pull in your belly as far as you can, then push it out all the way. Repeat this with a regular rhythm as many times as you can, immediately after a meal. Over a period of weeks or months, your abdominal muscles will become stronger and stronger, permitting progressively more repetitions before you tire. Eventually shoot for several hundred repetitions—the more the better. This

---

* Such as Rockwell Compounding Associates, (800) 829-1493.

should require less than 4 minutes of your time per hundred reps, a small price to pay for an improvement in your blood sugar profiles.

Another patient discovered an exercise that I call the "back flex." Sit or stand while bending backward as far as you can. Then bend forward about the same amount. Repeat this as many times as you can tolerate.

Although these exercises may sound excessively simple, even silly, they have helped some people with gastroparesis.

Chewing Gum Can Make a Big Difference

The act of chewing produces saliva, which not only contains digestive enzymes but also stimulates muscular activity in the stomach and tends to relax the pylorus. Many of the modern "sugarless" chewing gums contain only 1 gram of xylitol per piece and so will have little effect upon your blood sugar. Chewing gum for at least 1 hour after meals is a very effective treatment for gastroparesis outside of major dietary changes. Don't chew one piece after another, because the grams of sugar can add up.

Meal Plan Modifications Utilizing Ordinary Foods

For some of us, changes in our meal plans will prove more effective than medication. The problem is that such changes are unacceptable to many patients. We usually proceed from most to least convenient in six stages:

1. Drinking at least two 8-ounce glasses of sugar-free, caffeine-free fluid while eating, and chewing slowly and thoroughly
2. Reducing or eliminating dietary fiber, or first running fiber foods through a blender until nearly liquid
3. Virtually eliminating unground beef, veal, pork, and fowl and also eliminating shellfish
4. Reducing protein at supper
5. Eating four or more small daily meals, instead of three larger meals
6. Introducing semiliquid or liquid meals

In the paretic stomach, soluble fiber (gums) and insoluble fiber can form a plug at the very narrow pyloric valve (see Figure 22-1). This is no problem for the normal stomach, where the pyloric valve is wide open. Many patients with mild gastroparesis have reported better relief of fullness and improved blood sugar profiles after modifying their diets to reduce fiber content or to render the fiber more digestible. This means, for example, that mashed cooked vegetables must be substituted for salads, and high-fiber laxatives such as those containing psyllium (e.g., Metamucil) should be avoided. Acceptable vegetables might include avocado, summer squash, zucchini, or mashed pumpkin (sweetened, if you like, with stevia and flavored with cinnamon). It also means that you would have to give up one of our alternatives to toast at breakfast—bran crackers. You might want to try cheese puffs (see page 187) instead.

Most people in the United States like to eat their largest meal in the evening. Furthermore, they usually consume their largest portion of meat or other protein food at this time. These habits make control of fasting blood sugars very difficult for people with gastroparesis. Apparently animal protein, especially red meat, tends to plug up the pylorus if it's in spasm. An easy solution is to move most of your animal protein from supper to breakfast and lunch. Many of my patients have observed remarkable improvements when they do this. We usually suggest a limit of 2 ounces of animal protein, restricted to fish, ground meat, cheese, or eggs, at supper. This is not very much. Yet people are usually so pleased with the results that they will continue with such a regimen indefinitely (of course, as protein is shifted from one meal to another, doses of premeal insulin or ISAs must also be shifted). With a reduction of delayed overnight stomach-emptying, the bedtime dose of a longer-acting insulin or ISA may have to be reduced so that fasting blood sugars will not drop too low.

Some people find that by moving protein to earlier meals, they increase the unpredictability of blood sugar after these meals. For such a situation, we suggest, for those who do not use insulin, four or more smaller meals each day, instead of three larger meals. We try to keep these meals spaced about 4 hours apart, so that digestion and doses of ISAs for one meal are less likely to overlap those for the next meal. This is usually impractical for those who take preprandial insulin. Remember, you must wait 5 hours after your last shot of preprandial insulin before correcting elevated blood sugars.

Both alcohol and caffeine consumption can slow gastric emptying, as can mint and chocolate. These should therefore be avoided, especially at supper, if gastroparesis is moderate or severe.

Semiliquid or Liquid Meals

A last resort for gastroparesis is the use of semiliquid or liquid meals. I say "last resort" because such a restriction takes much of the pleasure out of eating, but it may be the only way to ensure near-normal blood sugars. With this degree of blood sugar improvement, the gastroparesis may slowly reverse, as mine did. The restriction can then eventually be removed. In this section I'll give you some ideas that you can use to create meal plans using semiliquid foods that still follow our guidelines.

Baby food. Low-carbohydrate vegetables and nearly zero carbohydrate meat, chicken, and egg yolk protein meals are readily available as baby food. Remember to read the labels. Also remember that for a typical protein food, 6 grams of protein on the label corresponds to about 1 ounce of the food itself by weight. To avoid protein malnutrition, a sedentary person should consume at least 0.8 gram of protein for every 2.2 pounds (1 kg) of ideal body weight. Thus, a slim person weighing 150 pounds (68 kg) should consume at least 54 grams of protein daily. This works out to about 8 ounces of protein foods. People who are still growing or who exercise vigorously must consume considerably more than 0.8 gram per 2.2 pounds of ideal body weight.

When vegetables that only slowly raise blood sugar are ground or mashed, they can raise blood sugar more rapidly. So how can we justify using baby food? The answer is that we recommend baby food only for people whose stomach already empties very slowly. Thus even with baby food your blood sugar may still have difficulty keeping pace with injected regular insulin. Later in this chapter I will show you some tricks for circumventing this problem.

Below is a brief list of some typical baby foods that can be worked into the meal-planning guidelines set forth in Chapters 10 and 11. Do not exceed those guidelines for carbohydrate, since most of the Laws of Small Numbers still apply, even if you have gastroparesis.

Vegetables	Carbohydrate
Beech-Nut green beans (4-ounce jar)	9 grams
Beech-Nut garden vegetables (4-ounce jar)	10
Heinz butternut squash (3.84-ounce jar)	9

Meats—Strained	Protein
Beef (3-ounce jar)	2.25 ounces
Chicken (3-ounce jar)	2.25
Ham (3-ounce jar)	2.25
Egg yolks (3-ounce jar)	1.5 (plus 1 gram carbohydrate)

Unflavored whole-milk yogurt. Some brands of whole-milk yogurt, such as Erivan, Brown Cow Farm, Stonyfield Farm, and Fage, have no added sugars or fruits. As noted previously, Erivan is sold at health food stores and the others at supermarkets throughout the United States. Again, always specify "whole-milk, unflavored." Remember that "low-fat" dairy foods usually contain more carbohydrate than the whole-milk product.

Erivan yogurt contains 11 grams carbohydrate and 2 ounces protein per 8-ounce container. Stonyfield Farm and Brown Cow Farm both contain 12 grams carbohydrate and 1½ ounces protein per 8-ounce serving. A 7-ounce container of Fage has only 6 grams carbohydrate and 2⅓ ounces protein.

Bland foods like plain yogurt can be made quite tasty by adding a flavor extract, the powder from truly sugar-free gelatin (i.e., without maltodextrin), Crystal Light powder, DaVinci sugar-free syrup, or stevia with cinnamon. The amounts used should suit your taste.

Whole-milk ricotta cheese. While not as liquid as yogurt or baby food, ricotta cheese goes down better than solid foods. It can also be put into a blender with some water or cream to render it more liquid. Each 8-ounce serving of ricotta contains about 8 grams carbohydrate and 2 ounces protein. To my taste, ricotta is a very bland food, but when flavored with cinnamon and stevia, it can be a real treat—a meal that tastes like a dessert.

Liquid meals. When semiliquid meals are not fully successful, the last resort is high-protein, low-carbohydrate liquid meals. These are sold in health food stores for use by bodybuilders. Use only those made from egg white proteins or whey, if you wish to be assured of all the essential amino acids. Similar products made from soy protein may or may not contain these in adequate amounts. Soy may contain sterols similar to estrogen. A recent study by *Consumer Reports,* however, disclosed that of fifteen protein drinks tested, three contained levels of the toxic substances arsenic, lead, mercury, and cadmium in excess of U.S. Pharmacopeia guidelines. The study also points out that California is the only state that requires labeling to disclose toxic levels of such substances in food products. This implies a likelihood that protein drinks made in California are less likely to be contaminated.

Possible Last Resorts for Treating Gastroparesis

One of my patients claims that a costly new treatment has helped considerably both her gastroparesis and her neuropathic pain. It involves the application of small electric currents to acupuncture points on her limbs and is called STS therapy. The electronic device is designated model STS and is manufactured by Dynatronics of Salt Lake City, (800) 874-6251, www.dynatronics.com. It costs about $5,000 and the treatment must be performed for 45 minutes every day. Its effects begin after about two months, and it may actually facilitate the healing of damaged nerves. This device should not be used near an insulin pump or continuous glucose monitor or by people with implanted electrical devices.

Another costly option is electrical gastric stimulation. This involves surgical implantation through the skin of two electrodes that contact the muscular wall of the stomach. The connecting wires enter a control box that can be kept in a pocket or on a belt. The control unit can be set to stimulate the stomach muscles after each meal.

For updates on innovations for gastroparesis, contact the Gastroparesis Patient Association for Cures and Treatments at (888) 874-7228, www.g-pact.org.

TREATING LOW BLOOD SUGARS WHEN YOUR STOMACH IS SLOW TO EMPTY

A patient from Indiana with a hiatal hernia once told me, "These Dextrotabs don't raise my blood sugar one bit. What really works is one stick of that sugar-free chewing gum" (because chewing the gum encourages the stomach to empty a meal that may be sitting there).

Her comment illustrates a major hazard associated with any condition that retards stomach-emptying (gastroparesis, ulcers, and so on): treating hypoglycemia rapidly is nearly impossible. Note the qualifier, "nearly." There are some tricks to circumvent the problem.

If your hypoglycemia occurred because your last meal is still sitting in your stomach, you might thereafter try some chewing gum to help it empty.

Since chewed glucose tablets can take several hours to leave your stomach, you should suck them or, preferably, try a liquid glucose solution, such as Dex4 Liquid Blast. This is available under various brand names at most pharmacies in the United States and Canada and may appear shortly in the U.K. In other countries, ask for a glucose tolerance test beverage. One 2-ounce bottle of Dex4 liquid contains 15 grams of glucose and will raise a 140-pound person's blood sugar about 75 mg/dl. One teaspoon (1.27 grams glucose) will raise it 6 mg/dl. As with glucose tablets, the blood sugar effect is inversely proportional to body weight. See Table 20-1 (page 342) to calculate how much these amounts will raise your blood sugar. If you don't have a medicine spoon handy and are in a hurry, assume that one swallow from the bottle is equivalent to 3 teaspoons.

If you're traveling and forget to bring along a bottle of your glucose tolerance test beverage, get some lactose-free milk. This product has been treated with an enzyme that converts the lactose to glucose. In the United States, the most widely marketed brand is Lactaid. Every 4 ounces contains 6 grams of glucose. Remember, however, that Lactaid will spoil after a few days if not refrigerated.

Even if you've used one of these liquid glucose products, you can speed up the action by chewing gum, by doing the back-flex and stomach exercises described earlier in this chapter, and/or, prior to drinking, by using some of the medications mentioned earlier.

MODIFICATIONS OF PREPRANDIAL INSULIN TO ACCOMMODATE GASTROPARESIS

It takes a while for your physician to select and fine-tune a program to improve stomach-emptying. In the meantime, it's possible to reduce the frequency and severity of postprandial hypoglycemia. To do this, you must slow the action of preprandial insulin to match more closely the delay you experience in digesting your meals. If you are using regular insulin to cover meals, your physician may want you to inject immediately before eating, instead of the usual 40–45 minutes before. If regular still works too rapidly for your slow digestion, you may be asked to take it in the middle of or after your meal. Alternatively, you might substitute 1 or more units of NPH insulin for 1 or more units of regular in your syringe, to slow the action. If, for example, you are asked to inject a preprandial mixture containing 4 units of regular and 1 unit of NPH, you would draw the 4 units of regular into the syringe in the usual manner (see page 269). Then insert the needle

into the vial of NPH and shake the vial and syringe together vigorously a few times, as illustrated in Figure 16-6 (page 271). Immediately but carefully draw 1 unit of NPH into the syringe. Now remove
the needle from the vial and draw in about 5 units of air. The exact
amount of air is not important. The air bubble will act a bit like the
metal ball in a can of spray paint to help mix the insulins. Invert
the syringe a few times to permit the air bubble to move back and
forth, thereby mixing the two insulins. (This is the only situation in
which it is acceptable to mix two different insulins in the same
syringe.) Once you have found a ratio of NPH to regular that works,
you can premix a vial of this concoction using the method described
on page 287, but substituting NPH for the diluting fluid.

Now you can inject the contents of the syringe, including the air.
The air will dissolve in your tissue fluids and cannot do any harm.

If this process confuses you, don't worry. Your physician or diabetes educator should demonstrate it for you and check your technique.

If you use this procedure to slow down your preprandial dose of
regular insulin, it'll keep working for an unknown period of time well
beyond the usual 5 hours. If you routinely correct elevated blood sugars with additional shots of rapid-acting insulin as described on page
318, you now have a real problem. When do you correct an elevated
blood sugar?

The answer is actually simple. Under these conditions, if you add
NPH to regular before *every* meal, you are limited to correcting a high
blood sugar only once daily—when you arise in the morning. This
will be about 12 hours after your suppertime shot of the regular-NPH
mixture. Twelve hours is more than enough time for the mixture to
finish acting.

If you only use the NPH mixture before dinner, then you may safely
continue to correct elevated blood sugars before breakfast and lunch
(after waiting the usual 5 hours or more).

*Do not use any most-rapid insulin instead of regular to cover
meals if you have delayed stomach-emptying.* The reasoning here
should be self-evident. Feel free, however, to use a most-rapid insulin
to bring down an elevated blood sugar using the methods previously
mentioned. The only premeal insulin should be regular or regular
mixed with NPH.

IT MAY BE POSSIBLE TO HEAL THE VAGUS NERVE EVEN IF BLOOD SUGARS ARE NOT KEPT VIRTUALLY NORMAL

Remember the insulin-mimetic antioxidants R-alpha lipoic acid (R-ALA) and evening primrose oil (EPO)? Well, studies in the United States and Germany have shown them to heal the nerves involved in painful diabetic neuropathy of the feet. These studies achieved their results in a matter of months, without any attempt to control blood sugars. More recent brief studies have actually brought about partial healing of the vagus nerve. The studies that I read, however, utilized very high doses of one of these agents (25,000 mg of alpha lipoic acid), administered intravenously on a number of occasions. A few naturopathic physicians in the United States and many in Europe administer such treatment. I'm not set up to do this, but I do ask my patients to take large oral doses of R-alpha lipoic acid and EPO, as outlined in Chapter 15. As indicated in that chapter, I suggest biotin supplementation whenever R-alpha lipoic acid is used. The problem here is that at the doses listed on page 254 (1,800 mg R-ALA daily), users must take 18 pills a day over and above whatever other medications or supplements they may be taking. Nevertheless, I sometimes prescribe these supplements for those who can afford them in the hope that vagal healing can be accelerated, although I don't really expect a miracle.

As mentioned in Chapter 2, many diabetics have another endocrine disorder, hypothyroidism. Since diminished production of thyroid hormones can cause neuropathy even in nondiabetics, it would be appropriate for diabetics with neuropathy of the vagus nerve (gastroparesis) to be tested for thyroid insufficiency. If this turns out to be present, the treatment is usually 1–3 pills daily. This may be an easy cure for gastroparesis, if it is not caused by high blood sugars.

THOUGH "CURABLE," GASTROPARESIS IS SERIOUS BUSINESS

Don't hesitate to use combinations of the medications and other treatments for gastroparesis that I have covered in this chapter. The more methods you find that will work for you, the better the likely outcome.

There is one exception to this rule: *do not use both domperidone and metoclopramide.* Use only one or the other, as they both work by the same mechanism and their potential for adverse effects will increase with the combined dosage.

The effects upon blood sugar of even asymptomatic (symptom-free) delayed stomach-emptying from any cause can be dramatic. Don't think that because you have no symptoms you're free from its effects upon blood sugar. If you're uncertain, ask your physician to perform an R-R interval study. If you're following the guidelines of this book and your blood sugars are still unpredictable, suggest that he or she read this chapter.

> I will personally answer questions from readers for
> one hour every month. This free service is available by
> visiting www.askdrbernstein.net.

23

Routine Follow-up Visits to Your Physician

Taking responsibility for the care of your own diabetes may free you from habits that have been with you for many years. It also requires the establishment of new habits, such as exercise and blood sugar self-monitoring, that are easier to abandon than to follow.

Once your blood sugars have become controlled, it may take only a few months for you conveniently to forget about the pain you used to have in your toes, or the parent or friend who lost a leg or vision due to complications of diabetes, and so on. As time goes on, you will find that with diabetes, as with life in general, you will gradually tend to do what is easiest or most enjoyable at the moment. This backsliding is quite common. When I haven't seen a patient for six months, I'll usually take a meal history and find that some of the basic dietary guidelines have been forgotten. Concurrently blood sugar profiles, HgbA$_{1C}$ levels, lipid profiles, and even fibrinogen levels may have deteriorated. Such deterioration can be short-circuited when I see patients every two months. We all need a little nudge to get back on track, and it seems that a time frame of about two months does the trick for most of us. I was not the first diabetologist to observe this, and your physician may likewise want you to be in touch with him at similar intervals.

Dosage requirements for insulin or ISAs may change over time, whether due to weight changes, to deterioration or improvement of beta cell output, or just to seasonal temperature changes. So there's an ongoing need for readjustment of these medications. Again, two-month intervals are appropriate.

What are some of the things that your physician may want to consider at these follow-up visits?

First of all, your doctor should try to answer any new questions that you may have. These may cover a host of subjects, from something you read in the newspaper to new physical complaints or dissatisfaction with your diet. Write down your questions in advance, so that you won't forget them.

Your physician will, of course, want to review your blood sugar data sheets covering a period of at least two weeks. It makes no sense for your doctor to review prior data, as that is old history. If he or she wants to adjust your medications or meal plan, the changes should be based upon current information. Remember, however, that the data must be complete and honest. This means, for example, that if you spent a few hours shopping or overate, it should be noted on your data sheet. It doesn't make sense, and can be dangerous, for your doctor to change your medications based upon high blood sugars caused by a few unrecorded dietary indiscretions.

At each visit your HgbA$_{1C}$ should be checked. You need not be fasting for this test. Up-to-date physicians are now performing this test in the office using a small drop of finger-stick blood. Results can be had in about 6 minutes.

At least once annually, your physician may want to review blood and urine studies for kidney function, VAP lipid profile, and perhaps even thyroid function. If she has prescribed certain medications, she may even want liver function tests. It is wise to have blood drawn about two weeks in advance of a visit so that the results will be ready for review at the visit. If fasting bloods are required, don't eat breakfast. If you skip breakfast, be sure also to skip your preprandial insulin or ISA if you usually use these medications to cover breakfast. Do not omit glucose tablets or rapid-acting insulin needed to correct low or elevated blood sugars. Also remember to take your basal dose of ISA or long-acting insulin, as their purpose is merely to hold blood sugar level while fasting. Your physician may also want to perform other blood tests from time to time, such as a blood count and a chemical profile.

A partial physical examination, including weight, should be performed every two months. Usually the most important element of these visits should be examination of your feet. Such an examination is not merely to look for injuries, blisters, and so on. Equally important is the discovery of dry skin, athlete's foot, pink pressure points on the skin from ill-fitting shoes, ingrown or fungus-infected toenails, and calluses. Your shoes should also be examined for areas where they have been stretched by prominences on your toes, suggesting that they are smaller than your feet. Any of these can cause or may indicate problems that could lead to ulcers of the feet and should be corrected. Dry skin is best treated with daily applications of animal or vegetable oil such as vitamin E oil, olive oil, emulsified lanolin, mink oil, emu oil, or any proprietary oil or lotion other than mineral oil. The cure for ill-fitting shoes is new shoes (possibly custom-made) that have a wide toe box with a deep rise. Calluses frequently require the purchase of custom orthotics that redistribute the pressure on the bottoms of your feet. Grinding off calluses is not the solution, as calluses are a symptom, not a cause, of excess pressure. Their removal or filing down is the most common cause of amputations in patients that I see at my hospital's wound care clinic.

Resting blood pressures, repeated every few minutes until the lowest reading is obtained, are mandatory at every visit if your blood pressure is even slightly elevated. If your blood pressure is usually normal, it should be checked every twelve months anyway.

Over the course of a year or two, other aspects of physical examination should be performed. The tests need not be done all at one visit, but may be staggered. These include oscillometric studies of the blood circulation in your legs, an electrocardiogram (EKG), tests for sensation in your feet, and a complete eye exam. The eye exam should include pupillary reflexes, visual acuity, intraocular pressure, the Amsler grid test, a test for double vision, and examination of your lenses, anterior chambers, and retinas through dilated pupils. This last exam must be performed with certain specialized equipment that should include direct and indirect ophthalmoscopes and a slit lamp. If your physician is not so equipped, or if he has previously found potential vision-threatening changes in your eyes, you should be referred to an ophthalmologist or retinologist.

If your initial physical exam disclosed diabetic complications such as early signs of neuropathy, carpal tunnel syndrome, or Dupuytren's contractures, examination for these complications should be periodically repeated. The R-R interval study should be repeated every eighteen months, even if it was initially normal.

The best treatment for the complications of diabetes is prevention.

The second best treatment is detection in the very early stages, while reversal is still possible. For these and the reasons mentioned above, I strongly recommend contact with your physician every two months, or at least every three months.

I will personally answer questions from readers for one hour every month. This free service is available by visiting www.askdrbernstein.net.

24

What You Can Expect from Virtually Normal Blood Sugars

I am convinced from my personal experience, from the experiences of my patients, and from reading the scientific literature, that people with normal blood sugars do not develop the long-term complications of diabetes. I am further convinced that diabetics with even slightly elevated blood glucose profiles may eventually experience some of the long-term consequences of diabetes, but they will develop more slowly and likely be less severe than for people with higher blood sugars. In this chapter, I will try to describe some of the changes that I and other physicians have observed when the blood sugars of our patients dramatically improve.

MENTAL CHANGES

Most common, perhaps, is the feeling of being more alert and no longer chronically tired. Many people who "feel perfectly fine" before their blood sugars are normalized comment later that they had no idea that they could feel so much better.

Another common occurrence relates to short-term memory. Very frequently patients or spouses will refer to a patient's "terrible memory." When I first began my medical practice, I would ask patients to phone me at night with their blood sugar data for fine-tuning of medications. My wife, a physician specializing in psychoanalytic medicine, sometimes overheard my end of the conversation and would comment, "That person has a dementia." Weeks later, she would again hear my end of a conversation with the same individual, and would comment on the great improvement of short-term memory. This became so common that I introduced an objective test for short-term memory into the neurologic exam that I perform on all new patients.* About half my new patients indeed display this mild form of dementia, which appears to lift after several months of improved blood sugar. The improvement is usually quite apparent to spouses. This also occurs with low-thyroid patients after their hypothyroid condition has been corrected.

IMPROVEMENT IN DIABETIC NEUROPATHIES

Diabetic neuropathies seem to improve in two phases—a rapid partial improvement that may occur within weeks, followed by sustained very slow improvement that goes on for years if blood sugars continue to remain normal. This is most apparent with numbness or pain in the toes. Some people will even comment, "I know right away if my blood sugar is high, because my toes feel numb again." On the other hand, several patients with total numbness of their feet have complained of severe pain after several months of near-normal blood sugars. This continues for a number of months and eventually resolves as sensation returns. It is as if nerves generate pain signals while they heal or "sprout." The experience may be very frightening and distressing if you haven't been warned that it might occur.

Erectile dysfunction affects about 65 percent of diabetic males, and is the result of years of elevated blood sugars. It may be defined as an inability to maintain a rigid enough penile erection for adequate time to perform intercourse. It usually results from neuropathy, blocked blood vessels, or both. We can perform simple tests to determine which of these causes predominates. When the problem is principally neurologic, I frequently hear the comment, sometimes after only a few weeks of near-normal blood sugar profiles, "Hey, I'm able to have intercourse again!" Unfortunately, this turnaround appears to occur only if the man was able to attain at least partial erections before. If at the original interview, I'm told, "Doc, it's been dead for years," I know recovery is unlikely. If testing shows that the problem was due pri-

* I recite six digits (Sam Spade's license number) and ask the patient to repeat them in reverse order.

marily to blocked blood vessels, I never see improvement. Note, however, that it's normal to be unable to have erections when blood sugars are too low, say below 75 mg/dl.

Another remarkable change relates to autonomic neuropathy and associated gastroparesis. I have documented major improvement in R-R interval studies in many patients, and total normalization in a few. Along with this, we see reduction in signs and symptoms of gastroparesis. Usually such improvement takes place over a period of years. Although it occurs most dramatically in younger people, I've also seen it occur in seventy-year-olds.

VISUAL IMPROVEMENTS

Diplopia, or double vision, is caused by neuropathy of the nerves that activate the muscles that move the eyes. It is a very common finding in the physical examination that I perform, but rarely severe enough to be noticed by patients on a day-to-day basis. Here again, when testing is redone after a few years, we find improvement or even total cures with blood sugar improvement.

Vacuoles are tiny bubbles in the lens of the eye and are thought to be precursors of cataracts. I have seen a number of these vanish after a year or two of improved blood sugars. I have even seen the disappearance of small "spokes" on the lens that signify very early cataracts.

I've seen mild cases of glaucoma cured by normalization of blood sugars, as well as retinal hemorrhages, macular edema, and microaneurysms.

OTHER IMPROVEMENTS

Improvements in risk factors for heart disease, such as mild hypertension, elevated cholesterol/HDL ratios, triglycerides, and fibrinogen levels, are commonplace. They usually can be observed after about two months of sustained normal or near-normal blood sugars and continue to improve for about one year.

Similarly, improvements in early changes noted on renal risk profiles are often obtained, usually after one or two years, but sometimes after a few months.

It has long been known that elevated blood sugars adversely affect growth in children and teenagers. As blood sugars approach normal, children with delayed growth rapidly return to their pre-diabetic growth curves. I, unfortunately, missed this opportunity because I was thirty-nine years old when I finally figured out how to normalize my blood sugars. I did have, however, the joy of watching my nondiabetic son and some of my young diabetic patients become giants in comparison to me.

Most dramatic and commonplace is the feeling of satisfaction and control that nearly everyone experiences when they produce normal or nearly normal blood sugar profiles. This is especially true for individuals who had already been taking insulin, but appears also to occur in those who do not take insulin.

In the late 1970s, the methods of this book were used at Rockefeller University to normalize blood sugars in a group of type 1 diabetics. They were initially tested by a psychiatrist using the Hamilton depression scale. The starting score for the group was in the "severely depressed" range. This dropped to normal after the patients became the masters of their blood sugars.

Last but not least is the feeling that we are not doomed to share the fate of others we have known, who died prematurely after years of disabling or painful diabetic complications. We come to realize that with the ability to control our blood sugars comes the ability to prevent the consequences of high blood sugars.

I have long maintained that diabetics are entitled to the same blood sugars as nondiabetics. But it is up to us to see that we achieve this goal.

Please read Appendices A–E on pages 499–503.

I will personally answer questions from readers for one hour every month. This free service is available by visiting www.askdrbernstein.net.

Your Diabetic Cookbook

RECIPES

25

Recipes for Low-Carbohydrate Meals

The recipes that follow are in and of themselves wonderful examples of how you can eat well with very little fast-acting carbohydrate. They are, however, not intended as the end-all and be-all for diabetic nutrition. As you learned in Chapters 9–11, developing a meal plan is at its foundation science, but there is also art involved. The science offers you the metabolic and nutritional underpinnings of what should and should not be in your meal plan. The art portion is the negotiation that has to take place between you and your physician, and between your nutritional needs and your lifestyle, especially your tastes and the time you have to spend on cooking. You can do well with these recipes, but you can also do well by adjusting these recipes to your own tastes.

The recipes were developed by two quite talented but different chefs. Karen A. Weinstock, who wrote most of the newer recipes in this book, is herself a type 1 diabetic. She is also a nutritional health care provider. For more than twenty-five years, she has taught cooking to individuals, with the goal of maximizing health through diet. When she was diagnosed with type 1 diabetes many years ago, her sense of healthy eating went into a tailspin, as her own diet, like that of most Americans—even those who "know food"—included an excess of refined and fast-acting carbohydrate. After many years of unsuccessfully regulating her own blood sugar levels, she met me. She says, "This program saved my life by providing me with the necessary guidelines and practical how-tos to live a normal life as a diabetic."

Her goal in creating recipes for this book was to provide the diabetic community with delicious gourmet meals based on our program and her own nutritional expertise. She says, "It is my hope that you can enjoy both preparing and eating these meals while maintaining healthy blood sugar levels." The recipes she created are identified by the initials KW at the end. The recipes identified by the initials TA were created by Timothy J. Aubert, CWC, for the first edition of this book.

USING THE RECIPES

All the recipes are, in one sense, a guide to how you can incorporate into your diet foods you may not have considered eating, and how you can use low-carbohydrate foods and protein to arrive at tasty approximations of foods from the high-carbohydrate world.

You can use the recipes exactly as written and trust that they will play a significant role in assisting you with blood sugar normalization; or you can play with them and customize them to suit your own tastes and dietary guidelines. It is best, however, unless you are a seasoned cook, to try the recipes first as they are written, and then make adjustments if they seem warranted. Changes in herbs and spices or including slightly more of the whole-plant vegetables listed in "So What's Left to Eat?" beginning on page 157 are not likely to alter blood sugars significantly, but you should follow carbohydrate and protein content guidelines and check your blood sugars to make sure. If a recipe calls for less carbohydrate than required by your meal plan, add some vegetables, salad, bran crackers, et cetera, to the meal to make up the difference. Refer to Chapter 10 for some typical suggestions.

If you've flipped straight to these recipes without gaining a good understanding of how to follow a meal plan, stop and at least read Chapters 9–11. Look especially at the box entitled "No-No's in a Nutshell," on page 160. Then look at the list of vegetables on page 158; it's likely that any vegetable not listed in that section is not suitably low in fast-acting carbohydrate. Remember that ½ cup of diced or sliced cooked low-carbohydrate vegetables (or ¼ cup mashed) is approximately equivalent to 6 grams carbohydrate, as is 1 cup of mixed salad. Assume that ⅔ cup of whole cooked vegetables is also equivalent to about 6 grams of carbohydrate.

Throughout these recipes the abbreviation CHO is used for carbohydrate (CHO stands for carbon, hydrogen, and oxygen, the elements that make up carbohydrates) and PRO is used for protein. Each recipe shows the number of servings provided and the approximate grams of carbohydrate and ounces of protein in each serving. (If you are adapting these recipes or creating your own and consulting food value books, remember our rule of thumb: divide by 6 to convert grams of protein to ounces of a raw protein food; divide by 4 for ounces of a cooked protein food.)

PREPARING POWDERED ARTIFICIAL SWEETENERS

As you know, the paper packets containing granulated, so-called sugar-free sweeteners usually contain about 96 percent glucose, maltodextrin, or other sugar, making them inappropriate for diabetics. You can prepare your own granulated sweetener for use in some of the following recipes by crushing or grinding aspartame, Splenda, or saccharin *tablets* (not packets) in one of the following ways:

- in a mortar and pestle
- between two spoons
- in a pepper mill
- in a small electric coffee grinder

You can also dissolve the crushed tablets in a small amount of hot water (unless the recipe calls for powdered sweetener).

Aspartame (but not saccharin) will lose its taste if added to food before cooking, so it must be used only after cooking. You may prefer to use stevia, since it is sold as powder or liquid and is not degraded by heat. Make sure that you purchase only powdered stevia that does not contain maltodextrin.

GG SCANDINAVIAN BRAN CRISPBREAD

Several recipes contain these bran crackers. Their source appears on page 164. Each cracker contains 3 grams carbohydrate and 1 gram (1/6 ounce) protein.

MORE RECIPES

My book *The Diabetes Diet,* also published by Little, Brown, has a hundred new low-carbohydrate recipes for breakfast, lunch, and dinner designed specifically for facilitating blood sugar control.

SAUCES

ITALIAN-STYLE RED SAUCE

6 servings, about ½ cup each   Per serving: 5.6 gm CHO, <0.5 oz PRO

	CHO (gm)	PRO (gm)
3 cups diced red bell pepper	27.6	3.6
1 Tbsp olive oil	—	—
¼ cup chopped fresh basil	0.4	0.2
2 cloves garlic, minced	2.0	0.4
1 cup College Inn chicken broth	—	1.0
⅓ cup heavy cream	2.2	1.6
½ tsp salt	—	—
⅓ tsp black pepper	—	—
½ tsp dried oregano	1.0	0.2
½ tsp stevia powder (without maltodextrin)	—	—
2 Tbsp grated Parmesan cheese	0.4	4.2

In a saucepan, bring a quart of water to a boil. Add diced pepper, cover, and simmer for 20 minutes. Drain liquid from pepper by pouring through a colander. Add pepper to food processor work bowl and puree for 2–3 minutes. The finished texture of the puree will contain some pulp. Heat olive oil in a saucepan over a low flame. Add basil and garlic. Sauté on a low flame until the aroma is released, 3–4 minutes. Stir in the pepper puree, chicken broth, and heavy cream. While stirring, add remaining seasonings except for grated cheese. Simmer the sauce uncovered for 40 minutes. Add grated cheese to sauce just before serving.

This sauce can be used in many recipes that call for a red sauce, such as meat loaf or stuffed cabbage. It will keep in the refrigerator for 4–5 days. It may be stored in the freezer for 2–3 months. KW

RED PEPPER COCKTAIL SAUCE

16 servings, about 1 Tbsp each   Per serving: 1.2 gm CHO, <0.1 oz PRO

	CHO (gm)	PRO (gm)
2 cups diced red bell pepper	18.4	2.4
¼ tsp salt	—	—
½ tsp stevia powder (without maltodextrin)	—	—
2 tsp white horseradish	—	—
1 Tbsp Worcestershire sauce	1.0	—
1 Tbsp cider vinegar	—	—
Hot sauce to taste	—	—

In a saucepan, bring a quart of water to a boil. Add diced red pepper and cover the pot. Reduce heat to a simmer and cook for 15 minutes. Drain water from pepper and put them into a blender. Blend pepper to a pureed consistency. Pour puree into a glass bowl and refrigerate for 30 minutes.

Remove the chilled pepper puree from the refrigerator. Add the salt and stevia to the puree and combine. A whisk is helpful here. Add horseradish, Worcestershire sauce, vinegar, and hot sauce. Serve this sauce with chilled shrimp or other seafood.

The sauce will keep in the refrigerator for 2–3 days in a glass jar. It may be stored in the freezer for 2–3 months. KW

RUSSIAN DRESSING

24 servings, 1 Tbsp each   Per serving: <1 gm CHO, <0.1 oz PRO

	CHO (gm)	PRO (gm)
1½ cups diced red bell pepper	13.8	1.8
¾ cup mayonnaise	—	—
1 Tbsp canola oil	—	—
1 tsp Worcestershire sauce	0.3	—
½ tsp stevia powder (without maltodextrin)	—	—
¼ tsp black pepper	—	—
2 Tbsp diced sour dill pickle	0.5	—

In a saucepan, bring 1 quart of water to a boil. Add bell pepper and cover. Reduce heat to simmer for 10 minutes. Drain in a colander and discard cooking liquid. Add bell pepper to the work bowl of a food processor. Chop for 2–3 minutes. The consistency should be smooth, but some of the fiber will remain. Add the mayonnaise, oil, and Worcestershire sauce. Blend together for a moment. Add the stevia and black pepper and blend again. Scrape mixture from the work bowl into a glass bowl. Fold in diced pickle.

This dressing will keep in the refrigerator for 10–14 days. (Don't try to freeze.) Store in an airtight container. KW

DIJON MUSTARD BUTTER

12 servings, 2 Tbsp each   Per serving: 0.7 gm CHO, <0.1 oz PRO

	CHO (gm)	PRO (gm)
2 Tbsp minced shallots	3.4	0.6
1¼ cups (2½ sticks) butter, softened	—	2.5
3 Tbsp Dijon mustard	3.0	—
1 tsp lemon juice	0.43	0.03

1 Tbsp Worcestershire sauce	1.0	—
Tabasco sauce to taste	0.5	—

Sauté shallots in 1 teaspoon of the butter. In a food processor, combine shallots with all other ingredients until smooth. Place on parchment paper or on plastic wrap. Roll butter in the paper or wrap until you have a 1-inch-diameter cylinder. Refrigerate until butter is needed. Slice into ¼-inch pieces to use (3 slices = 1 tablespoon). TA

LEMON BUTTER

4 servings, 2 Tbsp each   Per serving: 0.7 gm CHO, <0.1 oz PRO

	CHO (gm)	PRO (gm)
½ cup (1 stick) unsalted butter, softened	—	1.0
2 Tbsp lemon juice	2.6	0.2
Salt and white pepper to taste	—	—

In a food processor, combine all ingredients until smooth. Roll butter into a 1-inch-diameter cylinder as directed for Dijon Mustard Butter, above, and refrigerate until needed. Slice into ¼-inch pieces to use (3 slices = 1 tablespoon). TA

LEMON PEPPER BUTTER

4 servings, 2 Tbsp each   Per serving: 0.7 gm CHO, <0.1 oz PRO

	CHO (gm)	PRO (gm)
½ cup (1 stick) butter, softened	—	1.0
2 Tbsp lemon juice	2.6	0.2
⅛ tsp salt	—	—
⅛ tsp white pepper	—	—
Lemon pepper seasoning to taste	—	—

In a food processor, combine all ingredients until smooth. Roll butter into a 1-inch-diameter cylinder as directed for Dijon Mustard Butter, above, and refrigerate until needed. Slice into ¼-inch pieces to use (3 slices = 1 tablespoon). TA

GINGER SCALLION BUTTER

12 servings, 2 Tbsp each   Per serving: 0.5 gm CHO, <0.1 oz PRO

	CHO (gm)	PRO (gm)
1¼ cups (2½ sticks) butter, softened	—	2.5
4 minced scallions	1.85	0.45
¼ tsp minced garlic	0.5	0.08
½ tsp minced fresh ginger	0.15	0.01

	CHO	PRO
1 Tbsp minced parsley	0.6	0.3
1 Tbsp soy sauce	2.0	2.0
1 Tbsp lemon juice	1.3	0.1

In a food processor, combine all ingredients until smooth. Roll butter into a 1-inch-diameter cylinder as directed for Dijon Mustard Butter, above, and refrigerate until needed. Slice into ¼-inch pieces to use (3 slices = 1 tablespoon). TA

TARRAGON BUTTER

12 servings, 2 Tbsp each   Per serving: 1.7 gm CHO, <0.5 oz PRO

	CHO (gm)	PRO (gm)
¾ cup white wine	7.2	0.6
1 bay leaf	0.3	0.1
7 black peppercorns, crushed	0.7	0.1
3 Tbsp tarragon vinegar	—	—
2 Tbsp minced shallots	4.8	0.7
1 cup heavy cream	6.6	4.9
¾ cup (1½ sticks) butter, softened	—	1.5
½ tsp chopped fresh tarragon	0.8	0.4
Pinch of salt and white pepper	—	—

Combine wine, bay leaf, crushed peppercorns, vinegar, and shallots in a nonreactive pan. Bring to a boil and reduce to about 2 tablespoons. Strain, removing bay leaf and crushed peppercorns. Reduce cream by half in a separate pan and add to the wine reduction. Gradually whisk in the butter over low heat. When all the butter is dissolved, add the chopped fresh tarragon and season to taste. TA

SPICY MUSTARD SAUCE

16 servings, 2 Tbsp each   Per serving: 2.3 gm CHO, <0.5 oz PRO

	CHO (gm)	PRO (gm)
½ cup minced shallots	19.2	2.8
¼ cup cider vinegar	—	—
1 tsp black peppercorns, cracked	1.4	0.2
1 bay leaf	0.3	0.1
1 cup dry white wine	9.6	—
1 cup heavy cream	6.6	4.9
1½ cups (3 sticks) unsalted butter, softened	—	3.0
Dijon-style mustard to taste	—	—
Creole mustard (or any other spicy mustard) to taste	—	—

418 *Your Diabetic Cookbook*

Combine the first 5 ingredients in a small nonreactive saucepan and reduce to ⅓ cup. Add heavy cream and reduce mixture by half. Strain and return to the stove. Cut softened butter into small pieces and slowly add to the sauce while whisking. After all the butter is incorporated, add the mustard to taste. TA

BREAKFAST FOODS

Breakfast is the meal where you may find you miss carbohydrates the most. No more home fries or hash browns, toast, pancakes, French toast, waffles, cereals, and the like. The recipe suggestions that follow can put some zip back into breakfast while keeping carbohydrates way down.

MUSHROOM OMELET WITH BACON

1 serving   Per serving: 3.1 gm CHO, 2.8 oz PRO

	CHO (gm)	PRO (gm)
2 slices bacon	—	4.0
1 fresh mushroom, sliced	1.5	0.35
Butter to taste	—	—
2 eggs	1.2	12.0
1 Tbsp heavy cream	0.4	0.3
Salt and black pepper to taste	—	—

Pan-fry bacon and remove to paper towel to drain. Sauté sliced mushroom in butter for 2–3 minutes. In a small bowl, mix eggs with cream, then add to mushrooms. Cook eggs without stirring for 2 minutes, or until desired firmness. Season with salt and pepper to taste. Roll or fold omelet and turn out on a plate. Serve with the bacon. TA

SCRAMBLED EGGS WITH ONIONS, PEPPERS, AND STRIPPLES

1 serving   Per serving: 5.3 gm CHO, 2.4 oz PRO

	CHO (gm)	PRO (gm)
2 slices Stripples (soy bacon)	2.0	2.0
2 eggs	1.2	12.0
1 Tbsp cream	0.4	0.3
Butter to taste	—	—
1 Tbsp minced onion	0.9	0.3
1 Tbsp minced green bell pepper	0.8	—
Salt and black pepper to taste	—	—

Microwave Stripples and set aside. Combine eggs and cream thoroughly in a small bowl. Heat butter in sauté pan, add eggs, and cook for 1 minute. Add minced onion and green pepper. Season with salt and pepper to taste and cook to desired consistency. TA

HAM AND CHEESE OMELET

1 serving   Per serving: 3.6 gm CHO, 6 oz PRO

	CHO (gm)	PRO (gm)
2 eggs	1.2	12.0
1 Tbsp cream	0.4	0.3
Butter to taste	—	—
1 slice (2 oz) ham, diced or julienned	—	18.0
2 oz cheese, grated or sliced thin	2.0	12.0
Salt and black pepper to taste	—	—

Mix together eggs and cream in a small bowl. Heat butter in sauté pan and cook egg mixture 1–2 minutes without stirring. Place ham and cheese on top and season to taste with salt and pepper. Either roll or fold the eggs and cook to desired consistency. TA

MEAT AND EGG OPEN SANDWICH

This recipe was developed by Amy Z. Kornfeld and Hank Kornfeld.
You may substitute 2 slices ham, turkey, or salami for the sausage.

1 serving   Per serving: 8 gm CHO, 5 oz PRO

	CHO (gm)	PRO (gm)
2 sausage patties, 1 oz each	—	12.0
1 Tbsp butter or 1 tsp vegetable oil	—	—
2 eggs	1.2	12.0
2 GG Scandinavian Bran Crispbreads	6.0	2.0
2 slices cheese (about ¾ oz total)	0.8	4.0

Brown sausage and drain off fat. Keep warm in 250°F oven. Heat butter or oil in a nonstick skillet until water drops sprinkled on surface skitter across. Break eggs into pan. Fry eggs for 2–3 minutes over medium heat. If desired, flip them over and fry for another minute or so. Put crispbreads on an ovenproof plate and place eggs on top. Cover with sausage and top off with cheese. Warm briefly in oven to melt cheese. TA

FRENCH BRAN TOAST

This is another recipe from Amy Z. Kornfeld and Hank Kornfeld.

1 serving   Per serving: 7 gm CHO, *1.4 oz* PRO

	CHO (gm)	PRO (gm)
2 GG Scandinavian Bran Crispbreads	6.0	2.0
2 tsp water	—	—
1 egg or egg substitute	0.6	6.0
¼ tsp cinnamon	—	—
⅛ tsp nutmeg	—	—
⅛ tsp vanilla extract	—	—
Artificial maple or fruit-flavored extract to taste	—	—
1 Tbsp cream	0.4	0.3
1 tsp vegetable oil	—	—
Melted butter to taste	—	—
1 or more Equal tablets, crushed, or pinch of stevia powder (without maltodextrin)	—	—

Soak crispbreads in 2 teaspoons water for 5 minutes, or just long enough to soften. Meanwhile, in a broad shallow bowl beat egg or egg substitute with cinnamon, nutmeg, vanilla, and other flavor extract. Add cream and beat gently. Place softened crispbreads in egg mixture for 1–2 minutes. Heat nonstick skillet until water droplets sprinkled on surface skitter across. Add oil to skillet and spread it around with a folded paper towel. Place egg-soaked crispbreads in pan and cook over medium heat for about 3 minutes per side. When done remove from pan, pour on melted butter, and sprinkle with crushed Equal tablets or stevia.

PANCAKES

Amy Z. Kornfeld and Hank Kornfeld also suggested this substitute for traditional pancakes.

1 serving   Per serving: 7 gm CHO, *1.4 oz* PRO

	CHO (gm)	PRO (gm)
2 GG Scandinavian Bran Crispbreads	6.0	2.0
1 egg, beaten	0.6	6.0
⅛ tsp nutmeg	—	—
¼ tsp cinnamon	—	—
⅛ tsp vanilla extract	—	—
Artificial vanilla, orange, or almond extract to taste	—	—
1 Tbsp cream	0.4	0.3

1 tsp vegetable oil	—	—
Melted butter to taste	—	—
1 or more Equal tablets, crushed, or pinch of stevia powder (without maltodextrin)	—	—

Grind crispbreads in blender, food processor, or electric coffee grinder to a flourlike consistency. Combine egg, nutmeg, cinnamon, vanilla, other flavor extract, and cream in bowl. Add ground crispbreads and mix. Heat nonstick skillet. When hot, add oil to skillet and spread it around with a paper towel. Add one-quarter of batter to skillet. Cook for 2 minutes. Turn carefully and cook other side for another 2 minutes, to produce first pancake. Repeat 3 times to produce 3 more pancakes. Cover with melted butter. Sprinkle pancakes with crushed Equal tablets or stevia.

SOUPS

ACORN SQUASH BISQUE

4 servings, about 1 cup each   Per serving: 8 gm CHO, <0.5 oz PRO

	CHO (gm)	PRO (gm)
1 small (1 lb) acorn squash (see Note)	21.4	1.6
1 Tbsp butter	—	—
2 stalks celery, thinly sliced diagonally (set aside leaves for garnish)	3.0	0.6
1 small leek, cleaned and thinly sliced diagonally	4.0	0.4
⅓ tsp salt	—	—
½ cup heavy cream	3.3	2.5
1¾ cups water	—	—
¼ tsp cinnamon	0.4	—

Quarter the acorn squash and scrape out the seeds. Use some caution when cutting the squash—the skin can be tough and the flesh is dense, so work your knife in gradually as you cut.

In a large saucepan, bring 5 cups of water to a boil. Add squash and simmer until tender, about 15 minutes. Drain liquid from squash and allow to cool. Scoop pulp from the outer peel into the work bowl of your food processor. Discard peel. Puree cooked squash in the food processor until liquefied. This should yield about 1 cup of squash puree (any more will increase the carbohydrate count).

In the same saucepan, add butter and sauté celery and leeks with salt for 5–7 minutes, or until wilted. Add squash puree, heavy cream, and water and stir well. Heat on a low flame for 10 minutes. Stir in cinnamon, garnish with the fresh celery leaves, and serve warm.

The bisque will keep in the refrigerator for 2–3 days. It may be stored in the freezer for 1 month.

This is a recipe that, because of its texture, can be fairly easily digested by those who suffer from gastroparesis.

Note

Acorn squash has a wonderful flavor, very close to sweet potatoes, with lots of carotenoids but with considerably less fast-acting carbohydrate. You can substitute canned pumpkin for the squash, but be sure to read food labels and ensure that what you buy doesn't have added sugar (it doesn't as long as the only ingredient is pumpkin). KW

CUCUMBER SOUP

4 servings, about ¾ cup each   Per serving: 3.9 gm CHO, <0.5 oz PRO

	CHO (gm)	PRO (gm)
1 whole cucumber, peeled and sliced	8.3	2.1
½ cup chopped fennel	6.3	1.1
1 Tbsp whole-milk yogurt	0.75	0.75
½ cup cold water	—	—
½ tsp chopped fresh dill	—	—
Lemon pepper seasoning to taste	—	—

In a blender combine sliced cucumber, fennel, yogurt, water, and dill. Puree until smooth, season with lemon pepper seasoning, and serve. TA

ZUCCHINI SOUP

3 servings, about 1½ cups each   Per serving: 3.2 gm CHO, <0.5 oz PRO

	CHO (gm)	PRO (gm)
4 medium zucchini, cleaned and sliced	4.0	3.5
1½ Tbsp chopped onion	1.35	0.15
1 Tbsp butter	—	0.1
3 Tbsp hot water	—	—
1 cube Knorr chicken bouillon, crushed	2.0	0.8
Salt, black pepper, and garlic powder to taste	—	—
⅓ cup heavy cream	2.2	1.63

In a 2-quart pan, sauté zucchini and onion in butter until tender. Transfer vegetables to a blender and puree. Add hot water and crushed bouillon cube; blend for 1–2 minutes. Season with salt, pepper, and garlic powder to taste. Serve hot or cold. Add cream to individual portions, about 2 tablespoons per serving. TA

CHICKEN EGG-DROP SOUP WITH SCALLIONS

4 servings   Per serving: 3.5 gm CHO, 2.3 oz PRO

	CHO (gm)	PRO (gm)
2 large eggs	1.2	12.4
4 cups College Inn chicken broth	—	4.0
½ cup finely chopped scallions	3.7	0.9
6 oz cooked chicken breast fillet, shredded (see Note 1)	—	54.0
1 Tbsp soy sauce	2.0	2.0
1 Tbsp arrowroot powder (see Note 2)	7.0	—
2 Tbsp cold water	—	—

In a mixing bowl, crack open eggs and whisk together with ½ cup of the chicken broth. Place this mixture in the refrigerator. Place the remaining 3½ cups chicken broth in a saucepan. Bring liquid to a low boil. Add scallions, shredded chicken, and soy sauce. Reduce heat and simmer 3–5 minutes. Remove egg mixture from the refrigerator. Slowly add egg mixture to the soup, while stirring the soup constantly. As you stir in the egg, it will feather out and thicken. Dissolve arrowroot powder in cold water in a small bowl. Stir this into the soup. Cook for 3–5 minutes with a lid. Serve warm.

This recipe will keep in the refrigerator for 4–5 days. It may also be stored in the freezer for 2–3 months.

Notes

1. Leftover cooked chicken works best for this recipe. It is easiest to shred chicken when it is cold, using a fork or tongs.

2. Arrowroot powder (also called arrowroot flour) is a thickening agent used like cornstarch. It must be dissolved in a small amount of cold water before being added to warm ingredients. KW

SEAFOOD CHOWDER TRIO

6 servings   Per serving: 2.9 gm CHO, 2.8 oz PRO

	CHO (gm)	PRO (gm)
⅓ lb shrimp in their shells	0	31.6
3 cups water	—	—
2 Tbsp butter	—	—
½ cup thinly sliced button mushrooms	4.0	1.7
1 stalk celery, diced	1.5	0.3

½ tsp dried tarragon	0.4	—
1 bay leaf	—	—
1 tsp salt	—	—
⅓ tsp black pepper	—	—
½ lb scrod, cod, or other firm white fish	—	40.4
½ cup heavy cream	3.3	2.4
½ cup dry white wine	4.8	—
⅓ lb bay scallops	3.6	25.3

To clean shrimp, rinse in a colander under cold running water. Remove shells and set them aside. They will be used for the soup stock. Remove the vein along the back and discard it. Cut shrimp into small bite-sized pieces and set aside. Place shells in a saucepan with 3 cups of water. Bring to a boil and simmer for 10 minutes. Strain out shells and return stock to saucepan. In a skillet, heat butter on a low flame. Add mushrooms, celery, tarragon, bay leaf, salt, and black pepper. Sauté for 3–5 minutes. Meanwhile, add scrod, heavy cream, and white wine to the seafood stock. Add the cooked vegetables from the skillet. Turn on heat under saucepan and bring chowder to a low boil. The scrod will fall apart as it cooks, so there is no need to cut it. Reduce heat and simmer covered for 15 minutes. Add scallops and shrimp to chowder. Cook for 3–5 minutes. Remove bay leaf, adjust seasoning, and serve warm.

The chowder will keep in the refrigerator for 3–4 days. It may also be stored in the freezer for 1 month. KW

SALADS

CURRIED CHICKEN SALAD WITH JICAMA

4 servings   Per serving: 3 gm CHO, 4 oz PRO

	CHO (gm)	PRO (gm)
1 lb chicken breasts, boned and skinned	—	96.0
1 stalk celery, diced	1.5	0.3
½ cup coarsely grated jicama (see Note)	5.3	0.4
½ cup diced green bell pepper	4.6	0.6
3 Tbsp cider vinegar	—	—
3 Tbsp mayonnaise	—	—
⅓ tsp salt	—	—
½ tsp black pepper	—	—
¼ tsp stevia powder (without maltodextrin)	—	—
½ tsp curry powder	0.6	0.1

To cook chicken breasts, steam them until tender and no longer pink inside, 12–15 minutes. Allow to cool before slicing. Cut chicken breasts into bite-sized chunks.

In a medium-sized glass mixing bowl, combine chicken and celery, jicama, and green pepper. Add vinegar and mayonnaise and mix thoroughly. Add salt, black pepper, stevia, and curry power to chicken salad. Blend in all seasoning by evenly coating the ingredients. Serve chilled or at room temperature.

Note

If you're not familiar with jicama, it has brown skin like a potato and is shaped something like a turnip. Its flesh has a pleasing crunch, almost like a crisp apple. When purchasing jicama, which is available these days in most supermarkets, make sure the skin is firm without bruises. The small variety, about the size of an orange, is the best for its taste and texture. kw

ROASTED EGGPLANT SUMMER SALAD

4 servings   Per serving: 9.4 gm CHO, *0.5 oz* PRO

	CHO (gm)	PRO (gm)
1 eggplant, about 1¼ lb, peeled and cut into 1½-inch cubes	27.8	4.67
¾ tsp salt	—	—
5 Tbsp olive oil	—	—
¼ tsp dried oregano	0.2	—
2 cloves garlic, minced	2.0	0.2
¼ tsp black pepper	—	—
1 oz (¼ cup) crumbled feta cheese	1.0	5.0
2 Tbsp lemon juice	2.6	0.2
1 small head of Boston lettuce, washed, dried, and lightly shredded	3.8	2.1

Preheat oven to 425°F. Rub eggplant chunks with salt and allow to stand for 10 minutes. With a paper towel, pat dry any surface moisture (this helps to remove the bitter taste). In a large mixing bowl, combine the eggplant, 4 Tbsp olive oil (set aside 1 Tbsp olive oil for final seasoning), oregano, garlic, and black pepper. Mix thoroughly and place in a 9 × 13 baking dish. Bake uncovered for 45 minutes. Remove from oven and allow to cool. Sprinkle with feta cheese, lemon juice, and 1 Tbsp olive oil before serving on a bed of Boston lettuce. Serve chilled or at room temperature. kw

MARINATED CUCUMBER SALAD
WITH FRESH DILL

4 servings   Per serving: 2.6 gm CHO, <0.5 oz PRO

	CHO (gm)	PRO (gm)
4 pickling cucumbers, sliced into ⅓-inch rounds	5.6	1.6
2 stalks celery, sliced into thin crescents	3.0	0.6
2 Tbsp diced red onion	1.8	0.6
1 Tbsp chopped fresh dill, or 1 tsp dried dill	0.1	1.0
½ tsp salt	—	—
½ tsp stevia powder (without maltodextrin)	—	—
3 Tbsp cider vinegar	—	—

In a large glass mixing bowl, combine cucumbers, celery, onion, and dill. To preserve the crunchiness of the vegetables, *lightly* mix the salt, stevia, and vinegar into them (a heavy hand while mixing will tend to soften the vegetables). Cover the salad and refrigerate for a minimum of 30 minutes before serving. The longer it marinates, the more "pickled" the flavor. Store the salad in the liquid to maintain its freshness. It will keep in the refrigerator for 3–4 days in an airtight container. KW

GREEN CABBAGE COLESLAW WITH LEMON ZEST

4 servings   Per serving: 5.8 gm CHO, <0.5 oz PRO

	CHO (gm)	PRO (gm)
4 cups shredded green cabbage	15.2	4.0
½ cup diced green bell pepper	4.6	0.6
½ cup coarsely chopped flat-leaf parsley	1.9	0.9
½ tsp salt	—	—
½ tsp grated lemon zest (see Note)	—	—
¼ tsp black pepper	—	—
½ tsp celery seeds	0.4	0.2
4 Tbsp cider vinegar	—	—
2 heaping Tbsp mayonnaise	1.0	—

In a large glass mixing bowl, combine cabbage, green pepper, and parsley. Add the salt. Work it into the fiber of the vegetables. The salt, as it dissolves and mixes with the greens, will draw moisture from the vegetables. Add the lemon zest, black pepper, celery seeds, and vinegar, then the mayonnaise. Mix thoroughly. Allow the coleslaw to stand about 30 minutes in the refrigerator before serving. It will keep in the refrigerator for 4–5 days in an airtight container.

Note

Lemon zest is the fragrant outer yellow part of the lemon peel. Don't grate below to the bitter, pulpy white. ĸw

POULTRY

GROUND TURKEY BURGERS WITH MARJORAM

4 servings   Per serving: 3.3 gm CHO, *5 oz* PRO

	CHO (gm)	PRO (gm)
1 oz (¼ cup) grated cheddar cheese	1.0	7.0
½ cup chopped scallions	3.7	0.9
½ cup diced green bell pepper	4.6	0.6
2 Tbsp minced elephant garlic (see Note)	2.0	—
1 egg	0.6	6.2
1 Tbsp olive oil	—	—
1 tsp dried marjoram	0.4	0.1
½ tsp salt	—	—
¼ tsp black pepper	0.9	—
1 lb ground turkey	—	105
Oil, to coat	—	—

In a small glass mixing bowl, combine cheese, scallions, green pepper, and garlic. In a separate, large mixing bowl, lightly whisk together egg, oil, and seasonings. Stir the vegetable mixture into the eggs, then add the ground turkey. Mix evenly and form into 4 thick patties. Handle the uncooked burgers delicately. At first they will seem fragile, but they will bind nicely once they start to cook.

Heat a large cast-iron skillet. Add oil and coat the bottom of the skillet, then place the patties in the skillet. Do not cover the skillet.

Start your cooking over medium-high heat, and after a few minutes reduce to medium-low. Cook for 12–15 minutes on the first side, then flip gently and cook another 12–15 minutes (you don't need to raise heat when you turn the patties). When burgers are done they will be firm to the touch. Check for doneness by cutting into the center of a burger with a paring knife. They should look evenly cooked, and the inside color should be white, not pink. These burgers can be served on a bed of lettuce with sliced cucumber and your favorite low- or no-carbohydrate condiment.

Note

Elephant garlic is usually available in natural food stores. If you can't find it, an equivalent amount of conventional garlic or shallots may be substituted without significantly altering the food count. ĸw

TURKEY MELT

2 servings   Per serving: 4.5 gm CHO, 1.8 oz PRO

	CHO (gm)	PRO (gm)
2 GG Scandinavian Bran Crispbreads	6.0	2.0
2 slices cooked turkey, 1 oz each	—	18.0
2 slices Stripples (soy bacon), cooked	2.0	2.0
2 slices cheese, ½ oz each	1.0	6.0

Place GG crispbreads in a small broiler pan and lay turkey and cooked Stripples on top. Cover with cheese. Place in a 325°F oven or toaster oven until cheese is thoroughly melted. Serve hot. TA

JALAPEÑO CHICKEN WITH BROCCOLI AND JACK CHEESE

4 servings   Per serving: 5.2 gm CHO, 5 oz PRO

	CHO (gm)	PRO (gm)
1 Tbsp cream of tartar	1.8	—
2 Tbsp cold water	—	—
2 Tbsp olive oil	—	—
2 Tbsp diced jalapeño pepper	2.0	—
½ cup diced red bell pepper	4.6	0.6
2 Tbsp minced shallots	3.4	0.6
3 chicken breast cutlets, 6 oz each, cut into thin strips	—	108.0
¼ tsp ground cumin	0.2	0.1
½ tsp salt	—	—
1 cup broccoli florets	7.8	6.4
1 oz (¼ cup) grated Monterey Jack cheese	1.0	6.0

In a small bowl, dissolve cream of tartar into cold water and set aside. Heat oil in a skillet over a low flame and sauté jalapeño pepper, red bell pepper, and shallots. Stir ingredients and cook for 2–3 minutes. Add chicken strips, cumin, and salt. Cover and cook for 5–7 minutes. Add dissolved cream of tartar to the chicken mixture, stirring as it thickens. Add broccoli florets and cook 3–4 minutes. Remove the skillet from the flame. Sprinkle with grated cheese and serve warm. KW

GRILLED CHICKEN WITH TARRAGON BUTTER

1 serving   Per serving: 3.8 gm CHO, 6.2 oz PRO

	CHO (gm)	PRO (gm)
1 Tbsp oil	—	—
1 Tbsp lemon juice	1.3	0.1

	CHO (gm)	PRO (gm)
1 tsp chopped fresh tarragon	1.6	0.8
Salt and black pepper to taste	—	—
½ chicken breast (6 oz)	—	36.0
1 Tbsp Tarragon Butter (page 417)	0.9	0.06

Combine oil, lemon juice, chopped tarragon, and salt and pepper. Pour mixture over chicken breast and let marinate for at least 15 minutes. Grill chicken to desired doneness. Top with pats of Tarragon Butter. TA

CHICKEN SHISH KEBAB WITH VEGETABLES

1 serving   Per serving: 6 gm CHO, 4.1 oz PRO

	CHO (gm)	PRO (gm)
4 oz chicken breast, cut into 1-inch cubes	—	24.0
1 oz yellow onion, cut into 1-inch squares	2.4	0.3
1 oz red bell pepper, cut into 1-inch squares	1.8	0.25
1 oz green bell pepper, cut into 1-inch squares	1.8	0.25
Salt and black pepper to taste	—	—

Thread chicken, onion, and pepper pieces alternately on skewer. Season with salt and pepper and grill until chicken is fully cooked. TA

CHICKEN DIJON

1 serving   Per serving: 0.35 gm CHO, 4 oz PRO

	CHO (gm)	PRO (gm)
4 oz chicken breast	—	24.0
Salt and black pepper to taste	—	—
1 Tbsp Dijon Mustard Butter (page 415)	0.35	0.02

Season chicken breast with salt and pepper. Grill, bake, or broil to desired doneness. Place chicken on plate, put pats of Dijon Mustard Butter on top, let melt, and serve hot. TA

LEMON CHICKEN

1 serving   Per serving: 0.35 gm CHO, 4 oz PRO

	CHO (gm)	PRO (gm)
4 oz chicken breast	—	24.0
Salt and black pepper to taste	—	—
1 Tbsp Lemon Butter (page 416)	0.35	0.025

Season chicken breast with salt and pepper. Grill, bake, or broil to desired doneness. Place chicken on a plate, put pats of Lemon Butter on top, and let melt. Serve hot. TA

BROILED CHICKEN SALAD

1 serving   Per serving: 1.9 gm CHO, 4 oz PRO

	CHO (gm)	PRO (gm)
4 oz chicken breast	—	24.0
2 Tbsp salad oil	—	—
1 Tbsp vinegar	—	—
1 Tbsp chopped onion	0.9	0.3
1 clove garlic, minced	1.0	0.2
Basil, parsley, chives, and salt and black pepper to taste	—	—

Grill or broil chicken. Cool and cut into ¼-inch strips. Combine oil, vinegar, onion, garlic, basil, parsley, chives, and salt and pepper. Serve cold over chicken strips.

Additional vegetables (up to ⅔ cup) or salad greens (up to 1 cup) may be chopped and added to taste. Be sure they are not on the No-No list on page 160, and make sure you add their CHO content to your computation. TA

GRILLED MARINATED DUCK BREAST

4 servings   Per serving: 1.3 gm CHO, 4.2 oz PRO

	CHO (gm)	PRO (gm)
4 duck breasts, 4 oz each	—	96.0
2 Tbsp soy sauce	4.0	4.0
3 Tbsp water	—	—
¾ tsp chopped fresh ginger	0.23	0.03
1 clove garlic, chopped	1.0	0.2
Salt and black pepper to taste	—	—

Trim duck breasts of visible fat, if necessary, and place in a large bowl. Combine all the remaining ingredients in a small bowl and pour over duck. Turn duck breasts over to evenly coat. Let duck marinate, refrigerated, for several hours or overnight, turning occasionally. Remove duck from marinade and grill or sauté, skin side down, until golden brown. Turn breasts over and cook 1–2 minutes more. Remove duck from grill or sauté pan. Duck should be medium-rare to medium. Slice on the diagonal to serve hot with vegetables or salad. TA

BEEF, LAMB, AND VEAL

Note that the serving size for most recipes in this section is 4 ounces protein. This does not imply any preference for this

*particular amount. In fact, many people will want more pro-
tein. If this is the case for you, simply eat a larger serving or
increase recipe ingredients proportionately.*

GRILLED CHEESEBURGER WITH CANADIAN BACON

1 serving   Per serving: 2 gm CHO, *4 oz* PRO

	CHO (gm)	PRO (gm)
2½ oz hamburger patty	—	15.0
Salt and black pepper to taste	—	—
1 slice cooked Canadian bacon (1 oz)	0.5	6.0
1 slice cheese (½ oz)	0.5	3.0
1 pickle slice	1.0	—

Season hamburger to taste and grill or fry until almost cooked to
desired doneness. Place Canadian bacon and cheese on top and let the
cheese melt. Serve with pickle. TA

GRILLED STEAK WITH MUSHROOM SAUCE

4 servings   Per serving: 2.3 gm CHO, *4 oz* PRO

	CHO (gm)	PRO (gm)
4 small steaks, 4 oz each	—	96.0
Salt and black pepper to taste	—	—
Oil, to coat	—	—
4 oz mushrooms, caps sliced, stems chopped	1.6	0.7
3 Tbsp butter	—	0.4
1 oz minced shallots	4.8	0.7
1 sprig thyme	0.45	0.05
½ bay leaf, crumbled	0.1	0.05
¼ cup dry red wine	2.4	—
¼ cup water	—	—

Preheat grill. Season steaks with salt and pepper, coat lightly with oil,
and set aside.

On medium to high heat, in a small saucepan, sauté sliced mushroom caps in butter until soft. Remove mushrooms and keep warm.
In the same saucepan, sauté shallots until shallots become translucent. Add the chopped mushroom stems and cook until moisture is
released. Add thyme, bay leaf, red wine, water, and salt and pepper to
taste. Simmer to reduce sauce by one-quarter.

While sauce is simmering, grill steaks to desired doneness.
Strain sauce, add the precooked mushroom caps, heat, and serve over
steaks. TA

MARINATED FLANK STEAK

5 *servings*   *Per serving: 0.4 gm* CHO, *8 oz* PRO

	CHO (gm)	PRO (gm)
2½ lb flank steak	—	240.0
2 cloves garlic, minced	2.0	0.4
½ cup olive oil	—	—
¼ cup red wine vinegar	—	—
¾ cup white wine vinegar	—	—
Salt and black pepper to taste	—	—

Place flank steak in a shallow glass baking dish. Combine remaining ingredients in a small bowl and mix well. Pour over steak and cover dish with plastic wrap. Marinate meat 12–24 hours, refrigerated, turning occasionally.

Remove steak from refrigerator about 1 hour before you are ready to cook it. When grill is hot, remove steak from marinade and grill approximately 8 minutes per side for medium-rare. To serve, carve in thin slices, cutting diagonally across the grain. TA

FILET MIGNON WITH GREEN AND BLACK PEPPERCORN SAUCE

2 *servings*   *Per serving: 2.2 gm* CHO, *4 oz* PRO

	CHO (gm)	PRO (gm)
8 oz filet mignon	—	48.0
1 Tbsp oil	—	—
Salt and black pepper to taste	—	—
¼ cup dry red wine	2.4	—
6 whole green peppercorns	1.0	—
6 whole black peppercorns	1.0	—
1 tablespoon butter	—	0.1

Preheat oven to 350°F. Lightly coat filet with oil and season with salt and pepper. Set aside.

Heat an oven pan on top of the stove. When very hot, place filet in it and sear on all sides. Place pan with filet in oven and bake (8 minutes for rare, 10–12 minutes for medium, or 15–18 minutes for well done). Remove pan from oven, place filet on a plate, and keep it warm.

Deglaze pan with wine on stovetop, scraping all drippings from bottom of pan. Add peppercorns. Simmer until liquid is reduced by one-quarter of original amount, then swirl in butter. Divide filet mignon into two equal portions, pour sauce over, and serve. TA

BROILED STEAK SALAD

1 serving   Per serving: 1.9 gm CHO, *4 oz* PRO

	CHO (gm)	PRO (gm)
4 oz lean steak	—	24.0
2 Tbsp oil	—	—
1 Tbsp vinegar	—	—
1 Tbsp chopped onion	0.9	0.3
1 clove garlic, minced	1.0	0.2
Basil, parsley, and salt and black pepper to taste	—	—

Grill or broil steak to desired doneness. Cool and cut into ¼-inch strips. Combine remaining ingredients thoroughly in a bowl, then add steak and mix. Correct the seasoning.

Additional vegetables (up to ⅔ cup) or salad greens (up to 1 cup) may be chopped and added to taste. Be sure they are not on the No-No list on page 160, and make sure you add their CHO content to your computation. TA

BEEF BURGUNDY STEW

4 servings   Per serving: 7.9 gm CHO, *5.3 oz* PRO

	CHO (gm)	PRO (gm)
1 Tbsp butter	—	—
1 lb beef stew cubes	—	122.4
1 bay leaf	—	0.1
2 stalks celery, chopped	3.0	0.6
½ cup sliced button mushrooms	4.0	1.7
1 cup turnip cut into large chunks	7.6	1.2
1 small celery root, peeled and quartered (4 oz) (see Note)	10.4	1.7
½ tsp salt	—	—
⅓ tsp black pepper	—	—
½ tsp dried tarragon	0.5	—
½ cup burgundy wine (dry red)	4.8	—
1 tsp arrowroot powder (see Note 2, page 423)	2.3	—
2 Tbsp cold water	—	—

Heat butter in a large heavy pot and brown cubes of beef for 3–5 minutes. Remove beef from pot and set aside. Add to the pot bay leaf, celery, mushrooms, turnip, and celery root. Sauté vegetables and add salt, black pepper, and tarragon. Cook on a low flame for 3–5 minutes. Return browned beef to pot, placing it on top of vegetables. Add wine, cover with a tight-fitting lid, and cook for 40 minutes over low heat. Thicken cooking liquid at the end of cooking time by dissolving arrowroot powder in cold water, then adding it to the stew. Stir continually as it thickens. Continue cooking the stew, covered, for 3–5 minutes. Remove bay leaf. Serve warm.

The stew will keep in the refrigerator for 4–5 days. It may also be stored in the freezer for 2–3 months.

Note

Celery root, or celeriac, can be found in most groceries, usually alongside jicama and other tuberous vegetables. It is a bulbous root about the size of an orange, with a brownish, gnarled, slightly hairy surface. Despite its appearance, it's quite tasty, with a mild celery flavor. KW

MANDARIN BEEF SAUTÉ

4 servings   Per serving: 1.2 gm CHO, *4.1 oz* PRO

	CHO (gm)	PRO (gm)
1 Tbsp roasted sesame oil (see Note 1)	—	—
½ tsp minced fresh ginger	0.15	0.02
⅓ tsp crushed red pepper flakes (optional)	—	—
⅓ cup sliced button mushrooms	2.6	1.13
1 lb thinly sliced lean beef (see Note 2)	—	96.0
1 Tbsp soy sauce	2.0	2.0
2 Tbsp cider vinegar	—	—

In a large heavy skillet, heat oil on a low temperature. Add ginger, red pepper flakes (if using), and mushrooms, then sauté for 2–3 minutes. Add sliced beef to the skillet and increase temperature to a medium-high setting. Stir continuously for 3–4 minutes. Stir in soy sauce and vinegar. Immediately remove skillet from burner and serve warm.

This recipe will keep in the refrigerator for 3–4 days. It will store in the freezer for 2–3 months.

Notes

1. Oriental-style roasted (dark) sesame oil is made from natural sesame seeds that are roasted before the oil is extracted. The taste is richer than that of the lighter variety. Either one can be used for this recipe.

2. Slice beef by holding the knife on a diagonal angle across the grain. A thin cut provides the best flavor for this quick cooking style. The meat is easier to slice if it's slightly frozen, and you get nicer slices. KW

LAMB SHISH KEBAB

4 servings   Per serving: 5 gm CHO, *4.2 oz* PRO

	CHO (gm)	PRO (gm)
1 lb lamb, cut into 1-inch cubes	—	96.0
Salt and black pepper to taste	—	—
4 oz yellow onion, cut into 1-inch squares	9.6	1.2
4 oz green bell pepper, cut into 1-inch squares	7.2	1.0
8 whole mushrooms	3.2	1.4
Oil, to coat	—	—

Preheat broiler or grill. Season lamb cubes with salt and pepper. On skewers alternate pieces of lamb, onion, green pepper, and whole mushrooms. Lightly brush with oil and broil or grill to desired doneness. TA

VEAL SCALLOPINI

1 serving   Per serving: 7 gm CHO, *6.8 oz* PRO

	CHO (gm)	PRO (gm)
6 oz veal cutlets for scallopini	—	36.0
Salt and black pepper to taste	—	—
2 Tbsp full-fat soy flour	3.8	3.6
2 Tbsp butter	—	0.3
1 tsp minced shallots	0.85	0.15
3 Tbsp white wine	1.8	—
3 Tbsp water	—	—
1 Tbsp chopped parsley	0.6	0.03

Season veal with salt and pepper and lightly coat with soy flour. Heat sauté pan and add 1 tablespoon butter. Sauté veal until golden brown on both sides. Remove from pan and keep warm. Add shallots to pan drippings and sauté briefly. Remove pan from heat and add white wine. Scrape bottom of pan to get all the drippings, add water, and simmer to reduce sauce slightly. Add the parsley and 1 tablespoon butter to finish the sauce. Season to taste. Place veal on a platter, pour sauce over veal, and serve. TA

PORK

PORK CHOPS WITH HORSERADISH SAUCE

2 servings   Per serving: 3 gm CHO, 3.7 oz PRO

	CHO (gm)	PRO (gm)
4 Tbsp grated fresh horseradish	1.6	1.8
¼ cup cider vinegar	—	—
¼ cup water	—	—
½ cup sour cream	4.0	3.2
1 egg yolk	0.3	2.8
½–1 Equal tablet, crushed, or stevia powder (without maltodextrin) to taste (optional)	—	—
Salt and black pepper to taste	—	—
2 small pork chops, about 4 oz each with bone	—	36.0

Soak horseradish in vinegar and water for 15 minutes or more. In the top of a double boiler, combine sour cream, egg yolk, crushed Equal tablet or stevia (if using), and salt and pepper to taste. Stir over, not in, hot water until thick and smooth. Drain horseradish in a strainer, pressing to remove excess liquid, and add to the sauce. Adjust seasoning, cover sauce, and keep warm.

Season pork chops with salt and pepper. Grill, bake, or broil to desired doneness and serve with warm horseradish sauce. TA

STIR-FRIED PORK WITH SWEET-AND-SOUR CABBAGE

1 serving   Per serving: 5.8 gm CHO, 4.3 oz PRO

	CHO (gm)	PRO (gm)
½ cup shredded red cabbage	2.1	0.5
½ cup shredded white cabbage	1.9	0.5
2 Tbsp water	—	—
½ cup bean sprouts	0.6	0.7
Pinch of cumin seeds	—	—
1 Tbsp cider vinegar	—	—
½–1 Equal tablet, crushed, or stevia powder (without maltodextrin) to taste	—	—
Salt and black pepper to taste	—	—
1 Tbsp oil	—	—
4 oz pork tenderloin, cut into ¼-inch strips	—	24.0
2 Tbsp dry white wine	1.2	—

In a large sauté pan or medium pot, combine red cabbage, white cabbage, and water. Cook over medium heat until the cabbage wilts. Add bean sprouts, cumin seeds, vinegar, and crushed Equal tablet or stevia to taste. Season with salt and pepper. Cook over low heat for 3–5 minutes, or until vegetables are tender. Cover and keep warm. In a medium sauté pan or wok, heat oil. Season pork strips with salt and pepper. Add to hot oil, and stir constantly to prevent scorching. When the pork is almost cooked through (this will take just 2–3 minutes), add white wine and cook another minute or so to let the alcohol boil away. Serve with the cabbage. TA

SEAFOOD

TUNA MELT

1 serving   Per serving: 8 gm CHO, 7.3 oz PRO

	CHO (gm)	PRO (gm)
1 can (5 oz) tuna fish	—	45.0
2 Tbsp mayonnaise	—	—
Black pepper to taste	—	—
2 GG Scandinavian Bran Crispbreads	6.0	2.0
2 oz cheese, sliced	2.0	12.0

Drain tuna and mix with mayonnaise and pepper. Mound tuna mix on GG crispbreads and top with cheese slices. Place in oven or toaster oven at 350°F until cheese is fully melted. TA

SALMON SALAD

3 servings   Per serving: 1.8 gm CHO, 4.4 oz PRO

	CHO (gm)	PRO (gm)
1 can (14.75 oz) salmon	—	78.0
1 stalk celery, chopped	1.5	0.3
¼ cup chopped onion	1.8	0.25
1 tsp chopped parsley	—	—
¼ pickle spear, chopped	1.0	—
Lemon pepper seasoning to taste	—	—
2–3 Tbsp mayonnaise	—	—
1 Tbsp prepared mustard	—	—
½ tsp minced chives	—	—
Salt and black pepper to taste	—	—

Place salmon in a large bowl with next 8 ingredients (celery through chives) and mix well. Season to taste with salt and pepper and chill. Serve cold. TA

STUFFED AVOCADO WITH CRABMEAT

2 servings   Per serving: 7.2 gm CHO, *3.7 oz* PRO

	CHO (gm)	PRO (gm)
6 oz crabmeat (see Note 1)	—	54.0
1 heaping Tbsp mayonnaise	—	—
1 tsp olive oil	—	—
1 Tbsp cider vinegar	—	—
½ tsp poppy seeds	—	—
⅓ tsp paprika	0.6	—
¼ tsp salt	—	—
1 stalk celery, diced	1.5	0.3
1 heaping Tbsp minced scallions	0.4	0.1
1 ripe Hass avocado (see Note 2)	12.0	4.8

Place crabmeat in a glass mixing bowl and gently break up any lumps with a fork. Add mayonnaise, olive oil, and cider vinegar. Mix together with a light hand (do not break up the fiber of the crabmeat; merely separate the flakes). Add poppy seeds, paprika, salt, celery, and scallions. Slice avocado in half and remove the pit. Using the tines of a metal fork, lightly score the inside surface of the avocado halves. Do not penetrate the pulp all the way to the skin. Fill each half with half the crabmeat mixture. Serve chilled or at room temperature.

You can store the crabmeat filling in the refrigerator for 2–3 days. Do not split and stuff the avocado until you are ready to serve it.

Notes

1. A variation of this recipe is to use other salad fillings in place of the crabmeat. Tuna or chicken salad would substitute nicely. Be sure to make the proper food count adjustments.

2. Hass avocados are a small variety with a thick, pebbly skin. They are ripe when slightly soft to the touch. KW

FIVE-SPICE SHRIMP WITH BEAN SPROUTS

2 servings   Per serving: 5.6 gm CHO, *4.5 oz* PRO

	CHO (gm)	PRO (gm)
1 Tbsp roasted sesame oil (see Note 1, page 434)	—	—
1 tsp minced fresh ginger	0.3	0.03
2 cups mung bean sprouts (see Note)	8.0	6.0
½ lb medium shrimp, cleaned	—	46.0
1 Tbsp soy sauce	2.0	2.0
½ tsp Chinese five-spice powder	—	—
2 Tbsp chopped scallions	0.8	0.2

In a large heavy skillet, heat oil on a low temperature. Add ginger and sauté for a minute or two, until it is fragrant. Don't let it burn. Add sprouts and shrimp to skillet. Raise heat to high and stir continuously. Add soy sauce and five-spice powder. Cook for 4–5 more minutes. Shrimp are done when they turn pink and are no longer translucent. Garnish with scallions at the end of the cooking time. Serve warm.

This recipe will keep in the refrigerator for 2–3 days in a tightly sealed container.

Note

Mung bean sprouts are sold packaged in the refrigerated section of the produce aisle. Check for a freshness date on the package. The sprouts should appear firm and dry with no liquid accumulated in the bag. Rinse sprouts briefly in a colander under cold water before using. KW

SCALLOPS PROVENÇAL

4 servings   Per serving: 5.0 gm CHO, *4.2 oz* PRO

	CHO (gm)	PRO (gm)
1 Tbsp butter	—	—
1 Tbsp minced shallots	1.7	0.3
½ cup leeks finely sliced diagonally	4.0	0.4
½ cup celery finely sliced diagonally	3.0	0.4
¼ tsp salt	—	—
⅛ tsp dried thyme	0.2	—
⅛ tsp dried tarragon	0.1	—
⅛ tsp dried rosemary	0.1	—
1 lb sea scallops (see Note 1)	10.8	96.0
4–6 leaves fresh basil, chiffonade cut (see Note 2)	0.1	0.1

In a medium skillet, heat butter on a low temperature. Add shallots, leeks, celery, salt, and dried herbs. Sauté for 2–3 minutes. Add the scallops to the skillet and cook over medium heat for 4–5 minutes. Scallops will be done when they are firm in texture and you see small splits on the top. Add shredded basil, cover the skillet, and immediately remove from heat. Set aside for 1–2 minutes. Serve warm.

Notes

1. If you substitute bay scallops (the small variety) for sea scallops, they tend to cook very quickly, so reduce the cooking time by a minute or two. The food counts will be the same.

2. A chiffonade cut is done by uniformly stacking the basil leaves on top of one another, rolling them into a tight pencil shape, and then slicing into thin diagonal strips. KW

GRILLED SALMON WITH LEMON
PEPPER BUTTER

1 serving   Per serving: 1.3 gm CHO, 8.0 oz PRO

	CHO (gm)	PRO (gm)
8 oz salmon steak	—	48.0
Oil, to coat	—	—
Salt and black pepper to taste	—	—
½ Tbsp lemon juice	0.65	0.05
2 Tbsp Lemon Pepper Butter (page 416)	0.65	0.05

Preheat grill or broiler. Coat salmon with oil and season with salt and pepper. Place salmon on heated grill or broiler pan and grill about 4 minutes per side. When the salmon is ready to be turned over, be careful not to break the meat apart. After the salmon is turned, pour lemon juice over it and finish cooking. Remove fish from grill and place on a heated plate. Cover with Lemon Pepper Butter and serve. TA

BLACK OLIVE CRUSTED SALMON

2 servings   Per serving: 4.5 gm CHO, 4.3 oz PRO

	CHO (gm)	PRO (gm)
2 GG Scandinavian Bran Crispbreads	6.0	2.0
6 small black olives, pitted	1.8	—
3 Tbsp chopped scallions	1.2	0.3
2 Tbsp butter, softened	—	2.0
⅓ tsp salt	—	—
¼ tsp black pepper	—	—
Canola oil, to coat baking tray and top of fish	—	—
2 small salmon steaks, 4 oz each	—	48.0

Check to make sure that the work bowl of your food processor is completely dry, then add the crispbreads and process for 1–2 minutes, making coarse-textured crumbs. Remove crumbs to a medium mixing bowl. Add olives, scallions, and butter to your food processor's work bowl (don't worry if there are still a few crumbs) and process for 1–2 minutes. Add salt and pepper and blend again. Transfer this mixture to the bowl with the crumbs. Blend these ingredients together evenly. Refrigerate this mixture until ready to use.

Place salmon steaks on an oiled tray for broiling. Lightly oil the top of the salmon. Broil salmon for 4–5 minutes. Remove tray from broiler. Turn salmon with a spatula. Remove black olive mixture from the refrigerator. Gently press the top of each salmon steak with 3 Tbsp of black olive coating. Place salmon back under broiler. Do not place it too close to the heat, because the crust will burn before the salmon cooks. Cook an additional 4–5 minutes. When the salmon is done it will easily flake apart with a fork. Serve warm.

The salmon will keep in the refrigerator, covered, for 2–3 days. ᴋᴡ

STEAMED SCROD WITH WATERCRESS AND GINGER

4 servings   Per serving: 5.1 gm ᴄʜᴏ, *4.1 oz* ᴘʀᴏ

	CHO (gm)	PRO (gm)
1½ cups thinly sliced (¼ inch) daikon radish or white turnip	7.5	1.5
1 cup sliced yellow summer squash	7.8	1.6
16 oz fresh scrod fillet (½ inch thick), cut into 4 pieces	—	96.0
¾ cup water	—	—
1 Tbsp roasted sesame oil (see Note 1, page 434)	—	—
¼ tsp grated fresh ginger	0.08	—
1 Tbsp soy sauce	2.0	2.0
1 tsp cream of tartar dissolved in ¼ cup cold water	0.6	—
2 Tbsp sesame seeds	1.8	4.2
½ bunch watercress, washed thoroughly and drained	0.6	1.2

In the bottom of a large skillet, layer first the daikon and then the yellow squash. Place the scrod on top of the vegetables. In a small mixing bowl, combine the water, sesame oil, ginger, and soy sauce and whisk together. Pour the mixture evenly over the fish and vegetables. Cover the skillet and bring the liquid to a boil, then reduce the heat. Simmer for 5–7 minutes. Stir the dissolved cream of tartar into the cooking liquid. Keep the flame low as the liquid thickens. Add the sesame seeds and watercress, cover skillet, and immediately remove from the heat. Allow the watercress to cook in the accumulated heat of the covered skillet as it sits for 3–4 minutes before serving. Use a slotted spoon or metal spatula to serve each portion of fish and vegetables. Serve warm. ᴋᴡ

PAN-FRIED SWORDFISH WITH
GINGER SCALLION BUTTER

1 serving   Per serving: 7.6 gm CHO, *4.8 oz* PRO

	CHO (gm)	PRO (gm)
¼ cup soy sauce	4.0	4.0
2 Tbsp dry white wine	1.2	0.1
¼ tsp minced garlic	0.25	0.05
1 tsp minced fresh ginger	0.3	0.2
2 scallions, minced	0.93	0.03
½ Tbsp lemon juice	0.65	0.05
4 oz swordfish steak	—	24.0
Salt and black pepper to taste	—	—
2 Tbsp butter	—	0.3
1 Tbsp Ginger Scallion Butter (page 416)	0.25	0.3

Combine first 6 ingredients (soy sauce through lemon juice) in a shallow glass bowl and place swordfish steak in it, turning to coat both sides. Allow the fish to marinate for 30 minutes. Remove swordfish and blot dry. Season with salt and pepper. Heat butter in a sauté pan over medium-high heat. When butter starts to foam, add fish and cook to desired doneness. Remove fish from pan and place on a heated plate. Serve with pats of Ginger Scallion Butter on top. TA

TROUT AMANDINE

1 serving   Per serving: 3.4 gm CHO, *5.2 oz* PRO

	CHO (gm)	PRO (gm)
5 oz trout fillet	—	30.0
Salt and black pepper to taste	—	—
2 Tbsp butter	—	0.3
2 Tbsp slivered almonds	1.72	1.68
1 Tbsp lemon juice	1.3	0.1
2 tsp chopped parsley	0.4	0.2

Season trout on both sides with salt and pepper. Sauté the trout in 1 tablespoon butter until almost cooked. Remove to a warm plate and keep warm (fish will continue cooking). Pour excess butter from sauté pan. Add 1 tablespoon butter and let brown slightly. Add the almonds and brown them. Just before serving, stir in lemon juice and parsley, and pour sauce over trout. TA

BLUEFISH WITH SPICY MUSTARD SAUCE

1 serving   Per serving: 2.3 gm CHO, *4 oz* PRO

	CHO (gm)	PRO (gm)
4 oz bluefish steak	—	24.0
Oil, to coat	—	—
Salt and black pepper to taste	—	—
2 Tbsp Spicy Mustard Sauce (page 417), warmed	2.3	0.11

Preheat grill or broiler. Lightly coat bluefish with oil and season with salt and pepper. Cook to desired doneness and serve topped with mustard sauce. TA

VEGETABLE ENTRÉES AND SIDE DISHES

MOUSSAKA À LA BERNSTEIN

6 servings   Per serving: 8.4 gm CHO, *4.3 oz* PRO

	CHO (gm)	PRO (gm)
3 Tbsp olive oil, approximately	—	—
1 medium eggplant, about 1 lb, peeled and sliced into ½-inch rounds	20.0	3.2
Salt and black pepper to taste	—	—
1 Tbsp minced garlic	3.0	0.6
½ cup diced red bell pepper	4.6	0.6
1 lb ground beef	—	96.0
1 tsp dried oregano	0.5	0.1
1 tsp ground cumin	0.9	0.4
2 Tbsp butter	—	—
½ cup thinly sliced turnip	4.1	0.6
1 cup whole-milk ricotta cheese	8.0	24.0
1 cup heavy cream	6.6	4.8
½ tsp paprika	1.2	0.3
2 eggs, lightly beaten	1.2	12.6
⅓ cup grated Parmesan cheese	—	11.0

Preheat oven to 375°F. In a large skillet, heat 2 Tbsp olive oil over a medium flame. Add eggplant slices, working in batches if necessary to avoid overcrowding. Sprinkle the eggplant with salt and pepper and brown for 5 minutes on a side. Remove from skillet. If working in batches, you may want to add a little more oil to the skillet before each new batch. When all the eggplant slices have been browned and removed, add 1 Tbsp olive oil to the skillet, along with the garlic and red pepper. Sauté for 2–3 minutes. Add ground beef, oregano, cumin, and salt and pepper to taste. Brown evenly.

In another large skillet heat butter on a low temperature. Layer turnip in skillet and sprinkle with salt and pepper. Brown for 5 minutes on each side. Use a spatula to flip turnip.

In a medium mixing bowl combine ricotta cheese, heavy cream, salt to taste, and paprika. Add eggs and blend together. In a lightly buttered 9 × 13 baking dish, layer eggplant, ground beef, and turnip. Pour ricotta cheese mixture over layered ingredients. Sprinkle casserole with grated Parmesan cheese. Place casserole in the oven and bake for 45 minutes. Serve warm.

The moussaka will keep in the refrigerator for 3–4 days. It may also be stored in the freezer for 2–3 months. It is convenient to package the casserole in individual servings if you are going to freeze it. KW

CREAMED SPINACH WITH NUTMEG

4 servings   Per serving: 8.6 gm CHO, <0.5 oz PRO

	CHO (gm)	PRO (gm)
2 lbs fresh baby leaf spinach (see Note)	27.2	0.9
1 Tbsp butter	—	—
⅓ tsp salt	—	—
¼ tsp black pepper	—	—
½ tsp nutmeg	0.6	—
1 cup heavy cream	6.6	4.8

Bring 4 quarts of water to a boil in a large pot. Add spinach and cook at a boil for 3–4 minutes. Drain spinach in a colander and rinse with cold water. Squeeze out the excess moisture from spinach. Place spinach on a cutting board and chop into bite-sized pieces. Melt butter in a nonreactive skillet. Add cooked spinach and season with salt, pepper, and nutmeg. Stir in the heavy cream. Reduce the flame and cook for 30 minutes. Do not cover the skillet; the spinach will release too much moisture and dilute the flavor. To avoid scorching the food, keep the flame at a low setting and stir frequently. You can also use a heat deflector (an inexpensive round metal disk, often with a wooden handle, that you can place between pot and burner while cooking) to prevent scorching. Serve warm.

The spinach will keep in the refrigerator for 3–4 days.

This dish is a good one for those who suffer from gastroparesis if the spinach is finely chopped.

Note

You can often buy spinach prewashed. Getting it this way will save some preparation time, as spinach can be very gritty and bunch spinach must be thoroughly washed. You can also use mature spinach leaves, but they should be stemmed and roughly shredded. KW

BAKED CHEDDAR CHEESE FRITTATA

4 servings   Per serving: 7.2 gm CHO, 2 oz PRO

	CHO (gm)	PRO (gm)
4 eggs	2.4	24.0
1 cup heavy cream	6.6	4.8
1 Tbsp butter	—	0.1
1 cup sliced button mushrooms	8.0	3.4
1 cup sliced red bell pepper	9.2	1.2
¾ tsp salt	—	—
¼ tsp dried oregano	0.3	—
¼ tsp cayenne pepper (optional)	0.4	0.1
½ cup (2 oz) grated cheddar cheese	2.0	14.0

Preheat oven to 375°F. Blend together eggs and heavy cream in a mixing bowl and set aside. In a 9-inch ovenproof skillet (see Note), melt butter over medium heat and sauté sliced mushrooms and bell pepper. Add salt, oregano, and cayenne pepper (omit if you don't care for spicy foods or suffer from gastroparesis) and cook for 3–5 minutes, until the mushrooms are tender and the bell pepper is wilted but not mushy. Add the egg and cream mixture to the sautéed vegetables. Cook on a low flame for 2–3 minutes. Sprinkle on grated cheddar cheese just before placing the skillet in the oven. Bake for 20 minutes uncovered. Serve warm or at room temperature.

This recipe works well as a light meal for lunch or supper. It will keep for 2–3 days refrigerated in an airtight container.

Note

If your skillet has a plastic handle, before baking, transfer the egg, cream, and vegetable mixture to a greased 9-inch round baking pan or pie plate, then sprinkle on the cheddar. KW

ROASTED FENNEL WITH ROSEMARY

8 servings   Per serving: 6.6 gm CHO, *<0.5 oz* PRO

	CHO (gm)	PRO (gm)
2 bulbs trimmed fennel (see Note), sliced into quarters lengthwise	34.2	5.8
1 cup leeks sliced into ½-inch diagonals	8.0	0.8
½ cup diced red bell pepper	4.6	0.6
3 Tbsp chopped black olives	4.0	—
4 Tbsp olive oil	—	—
½ tsp salt	—	—
½ tsp black pepper	0.9	—
1 tsp dried rosemary	0.8	0.1

Preheat oven to 425°F. In a large mixing bowl, gently toss together fennel, leeks, red pepper, and black olives. Add olive oil, salt, black pepper, and rosemary to the vegetables and mix ingredients together, taking care that all the vegetables are lightly coated with the oil and seasoning. In a baking tray, arrange the fennel first, placing cut sides down. Evenly distribute the remaining ingredients over the fennel. Bake the vegetables uncovered on the middle oven rack for 45 minutes. Serve warm.

The roasted vegetables will keep in the refrigerator for 4–5 days in an airtight container.

Note

Fennel resembles a smooth celery in color and shape but has a fragrance like anise or licorice. Its base is bulbous and it has featherlike strands in its center (its leaf looks a bit like dill). Select fennel that has smooth skin and does not appear wrinkled or dried out. Look for a large bulb, slightly smaller than a baseball. For this recipe trim away all parts of the vegetable but the bulb. KW

TURNIP "MASHED POTATOES" WITH FRESH CHIVES

4 servings   Per serving: 9.3 gm CHO, *<0.5 oz* PRO

	CHO (gm)	PRO (gm)
4 medium turnips, trimmed at the root and stem ends and quartered	33.6	4.9
⅓ tsp salt	—	—
2 Tbsp butter	—	—
½ cup heavy cream	3.3	2.4
¼ tsp black pepper	—	—
3 Tbsp finely chopped chives or scallions	0.3	0.3

In a medium saucepan, bring 3 quarts water to a boil. Add turnips and salt. Cover the pot and cook 30–40 minutes, or until tender when pricked with a fork. Drain turnips in a colander. While the turnips are still warm, put them into a large mixing bowl. Add butter and heavy cream. Using a potato masher, mash ingredients together. (If you would like a whipped texture you can use a food processor. Put the mixture into the food processor work bowl and blend for 2–3 minutes.) Add black pepper and chives or scallions. Serve warm as a vegetable side dish. This recipe's soft texture and mild flavor would nicely complement Steamed Scrod with Watercress and Ginger (page 441). kw

BAKED MUSHROOMS FLORENTINE

4 servings   Per serving: 8.4 gm CHO, *1.1 oz* PRO

	CHO (gm)	PRO (gm)
2 GG Scandinavian Bran Crispbreads	6.0	2.0
12 large white mushrooms (large enough to stuff)	16.0	6.8
4 cups fresh spinach leaves	8.0	6.4
3 strips crisp-cooked bacon, crumbled (optional)	—	6.0
2 Tbsp grated Parmesan cheese	0.4	4.2
1 Tbsp butter	—	—
1 tsp minced garlic	1.0	0.2
⅓ cup heavy cream	2.2	1.6

Preheat oven to 375°F. In the food processor work bowl, blend crispbreads into coarse crumbs. Remove the crumbs from the work bowl and set aside. With a paring knife remove the stems from the mushrooms. Keep the mushroom caps intact and set them aside. In the food processor, finely chop mushroom stems and spinach leaves. You may need to add the spinach in two portions because of its volume. Remove processed ingredients to a large mixing bowl and blend in the bacon (if using) and cheese. In a heavy skillet, heat butter on a low flame. Add garlic and spinach mixture. Stir in the heavy cream. Sauté for 4–5 minutes. Transfer ingredients to a mixing bowl. Spoon the filling into the mushroom caps. Sprinkle with crumbs. Lightly grease a baking tray. Place filled mushrooms on the tray and bake uncovered for 45 minutes. Serve warm.

The mushrooms will keep in the refrigerator for 3–4 days or in the freezer for about 1 month. kw

MEDITERRANEAN EGGPLANT STEW

6 servings   Per serving: 8.5 gm CHO, *3.5 oz* PRO

	CHO (gm)	PRO (gm)
1 Tbsp olive oil	—	—
1 Tbsp minced shallots	1.7	0.3
½ cup sliced button mushrooms	4.0	1.7
½ cup diced red bell pepper	4.6	0.6
2 medium eggplants, about 1 pound each, peeled and cut into large chunks	40.0	6.4
1 tsp salt	—	—
1 tsp dried oregano	0.5	0.1
½ tsp crushed red pepper flakes	0.6	—
1 lb ground turkey	—	96.0

Heat oil over low temperature in a Dutch oven. Add shallots, mushrooms, bell pepper, and eggplant. Add seasonings and stir ingredients together. Raise heat to medium. Vegetables will start to "sweat," or release liquid, as they cook. Continue stirring for 7–10 minutes, allowing some of this liquid to cook away. Add the ground turkey to the pot and stir gently to blend. Cover pot, lower the temperature, and allow to cook for 45 minutes. It is not necessary to stir the pot as long as the heat is low. Serve warm.

The stew will keep for 3–4 days in the refrigerator. It may also be stored in the freezer for 2–3 months. KW

STUFFED SAVOY CABBAGE WITH RED SAUCE

4 servings   Per serving: 11.3 gm CHO, *4.7 oz* PRO

	CHO (gm)	PRO (gm)
8 outer leaves Savoy cabbage (see Note)	6.0	—
2 GG Scandinavian Bran Crispbreads	6.0	2.0
1¼ lb lean ground beef	—	120.0
2 eggs	1.2	12.6
1 stalk celery, diced small	1.5	0.3
1 cup green bell pepper, diced small	9.2	1.2
½ tsp salt	—	—
1 tsp dried oregano	0.5	0.1
1½ cups Italian-Style Red Sauce (page 414)	16.8	0.9

Rinse the cabbage leaves under cold water. Bring 2 quarts of water to a boil in a stockpot. Add the cabbage leaves and cook at a boil for 4–5 minutes. Remove the leaves from the water and place in a colander to drain.

In the food processor work bowl, blend crispbreads into coarse crumbs. Combine the ground beef and eggs in a large mixing bowl. Add the crumbs, celery, bell pepper, salt, and oregano. Thoroughly mix all ingredients together, then divide the mixture into 8 portions.

Stuff the cabbage leaves one at a time. Place a leaf of cooked cabbage on a flat surface. Using a paring knife, remove about ½ inch from the bottom of the center rib, to make the leaf easier to roll. Place a portion of the meat and crumb mixture in the center of the leaf near the bottom. Fold the sides of the leaf over the filling. Starting at the bottom, roll up the leaf to enclose the filling. The finished roll should be about 2 × 3 inches. Continue in this fashion until all the leaves are stuffed.

Preheat oven to 375°F. Pour ¾ cup of the red sauce on the bottom of an 8 × 8 baking pan. Place cabbage rolls on the sauce seam side down. Pour the remaining red sauce over the cabbage. Bake uncovered for 1 hour. Serve warm.

The stuffed cabbage will keep in the refrigerator for 3–4 days. The rolls may also be stored in the freezer for 2–3 months.

Note
Savoy cabbage resembles the common variety of green cabbage in color and shape. Its leaves are thinner and have a lacy surface texture. You can substitute green cabbage if you are unable to find Savoy. Food counts will remain unchanged. KW

SPAGHETTI SQUASH FRITTERS / LATKES

4 servings, 3 fritters each   Per serving: 8.6 gm CHO, 1.2 oz PRO

	CHO (gm)	PRO (gm)
2 cups cooked spaghetti squash (see Note)	20.0	2.0
3 GG Scandinavian Bran Crispbreads	9.0	3.0
3 eggs	1.8	18.9
2 Tbsp grated Parmesan cheese	0.4	4.2
1 tsp paprika	1.2	0.3
½ cup coarsely chopped flat-leaf parsley	1.9	0.9
½ tsp salt	—	—
¼ tsp black pepper	—	—
1 cup canola oil	—	—

Prepare squash as described in Note. Measure 2 cups chopped pulp into a large mixing bowl and set aside. (Discard remaining pulp or save for another purpose.)

Blend crispbreads in the food processor work bowl for 2–3 minutes, until they are in coarse crumbs. Remove crumbs from work bowl and set aside. Combine eggs, cheese, paprika, parsley, salt, and pepper in the work bowl and blend together for 2–3 minutes.

Add egg-cheese mixture from work bowl to the cooked squash in the large mixing bowl. Stir to combine. Add crumbs to squash mixture and mix in evenly. Measure 2 Tbsp of mixture for each fritter. Shape them into patties about ⅓ inch thick.

Add the canola oil to a heavy skillet. Heat on medium-low flame. Test the cooking temperature by adding a drop of batter. You've got the right temperature when the batter cooks on the surface of the oil. Carefully lower the fritters into the oil a few at a time. Do not overcrowd. Cook for 4–5 minutes on each side. Place cooked fritters on paper towels to absorb excess oil.

Note

Spaghetti squash is an oblong, pale yellow squash. Its hard outer shell is not edible. The inside pulp separates into long spaghetti-like strands after cooking.

To cook the squash, slice it in half lengthwise. Remove the seeds. Oil a baking tray and place the squash cut side down on the tray. Bake at 375°F for 50 minutes. After the squash cools, scoop out the pulp. Coarsely chop the cooked squash before adding to fritter recipe. KW

BAKED ZUCCHINI WITH FRESH BASIL AND FETA CHEESE

4 servings   Per serving: 8.3 gm CHO, *0.7 oz* PRO

	CHO (gm)	PRO (gm)
2 Tbsp olive oil	—	—
1 cup diced red bell pepper	9.2	1.2
½ cup sliced button mushrooms	4.0	1.7
1 Tbsp minced garlic	3.0	0.6
½ tsp dried oregano	0.2	—
6 leaves fresh basil, chiffonade cut (see Note 2, page 440)	0.1	0.1
Pinch of salt	—	—
¼ tsp black pepper	—	—
2 medium zucchini	14.0	2.4
3 oz (¾ cup) crumbled feta cheese	3.0	12.0

Preheat oven to 375°F. In a heavy skillet, heat 1 Tbsp olive oil over low heat. Add bell pepper, mushrooms, garlic, oregano, basil, salt, and black pepper. Sauté for 3–5 minutes and set aside. Cut zucchini diagonally into ½-inch-thick slices. Coat a baking pan with 1 Tbsp oil and add zucchini, placing the cut sides down. Spoon the sautéed vegetable mixture over the zucchini. Sprinkle the crumbled feta cheese over vegetables. Cover the baking pan with foil and place in the oven. Bake for 45 minutes. The zucchini should be tender at the end of the baking time. Serve warm.

The baked zucchini will keep in the refrigerator for 4–5 days. It may also be stored in the freezer for 2–3 months. ĸw

PAN-FRIED TOFU WITH SWEET-AND-SOUR DIPPING SAUCE

4 servings   Per serving: 3.2 gm CHO, *2.3 oz* PRO

	CHO (gm)	PRO (gm)
1 lb firm tofu (see Note)	10.0	55.0
1 Tbsp canola oil	—	—
2 Tbsp prepared mustard	—	—
3 Tbsp mayonnaise	—	—
Scant ¼ tsp stevia powder (without maltodextrin)	—	—
½ tsp poppy seeds	0.3	—
1 Tbsp minced scallions	—	—
1 Tbsp minced sauerkraut, drained	0.5	—
1 Tbsp roasted sesame oil (see Note 1, page 434)	—	—
1 Tbsp soy sauce	2.0	2.0

Slice tofu into 4 thick slabs. Place the tofu on an absorbent kitchen towel. Fold the towel over the tofu and firmly press out the excess moisture for a few moments. Removing excess liquid helps tofu to brown. In a heavy skillet, heat oil over a low flame. Add the tofu and brown on each side for 5–7 minutes. The tofu will become a golden color. Do not cover the skillet. Combine remaining ingredients in a small mixing bowl and set aside. You will serve this sauce with the cooked tofu. Remove tofu from the skillet and serve warm.

The tofu and the sauce will keep in the refrigerator for 4–5 days.

Note

Tofu is made from soybeans that have been cooked and pressed into cakes. It's sold in the refrigerator case in many food stores. Check the expiration date for freshness before buying. Uncooked tofu should be stored in water in a sealed container and will keep in the refrigerator for 2–3 days. Cooked tofu will keep in the refrigerator for 4–5 days. ĸw

CELERY CHIPS

8 servings, about ¼ cup each   Per serving: 2.6 gm CHO, <0.1 oz PRO

	CHO (gm)	PRO (gm)
1 medium celery root (8 oz) (see Note, page 434)	20.8	3.4
2 Tbsp canola oil	—	—
⅓ tsp salt	—	—

Preheat oven to 425°F. Remove the thick peel from the celery root with a paring knife. Slice the root lengthwise into quarters. Slice into thin quarter-rounds. In a mixing bowl, combine celery root with oil and toss to evenly coat the slices. Add the salt and mix again. Place the celery root slices in a single layer on a baking tray. Bake for 30 minutes uncovered on the middle rack of the oven. Chips can be served immediately.

Allow chips to cool before storage. Place them in an airtight container in the refrigerator. They will keep for 2–3 days. Reheat them in a 425°F oven for 5–7 minutes before serving for a crunchy texture. KW

CREAMY STRING BEAN CASSEROLE WITH SAGE MUSHROOM SAUCE

6 servings   Per serving: 12.3 gm CHO, <0.6 oz PRO

	CHO (gm)	PRO (gm)
1 Tbsp olive oil	—	—
2 cups sliced button mushrooms	16.0	6.8
1 Tbsp minced shallots	1.7	0.3
¾ tsp ground sage	0.3	—
½ tsp salt	—	—
⅓ tsp black pepper	—	—
1 heaping Tbsp arrowroot powder (see Note 2, page 423)	7.5	—
1 cup College Inn chicken broth	—	1.0
½ cup heavy cream	3.3	2.4
4 cups chopped frozen string beans	39.2	9.6
1 cup Celery Chips (see previous recipe)	5.2	0.3

Preheat oven to 375°F. Heat oil over low temperature in a medium skillet. Add mushrooms, shallots, sage, salt, and black pepper. Sauté for 5–7 minutes. Dissolve arrowroot powder in chicken broth. Add this liquid and heavy cream to mushroom mixture in the skillet. The liquid will thicken as it heats. Stir the ingredients together for 3–5 minutes. Place the string beans in a layer on the bottom of a baking pan. Evenly pour the mushroom sauce over string beans. Layer celery chips on top. Bake uncovered for 45 minutes. Serve warm.

This recipe will keep in the refrigerator for 2–3 days. It may also be stored in the freezer for about 1 month. KW

PUREED CAULIFLOWER WITH CELERY ROOT

6 servings   Per serving: 8.8 gm CHO, <0.5 oz PRO

	CHO (gm)	PRO (gm)
½ tsp salt	—	—
1 bay leaf	—	—
1 medium celery root (8 oz), peeled and cut into large chunks (see Note, page 434)	20.8	3.4
1 small head cauliflower, cut into 1-inch pieces	31.2	13.2
1 Tbsp olive oil	—	—
½ tsp dried dill weed	0.6	—
1 Tbsp minced parsley	0.3	—

Add salt and bay leaf to 2 quarts water in a large saucepan. Bring liquid to a rolling boil. Drop in the celery root and cauliflower, reduce temperature, and simmer for about 30 minutes. Vegetables are ready when they are fork tender. Strain vegetables from cooking liquid and place in the work bowl of your food processor. Blend until they acquire a creamy texture (3–4 minutes). Add oil, dill, and parsley. Blend ingredients again for 1 minute. Serve pureed vegetables warm.

This recipe will keep in the refrigerator for 3–4 days. It may also be stored in the freezer for 2–3 months.

This recipe is helpful for gastroparesis. The soft texture and mild flavor of the pureed vegetables facilitate easier digestion when a low-bulk diet is recommended. KW

PAN-FRIED OKRA WITH TAMARI SCALLION GLAZE

4 servings   Per serving: 9.9 gm CHO, <0.5 oz PRO

	CHO (gm)	PRO (gm)
1 Tbsp olive oil	—	—
1 lb okra, trimmed and cut into ½-inch rounds (see Note 1)	24.4	6.4
1 cup diced yellow summer squash	10.0	—
1 tsp arrowroot powder (see Note 2, page 423)	2.3	—
½ cup cold water	—	—
1 Tbsp tamari or soy sauce	2.0	2.0
1 Tbsp minced scallions	0.4	0.1
½ tsp fresh ginger juice (see Note 2)	0.15	0.02

Heat oil over low temperature in a heavy skillet. Add okra and yellow squash. Raise the cooking temperature to medium-high. Stir continuously for 4–5 minutes. Dissolve arrowroot in cold water. Lower temperature under skillet, pour in arrowroot liquid, and stir as liquid thickens. Add tamari, scallions, and ginger juice. Cover the skillet and continue cooking for 4–5 minutes. Serve warm.

This recipe will keep in the refrigerator for 2–3 days.

Notes

1. Okra is a green, pod-shaped vegetable. Select okra that is firm to the touch and without discoloration or bruising. As it cooks, it releases a gelatinous liquid that is helpful as a thickening agent.

2. It is not necessary to peel the ginger before grating. First wash it with cold water to remove any surface dirt. Use the fine side of a box grater to pulp the ginger. Place the pulp in a garlic press (or in your hand) and squeeze out the liquid. Avoid adding the pulp to this recipe, because it is too fibrous. KW

AVOCADO SPREAD

2 servings   Per serving: 6.6 gm CHO, *<0.5 oz* PRO

	CHO (gm)	PRO (gm)
1 ripe Hass avocado (see Note 2, page 438)	12.0	4.8
1 Tbsp mayonnaise	—	—
1 Tbsp heavy cream	0.3	0.4
2 Tbsp cider vinegar	—	—
¼ tsp salt	—	—
1 Tbsp minced roasted red pepper	1.0	—
1 tsp minced fresh cilantro	—	—

Slice the avocado in half and remove the pit. Scoop out all of the pulp with a metal spoon and discard the skin. Place the pulp in the work bowl of your food processor. Add mayonnaise, heavy cream, vinegar, and salt. Blend together for 2–3 minutes. Remove the avocado mixture to a glass mixing bowl. By hand, mix in the roasted red pepper and cilantro. Serve the avocado spread either chilled or at room temperature. It is best served with low-carbohydrate crackers or as a dip with strips of raw vegetables such as red and green bell pepper, cucumber, yellow squash, zucchini, and celery.

The spread will keep in the refrigerator for 3–4 days in a tightly sealed glass container. KW

CHINESE-STYLE SCALLION PANCAKE

1 serving   Per serving: 8.6 gm CHO, 1.8 oz PRO

	CHO (gm)	PRO (gm)
1 GG Scandinavian Bran Crispbread, crumbled into fine crumbs	3.0	1.0
2 Tbsp full-fat soy flour	3.8	3.6
¼ tsp salt	—	—
¼ tsp Chinese five-spice powder	—	—
1 egg	0.6	6.0
2 Tbsp heavy cream	0.8	0.6
2 Tbsp water	—	—
1 Tbsp minced scallions	0.4	—
2 Tbsp canola oil	—	—

In a small mixing bowl, blend together crispbread crumbs, soy flour, salt, and five-spice powder. In a separate, medium-sized mixing bowl, combine the egg, heavy cream, water, and scallions. A whisk is useful here in blending the ingredients. Add the dry ingredients to the liquid ingredients and blend together thoroughly. Heat oil in a heavy skillet over medium temperature. Using a rubber spatula, scrape the batter from the bowl into the hot skillet. Use the spatula to spread out the batter before it sets in the skillet. Cook pancake for 3–4 minutes on each side. Serve the pancake warm as an accompaniment to Mandarin Beef Sauté (page 434) or another warm lunch or dinner entrée. Break off pieces and dip into the sauce of the entrée or eat by itself.

To make multiple pancakes, quadruple the recipe and use about ¾ cup batter per pancake. Leftover pancakes will keep for 3–4 days in a tightly sealed container in the refrigerator, and if you prepare them beforehand, you can heat them to warm in the microwave. They will keep in the freezer for 1–2 months. Do not freeze uncooked batter. KW

SAUTÉED KALE WITH CRIMINI MUSHROOMS

2 servings   Per serving: 8.4 gm CHO, <0.5 oz PRO

	CHO (gm)	PRO (gm)
5–6 large leaves kale (see Note 1)	11.2	4.0
1 Tbsp olive oil	—	—
1 tsp minced garlic	1.0	0.2
½ cup thinly sliced crimini mushrooms (see Note 2)	4.0	1.7
1 tsp soy sauce	0.6	0.6

In a large pot, bring 4 quarts of water to a rolling boil. Add kale and cook at a boil for 2–3 minutes. Remove kale from water and place in colander. Quickly rinse with cold water. Squeeze out excess moisture from leaves and place on cutting board. Cut off the stems and slice them into small pieces. Slice the leaves into bite-sized pieces (there should be about 2 cups). In a large skillet, heat oil on a low temperature. Add garlic and mushrooms and sauté for a minute or two. Then add kale leaves and stems to the skillet. Raise the temperature to medium-high and quickly sauté for 2–3 minutes, stirring frequently. Season with soy sauce and serve warm. Remove vegetables from hot skillet to avoid overcooking.

The kale will keep for 2 days in the refrigerator.

Notes

1. Select kale that has an even, dark green color. Any yellow color indicates a loss of nutritional value. Leafy greens are perishable and should be used quickly once purchased. Wash kale in a large bowl of cold water and rinse several times until the water runs clear. Leafy greens like beet tops, collards, turnip tops, and broccoli rabe are similar to kale in their selection and handling.

2. Crimini mushrooms are tan to dark brown in color. Select mushrooms that are dry to the touch, without any soft spots or discoloration. KW

QUICHES AND SOUFFLÉS

QUICHE LORRAINE

4 servings   Per serving: 12.2 gm CHO, *3.6 oz* PRO

	CHO (gm)	PRO (gm)
10 GG Scandinavian Bran Crispbreads, crushed	30.0	10.0
5 Tbsp butter, softened	—	0.7
5 slices bacon	0.16	9.8
1½ cups (6 oz) shredded Swiss cheese	6.0	36.0
½ cup chopped scallions	3.7	0.9
1 cup heavy cream	6.6	4.9
4 eggs, separated	2.4	24.0
¼ tsp nutmeg	—	—
¼ tsp salt	—	—
Black pepper to taste	—	—

Preheat oven to 350°F. To make crust, combine crushed crispbreads with softened butter. Press mixture into an 8-inch pie pan, making sure that it is of even thickness all over. Cook bacon until crisp. Let cool, then crumble. In a bowl, combine all other ingredients except the egg whites. Whip whites to soft peaks and then fold into mixture. Stir in the crumbled bacon. Pour into the cracker crust and bake for 30–40 minutes, or until top is light to golden brown. TA

CHEESE QUICHE

3 servings   Per serving: 14.2 gm CHO, 4.3 oz PRO

	CHO (gm)	PRO (gm)
10 GG Scandinavian Bran Crispbreads, crushed	30.0	10.0
5 Tbsp butter, softened	—	0.7
¼ cup grated Parmesan cheese	1.5	10.0
½ tsp dry mustard	—	—
¼ tsp salt	—	—
¼ tsp black pepper	—	—
¾ cup (3 oz) shredded Swiss cheese	3.0	18.0
¾ cup (3 oz) shredded cheddar cheese	3.0	18.0
3 eggs, separated	1.8	18.0
½ cup heavy cream	3.3	2.45

Preheat oven to 350°F. To make crust, combine crushed crispbreads with softened butter. Press mixture into an 8-inch pie pan, making sure that it is of even thickness all over. In a bowl, combine remaining ingredients except egg whites. Whip whites to soft peaks, then fold into the cheese mixture and pour into the cracker crust. Bake for 30–40 minutes, or until top is light to golden brown. TA

SPINACH SOUFFLÉ

6 servings   Per serving: 6.9 gm CHO, 2.9 oz PRO

	CHO (gm)	PRO (gm)
2 Tbsp butter	—	0.3
¼ cup full-fat soy flour	7.5	7.3
10 oz frozen chopped spinach, thawed, squeezed to remove excess moisture	10.0	8.0
¼ cup grated Parmesan cheese	1.5	10.0
1 clove garlic, minced	1.0	0.2
½ tsp salt	—	—
¼ tsp black pepper	—	—
1 tsp prepared mustard	—	—
1 cup milk	11.4	8.0
1½ cups (6 oz) shredded cheddar cheese	6.0	36.0
6 eggs, separated	3.6	36.0
½ tsp cream of tartar	0.6	—

Preheat oven to 350°F. Use a bit of the butter and soy flour to lightly grease and flour an 8-inch soufflé dish. In a large bowl, combine all ingredients except egg whites. Whip whites to soft peaks and then fold into the other ingredients. Pour the mixture into the greased and floured dish. Bake for 30–40 minutes, or until top is light to golden brown. TA

ZUCCHINI SOUFFLÉ

6 servings   Per serving: 7.1 gm CHO, *1.7 oz* PRO

	CHO (gm)	PRO (gm)
2 Tbsp butter	—	0.5
¼ cup full-fat soy flour	7.5	7.3
1 lb zucchini, sliced	15.2	6.4
1 medium onion, chopped	6.9	0.9
1 garlic clove, minced	1.0	0.2
¼ cup grated Parmesan cheese	1.5	10.0
¼ cup dry white wine	2.4	0.8
2 Tbsp minced parsley	0.4	0.2
1 Tbsp lemon juice	1.3	0.1
2 Tbsp diced pimiento	2.0	—
½ tsp cream of tartar	0.6	—
Pinch of nutmeg, or to taste	—	—
Salt and black pepper to taste	—	—
6 eggs, separated	3.6	36.0

Preheat oven to 350°F. Use a bit of the butter and soy flour to lightly grease and flour an 8-inch soufflé dish. Heat remaining butter in a sauté pan and sauté zucchini slices, onion, and garlic until zucchini becomes translucent. Put sautéed mixture into food processor and pulse to mince. Pour into a large bowl and add the rest of the soy flour and all remaining ingredients except the eggs. In a separate bowl, beat egg *yolks* until frothy. Blend into the mixture. In a separate bowl, beat egg *whites* into soft peaks. Carefully fold into the zucchini mixture and pour mixture into prepared soufflé dish. Bake for 30–40 minutes, until top is light to golden brown. TA

DESSERTS

CHOCOLATE VANILLA CHEESECAKE

8 servings   Per serving: 4.9 gm CHO, 1.8 oz PRO

	CHO (gm)	PRO (gm)
1 tsp butter	—	0.04
2 Tbsp full-fat soy flour	3.8	3.6
6 eggs, separated	3.6	36.0
6 Equal tablets, crushed, or stevia powder (without maltodextrin) to taste	—	—
1 lb cream cheese	11.2	36.8
1 cup sour cream	8.0	6.4
6 drops vanilla extract	0.6	—
¼ cup cocoa powder	12.0	4.0

Preheat oven to 350°F. Butter an 8- or 9-inch springform pan and dust with soy flour. In a large bowl, beat egg yolks with crushed Equal tablets or stevia until foamy. Add cream cheese, sour cream, and vanilla extract, and beat until fluffy. In a separate bowl, beat egg whites until stiff. Fold into cream cheese mixture. Pour half the mixture into the springform pan. Mix cocoa powder into remaining half, then spoon it over vanilla mixture already in pan. Bake until golden, about 25–30 minutes. TA

INDIVIDUAL CHOCOLATE SOUFFLÉS

4 servings   Per serving: 2.9 gm CHO, 1.8 oz PRO

	CHO (gm)	PRO (gm)
4 eggs, separated	2.4	24.0
4 Equal tablets, crushed, or stevia powder (without maltodextrin) to taste	—	—
8 oz cream cheese, cut into small pieces	5.6	18.4
1 Tbsp sour cream	0.5	0.4
1 Tbsp cocoa powder	3.0	1.0

Beat egg yolks with crushed Equal tablets or stevia until foamy. Add cream cheese, sour cream, and cocoa powder. Beat until very smooth. In a separate bowl, beat the egg whites until they form stiff peaks, then fold into the cream cheese mixture. Pour into individual soufflé cups and bake at 350°F for 15–20 minutes, or until golden brown. TA

RHUBARB PIE

6 servings   Per serving: 10.5 gm CHO, *0.7 oz* PRO

	CHO (gm)	PRO (gm)
10 GG Scandinavian Bran Crispbreads, crushed	30.0	10.0
5 Tbsp butter, softened	—	0.7
2 packets Jell-O brand unsweetened lemon pudding mix	13.0	—
1 cup sour cream	8.0	6.4
1 egg, separated	0.6	6.0
Equal tablets, crushed, or stevia powder (without maltodextrin) to taste	—	—
2 cups rhubarb cut into 1-inch pieces	11.2	2.4

Preheat oven to 350°F. To make crust, combine crushed crispbreads with softened butter. Press mixture evenly into an 8-inch pie pan. Combine lemon pudding mix, sour cream, egg yolk, and crushed Equal tablets or stevia. Beat until smooth. In separate bowl, beat egg white until stiff peaks form. Fold the egg white into pudding mixture. Put cut rhubarb into pie shell and cover with lemon pudding mixture. Bake for 25–30 minutes, or until golden brown. TA

BEIGNET

This recipe was created by my patient Elise Bahar when she was a nineteen-year-old fine arts student.

1 serving   Per serving: 2.9 gm CHO, *1.4 oz* PRO

	CHO (gm)	PRO (gm)
1 cup vegetable oil	—	—
1 egg	0.6	6.0
1 Tbsp full-fat soy flour	1.9	1.8
1 Tbsp heavy cream	0.4	0.3
Stevia powder (without maltodextrin) to taste	—	—
Cinnamon to taste	—	—

Heat vegetable oil for about 5 minutes in a 2-quart saucepan while you mix the batter. Beat egg, soy flour, cream, and stevia in a bowl until fully mixed. Drop a small amount of batter into hot oil. If the drop rises to the top, pour rest of batter into hot oil. Wait until edges of beignet are golden, then flip to other side. When edges are golden, remove beignet from oil and place on paper towel to drain. Sprinkle with cinnamon.

What About the Widely Advocated Dietary Restrictions on Fat, Protein, and Salt, and the Current High-Fiber Fad?

Most of this book is instructional, of the how-to variety. The intent of this appendix is to provide you with a little of the science that surrounds the program described in the rest of the book. With respect to a number of the issues raised in this section, I would also refer you again to Gary Taubes's award-winning article "The Soft Science of Dietary Fat," which is available at www.diabetes-book .com/articles/ssdf.shtml or in the March 3, 2001, issue of the journal *Science.* Another masterpiece by Taubes, "What If It's All Been a Big Fat Lie?," appeared as the cover article in the *New York Times Magazine* of July 2, 2002. It can be found at www.diabetes-book.com/cms/articles/ 3-advice-a-commentary/7416-what-if-its-all-been-a-big-fat-lie. I also recommend his book *Good Calories, Bad Calories* (Knopf, 2007), as well as the very informative *Trick and Treat* by Barry Groves (Hammersmith Press, 2008). Both books are available at Amazon.com.

I hope that I can cut through some of the myths that cloud diet and the treatment of diabetic complications so that you will have the why that supports the how-to. We've already discussed some of the myths. We'll look at the origins of those myths to try to give you as many of the facts as are available at this writing. If your only interest is in the how-to, feel free to skip this appendix.

Once you've started to follow a restricted-carbohydrate diet, you may find yourself pressured by well-meaning but uninformed friends or family, or even newspaper articles, to cease penalizing yourself and eat more "fun" foods—sweets, bread, pasta, and fruits. This chapter will provide you with specific scientific information that underpins my approach and will perhaps give you some ammunition for responding to this pressure. Even if you skip it now, you may want to come back to it later, or show it to your loved ones to lay their concerns to rest. As I don't expect most readers to be scientists, I've tried to keep all these explanations relatively simple. Some of the explanations may at this moment represent more theory than fact, but they're based on the latest information available to us.

Throughout the appendix I refer to the adverse effects of high serum insulin levels. This does not mean that insulin should not be injected to normalize blood sugars. It is the industrial doses of insulin commonly produced or injected to cover high-carbohydrate diets that cause problems. Furthermore, high blood sugars cause many more problems of much greater severity than do high insulin levels.

HOW DID THE COMMONLY PRESCRIBED HIGH-CARBOHYDRATE DIET COME ABOUT?

If, like me, you've had diabetes for a while, you've probably been told to cut way down on your dietary intake of fat, protein, and salt, and to eat lots of complex carbohydrate. You may even still read this advice in publications circulated to diabetic patients or touted by many (not all) dietitians and certified diabetes educators.

Why is such advice being promulgated, when the major cause of such diabetic complications as heart disease, kidney disease, high blood pressure, and blindness is high blood sugar?

When I first developed diabetes, in 1946, little was known about why this disease, even when treated, caused early death and such distressing complications. Prior to the availability of insulin, about twenty-five years earlier, people with type 1 diabetes usually died within a few months of diagnosis. Their lives could be prolonged somewhat with a diet that was very low in carbohydrate and usually high in fat. Most sufferers from the milder type 2 diabetes survived on this type of diet, without supplemental medication. When I became diabetic, oral hypoglycemic agents were not available, and many people were still following very low carbohydrate, high-fat diets. It was at about this time that diets very high in saturated fats, with supposedly resultant high serum cholesterol levels, were experimentally shown to correlate with blood vessel and heart disease in animals. It was promptly assumed by many physicians that the then-known complications of diabetes, most of which related to abnormalities of large or small blood vessels, were caused by the high-fat diets. I and many other diabetics were therefore treated with a high-carbohydrate, low-fat diet. This new diet was adopted in the mid-1940s by the American Diabetes Association (ADA) and the New York Heart Association, later by the American Heart Association (AHA), and eventually by other groups around the world. On the new diet, most of us had much higher serum cholesterol and triglyceride levels, and still developed the grave long-term complications of diabetes. Seemingly unaware of the importance of blood sugar control, the ADA raised the recommended carbohydrate content from 40 to 50 percent of calories, and then more recently to 60 percent. The ADA's most recent guidelines have backed off by vaguely stating that some diabetics may do better with less carbohydrate.

RECENT DEVELOPMENTS REGARDING RISK FACTORS FOR HEART DISEASE

In the past twenty years, research studies have generated considerable new information about heart disease and vascular (blood vessel) disease in general, and their relationship to diabetes in particular. Some of this recent information is summarized here.

A number of substances have been found in the blood which relate to risk of heart attacks and vascular disease. These include HDL (high-density lipoprotein), LDL (low-density lipoprotein), triglyceride, fibrinogen, homocysteine, C-reactive protein, ferritin (iron), and lipoprotein(a). High serum levels of dense, compact LDL particles, triglyceride, fibrinogen, homocysteine, C-reactive protein, ferritin, and lipoprotein(a) tend to be associated with increased cardiovascular risk, while high levels of HDL tend to protect from cardiovascular disease. Cholesterol is a component of both LDL and HDL particles. The fraction of total cholesterol found in LDL particles is considered an index of risk, while the fraction of cholesterol found in HDL particles is an index of protection. Nowadays, when we want to estimate the effects of lipids (fatty substances) upon the risk of coronary artery disease, we look at the ratio of total cholesterol to HDL and also at fasting triglyceride levels. Someone with high serum HDL can thus have a high total cholesterol and yet be at low statistical risk for a heart attack. Conversely, a person with low total cholesterol and very low HDL may be at high risk. A recent update of the very large Framingham Heart Study found no relationship between saturated fat and serum cholesterol and none between cholesterol and heart disease.

A large multicenter study (the Lipid Research Clinics Coronary Primary Prevention Trial) investigated the effects of a low-fat, high-carbohydrate diet versus a high-fat, low-carbohydrate diet on nondiabetic middle-aged men with elevated cholesterol levels. The study followed 1,900 people for seven years. Throughout this period, total cholesterol dropped only 5 percent from baseline in the low-fat group, but serum triglyceride went up about 10 percent! (Serum triglyceride rises very rapidly after a high-carbohydrate meal in nondiabetics, and moves up and down with blood sugar levels in most diabetics.) As with prior studies, no significant correlation was found between serum cholesterol levels and mortality rates. Furthermore, a study reported in the *Journal of the American Medical Association* in 1997 showed that a 20 percent increase in either saturated or monounsaturated dietary fat lowered the risk of stroke to one-eighth of what it was in individuals on lower-fat diets. Unsaturated fats showed no such benefit.

On average, diabetics with chronically high blood sugars have elevated levels of LDL (the "bad" cholesterol) and depressed levels of HDL (the "good" cholesterol), even though the ADA low-fat diet has now been in use for many years. Of great importance is the recent discovery that the forms of LDL that may harm arteries are small, dense LDL, oxidized LDL, and glycated LDL. All of these increase as blood sugar increases. In addition, independently of blood sugars, excessive serum insulin levels dictated by high-carbohydrate diets bring about increased production of the potentially hazardous small, dense LDL particles and enlargement of the cells lining the arteries. We now can measure the size distribution of these LDL subparticles as a routine laboratory test. Most labs report the benevolent large, buoyant LDL subparticles as "type A" and the small, dense LDL subparticles as "type B."

Under normal conditions, receptors in the liver remove LDL from the bloodstream and signal the liver to reduce its manufacture of LDL when serum levels rise even slightly. Glucose can bind to the surface of the LDL particle and also to liver LDL receptors, so that LDL cannot be recognized by its receptors. In people with high blood sugars, many LDL particles become glycosylated, and are therefore not cleared by the liver. This glycosylation is reversible if blood sugar drops. After about 24 hours, however, a rearrangement of electron bonds occurs in glycosylated proteins, so that the glucose can't be released even if blood sugar drops. This irreversible glycosylation is called glycation, and the affected protein molecules are said to be "glycated." They are also referred to as AGEs, or advanced glycation end products. These AGEs accumulate in the blood, where they can become incorporated into the walls of arteries, forming fatty deposits called atherosclerotic plaques. Since liver LDL production cannot be turned off by the glycosylated/glycated LDL (and also the presence of glycosylated/glycated LDL receptors), the liver continues to manufacture more LDL, even though serum levels may be elevated.

The proteins in the walls of arteries can also become glycosylated/glycated, rendering them sticky. Other proteins in the blood then stick to the arterial walls, causing further buildup of plaque.

Serum proteins glycosylate in the presence of glucose. White blood cells called macrophages ingest glycosylated/glycated proteins and glycosylated/glycated LDL. The loaded macrophages swell up, becoming very large. These transformed macrophages, loaded with fatty material, are called foam cells. The foam cells penetrate the now sticky arterial walls, causing disruption of the orderly architecture of the artery, and narrow the channel through which blood can flow.

The middle layer of the walls of large arteries contains smooth muscle cells that can invade the fatty coating (plaque) that foam cells create. They then prevent the plaque from breaking loose. When the nerves that control this smooth muscle die, as in diabetic autonomic neuropathy (caused by high blood sugars), the muscle layer dies and calcifies. It then cannot prevent plaque rupture. When a piece of ruptured plaque enters the blood it can block narrow vessels upstream and cause a heart attack or stroke.

In recent years, the tendency of blood to clot has come into focus as a major cause of heart attacks. People whose blood clots too readily are at very high risk for stroke, heart disease, and kidney disease. You may recall that one of the medical names for a heart attack is coronary thrombosis. A thrombus is a clot, and coronary thrombosis refers to the formation of a large clot in one of the arteries that feed the heart. People who have elevated levels of certain clotting precursors or depressed levels of clotting inhibitors in their blood are at high risk of dying from a heart attack. This risk probably far exceeds that caused by high LDL or low HDL. Some of the blood factors that enhance clotting include fibrinogen and factor VII. Another factor, lipoprotein(a), inhibits the destruction of small thrombi before they become large enough to cause a heart attack. All of these factors have been found to increase in people with chronically high blood sugars. Platelets, or thrombocytes, are particles in the blood that play major roles in the blocking of arteries and the formation of clots. These have been shown to clump together and stick to arterial walls much more aggressively in people with high blood sugars. What is exciting is that all of these factors, including sticky platelets, tend to normalize as long-term blood sugars improve.

Diabetics die from heart failure at a rate far exceeding that of people with normal glucose tolerance. Heart failure involves a weakening of the cardiac muscle so that it cannot pump enough blood. Most long-term, poorly controlled diabetics have a condition called cardiomyopathy. In diabetic cardiomyopathy, the muscle tissue of the heart is slowly replaced by scar tissue over a period of years. This weakens the muscle so that it eventually "fails." There is no evidence linking cardiomyopathy with dietary fat intake or serum lipids.

A fifteen-year study of 7,038 French policemen in Paris reported that "the earliest marker of a higher risk of coronary heart disease mortality is an abnormal elevation of serum insulin level." A study of middle-aged nondiabetic women at the University of Pittsburgh showed an increasing risk of heart disease as serum insulin levels increased. Other studies in nondiabetics have shown strong correlations between elevated serum insulin levels and other predictors of cardiac risk such as hypertension, elevated triglyceride, and low HDL. The importance of elevated serum insulin levels (hyperinsulinemia) as a cause of heart disease and hypertension has taken on such importance that a special symposium on this subject was held at the end of the 1990 annual meeting of the ADA. A report in a subsequent issue of the journal *Diabetes Care* quite appropriately points out that "there are few available methods of treating diabetes that do not result in systemic hyperinsulinemia [unless the patient is following a low-carbohydrate diet]." Furthermore, research published in the journal *Diabetes* in 1990 demonstrated that elevated serum insulin levels cause excessive leakage of protein from small blood vessels. This is a common factor in the etiology of blindness (via macular edema) and kidney disease in diabetics.

Although the AHA and the ADA have been recommending low-fat, high-carbohydrate diets for diabetics for many decades, no one had compared the effects on the same patients of low- versus high-carbohydrate diets until the late 1980s. Independent studies performed in Texas and California demonstrated lower levels of blood sugar and improved blood lipids when patients were put on low-carbohydrate, high-fat diets. It was also shown that, on average, for every 1 percent increase in HgbA$_{1C}$ (the test for average blood sugar over the prior four months), total serum cholesterol rose 2.2 percent and triglycerides increased 8 percent. A long-term study of 7,321 "nondiabetics" in 2006 showed that for every 1 percent increase in HgbA$_{1C}$ above 4.5 percent, the incidence of coronary artery disease increased 2.5-fold. The same study also showed that for every 1 percent increase in HgbA$_{1C}$ above 4.9 percent, mortality increased by 28 percent. Yet the ADA still advocates a target HgbA$_{1C}$ of 6.5–7 percent for selected diabetics, and higher for many others. No wonder I call diabetes an "orphan disease." The "authorities" who write the rules are not supporting our well-being.

The National Health and Nutrition Examination Follow-up Survey, which followed 4,710 people, reported in 1990 that "in the instance of total blood cholesterol, we found no evidence in any age-sex group of a risk associated with elevated values." That's right: they found no risk associated directly with elevated total cholesterol. On the same page, this study lists diabetes as by far the single most important risk factor affecting mortality. In males ages 55–64, for example, diabetes was associated with 60 percent greater mortality than smoking and double the mortality associated with high blood pressure.

The evidence is now simply overwhelming that elevated blood sugar is the major cause of the high serum lipid levels among diabetics and, more significantly, the major factor in the high rates of various heart and vascular diseases associated with diabetes. Many diabetics were put on low-fat diets for so many years, and yet these problems didn't stop. It is only logical to look to elevated blood sugar and hyperinsulinemia for the causes of what kills and disables so many of us.

My personal experience with diabetic patients is very simple. When we reduce dietary carbohydrate, blood sugars improve dramatically. After several months of improved blood sugars, we repeat our studies of lipid profiles and thrombotic risk factors. In the great majority of cases, I see normalization or improvement of abnormalities.* This

---

* If your physician finds all of this hard to believe, he or she might benefit from reading the seventy articles and abstracts on this subject contained in "Proceedings of the Fifteenth International Diabetes Foundation Satellite Symposium on Diabetes and Macrovascular Complications," *Diabetes* 45, supplement 3, July 1996. Also worth reading is "Effects of Varying Carbohydrate Content of Diet in Patients with Non-Insulin Dependent Diabetes Mellitus," by Garg et al., *Journal of the American Medical Association,* 1994; 271:1421–1428. Many studies comparing low-carbohydrate and low-fat diets are collected each year in the archives of the Nutrition and Metabolism Society, http://locarbvslofat.org. The low-carbohydrate diets invariably have shown reduced cardiac risk.

parallels what happened to me forty years ago when I abandoned the high-carbohydrate, low-fat diet that I had been following since 1946.

Sometimes, months to years after a patient has experienced normal or near-normal blood sugars and improvements in the cardiac risk profile, we will see deterioration in the results of such tests as those for LDL, HDL, homocysteine, and fibrinogen. All too often, the patient or his physician will blame our diet. Inevitably, however, we find upon further testing that his thyroid activity has declined. Hypothyroidism is an autoimmune disorder, like diabetes, and is frequently inherited by diabetics and their close relatives. It can appear years before or after the development of diabetes and is not caused by high blood sugars. In fact, hypothyroidism can cause a greater likelihood of abnormalities of the cardiac risk profile than can blood sugar elevation. The treatment of a low-thyroid condition is oral replacement of the deficient hormone(s) — frequently one pill daily. The best screening test is free T_3, tested by tracer dialysis. If this is low, then a full thyroid risk profile should be performed. Correction of the thyroid deficiency inevitably corrects the abnormalities of cardiac risk factors that it caused.

WHY IS PROTEIN RESTRICTION SO COMMON?

About 30 percent of diabetics develop kidney disease (nephropathy). Diabetes is the greatest single cause of kidney failure in the United States. Early kidney changes can be found within two to three years of the onset of high blood sugars. As we discussed briefly in Chapter 9, "The Basic Food Groups," the common restrictions on protein intake by diabetic patients derive from fear regarding this problem, and ignorance of the actual causes of diabetic kidney disease.

By looking at how the kidney functions, one can better understand the relative roles of glucose and protein in the kidney failure of diabetes. The kidney filters wastes, glucose, drugs, and other potentially toxic materials from the blood and deposits them into the urine. It is the urine-making organ. A normal kidney contains about 1 million microscopic blood filters, called glomeruli. Figure A-1 illustrates how blood enters a glomerulus through a tiny artery called the afferent (incoming) arteriole. This arteriole feeds a bundle or tuft of tiny vessels called capillaries. The capillaries contain tiny holes or pores that carry a negative electrical charge. The downstream ends of the capillaries merge into an efferent (outgoing) arteriole, which is narrower than the incoming arteriole. This narrowing results in high fluid pressure when blood flows through the capillary tuft. The high pressure forces some of the water in the blood through the pores of the capillaries. This water dribbles into the capsule surrounding the capillary tuft. The capsule, acting like a funnel, empties the water into a pipelike structure called the tubule. The pores of the capillaries are of such a size that small molecules in the blood, such as glucose and urea, can pass through with the water to form urine. In a normal kidney, large molecules, such as proteins, cannot readily get through the pores. Since most blood proteins carry negative electrical charges, even the smaller proteins in the blood cannot easily get through the pores, because they are repelled by the negative charge on each pore.

The glomerular filtration rate (GFR) is a measure of how much filtering the kidneys perform in a given period of time. Many diabetics with frequent high blood sugars and normal kidneys will initially have an excessively high GFR. This is in part because blood glucose draws water into the bloodstream from the surrounding tissues, thus

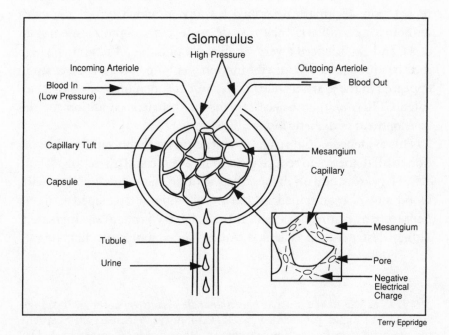

Terry Eppridge

Fig. A-1. *The microscopic filtration unit of the kidneys.*

increasing blood volume, blood pressure, and blood flow through the kidneys. A GFR that is one-and-a-half to two times normal is not uncommon in diabetics with high blood sugars prior to the onset of permanent injury to their kidneys. These people may typically have as much glucose in a 24-hour urine collection as the weight of 5 to 10 packets of sugar. According to an Italian study, an increase in blood sugar from 80 mg/dl to 272 mg/dl resulted in an average GFR *increase* of 40 percent even in diabetics with kidneys that were not fully functional. Before we knew about glycosylation of proteins and the other toxic effects of glucose upon blood vessels, it was speculated that the cause of diabetic kidney disease (nephropathy) was this excessive filtration (hyperfiltration).

The metabolism of dietary protein produces waste products such as urea and ammonium, which contain nitrogen.* It therefore had been speculated that in order to clear these wastes from the blood, people eating large amounts of protein would have elevated GFRs. As a result, diabetics have been urged to reduce their protein intake to low levels. However, studies by an Israeli group of nondiabetic people on high-protein (meat-eating) and very low protein (vegetarian) diets disclosed no difference in GFRs. Furthermore, over many years on these diets, kidney function was unchanged between the two groups. A report from Denmark described a study in which type 1 diabetics without discernible kidney disease were put on protein-restricted diets, and experienced a very small reduction in GFR and no change in other measures of kidney function. As long ago as 1984, a study appeared in the journal *Diabetic Nephropathy* demonstrating that elevated GFR is neither a necessary nor a sufficient condition for the development of diabetic kidney disease.

This evidence would suggest that the currently prevailing admonition to all diabetics to reduce protein intake is unjustified.

A Harvard study on diabetic rats showed the following: Rats with blood sugars maintained at 250 mg/dl rapidly developed diabetic nephropathy (kidney disease). If their dietary protein was increased, kidney destruction accelerated. At the same laboratory, diabetic rats

---

* A 1995 article in the journal *Nutritional Biochemistry*, 6:411–437, demonstrated that a higher-protein diet enables the kidneys to increase their capacity for net acid secretion as ammonium. In other words, it improved kidney function.

with blood sugars maintained at 100 mg/dl live full lives and never develop nephropathy, no matter how much protein they consume. Diabetic rats with high blood sugars and significant nephropathy have shown total reversal of their kidney disease after blood sugars were normalized for several months.

Other studies have enabled researchers to piece together a scenario for the causes of diabetic nephropathy, where glycosylation of proteins, abnormal clotting factors, abnormal platelets, antibodies to glycosylated proteins, and so on, join together to injure glomerular capillaries. Early injury may only cause reduction of electrical charge on the pores. As a result, negatively charged proteins such as albumin leak through the pores and appear in the urine. Glycosylated proteins leak through pores much earlier than normal proteins. High blood pressure, and especially high serum insulin levels, can increase GFR and force even more protein to leak through the pores. If some of these proteins are glycosylated or glycated, they will stick to the mesangium, the tissue between the capillaries. Examination of diabetic glomeruli indeed discloses large deposits of glycated proteins and antibodies to glycated proteins in capillary walls and the mesangium. As these deposits increase, the mesangium compresses the capillaries, causing pressure in the capillaries to increase (enlarging the pores) and larger proteins to leak from the pores. This leads to more thickening of the mesangium, more compression of the capillaries, and acceleration of destruction. Eventually the mesangium and capillaries become a mass of scar tissue. Independently of this, both high blood sugars and glycated proteins cause mesangial cells to produce type IV collagen, a fibrous material that further increases their bulk. Increase in mesangial volume has been found to be commonplace in poorly controlled diabetes even before albumin or other proteins appear in the urine.

Many studies performed on humans show that when blood sugars improve, GFR in slightly damaged kidneys improves and less protein leaks into the urine. When blood sugars remain high, however, there is further deterioration. There is a point of no return, where a glomerulus has been so injured that no amount of blood sugar improvement can revive it. Although this seems to be true for humans, blood sugar normalization has actually brought about the appearance of new glomeruli in rats.

Nowadays many diabetics who have lost all kidney function are treated by artificial kidneys (dialysis machines) that remove nitrogenous wastes from the blood. In order to reduce the weekly number of dialysis treatments, which are costly and unpleasant, patients are severely restricted in their consumption of both water and dietary protein. Instead of using large amounts of carbohydrate to replace the lost calories, many dialysis centers now recommend olive oil to their diabetics. Olive oil is high in monounsaturated fats, which are believed by some to lower the risk of heart disease.

Because the survival rate of diabetics on dialysis is so much lower than that of nondiabetics, some dialysis centers are now using low-carbohydrate, high-protein diets for their diabetic patients.

In summary: Diabetic nephropathy does not appear if blood sugar is kept normal. Dietary protein does not cause diabetic nephropathy, but can possibly (still uncertain) *slightly* accelerate the process once there has been major, irreversible kidney damage. Dietary protein has no substantial effect upon the GFR of healthy kidneys, certainly not in comparison to the GFR increase caused by elevated blood sugar levels.*

The May 1996 *Journal of the American Medical Association* published a summary of fifty-six studies demonstrating that in nondiabetics increased protein consumption actually lowered blood pressure.

By the way, it's been shown that dietary protein stimulates the production of the satiety hormone PYY, thereby inhibiting overeating.

RESTRICTIONS ON SALT INTAKE: ARE THEY REASONABLE FOR ALL DIABETICS?

Many diabetics have hypertension, or high blood pressure. Less than half of all people with hypertension will experience blood pressure elevations when they eat substantial amounts of salt for at least two

---

* Your physician might find informative the following articles on this subject: "Molecular and Physiological Aspects of Nephropathy in Type 1 Diabetes Mellitus," by Raskin and Tamborlane, *Journal of Diabetes and Its Complications,* 1996, 10:31–37; "The Effects of Dietary Protein Restriction and Blood Pressure Control on the Progression of Chronic Renal Disease," by S. Klahr et al., *New England Journal of Medicine,* 1994, 330:877–884; also, in the same issue of the *New England Journal of Medicine,* the editorial "The Role of Dietary Protein Restriction in Progressive Azotemia" (pp. 929–930). Another study, in the journal *Diabetes Care,* 25:425–430, in the year 2000, showed that obese people on a high-protein diet lost more fat and less muscle mass than those on a low-fat diet. They also showed more than double the reduction in LDL (the "bad" cholesterol).

months. This rarely occurs in those who are not already hypertensive. In fact, a study published in the *Journal of the American Medical Association* in May 2011 (305:1777–1785) showed that among nondiabetic, nonhypertensive individuals, there was no difference in the incidence of new hypertension over 7.9 years between the highest and lowest salt eaters. Furthermore, this study showed that cardiovascular mortality in the lowest salt consumers was five times that in the highest consumers. Hypertension accelerates glomerulopathy (destruction of the glomerulus) in people with chronically elevated blood sugars, but in type 1 diabetics, hypertension usually appears after, not before, the appearance of kidney damage as indicated by significant amounts of albumin in the urine. A study in the March 2011 issue of *Diabetes Care* showed that for type 2 diabetics, for every extra 2.3 grams of sodium (from salt) consumed, the risk of dying from all causes dropped by 28 percent. The following month, *Diabetes Care* published another study showing that type 1 diabetics who ate more sodium (salt) were less likely to develop kidney failure. Is it, therefore, appropriate to ask all diabetics to lower their salt intake?* Let us look at a few of the mechanisms involved in the hypertension that some diabetics experience.

People with advanced glomerulopathy will inevitably develop hypertension, in part because GFR is severely diminished. These people cannot make enough urine, and therefore they retain water. Excessive water in the blood causes elevated blood pressure. There are many other ways hypertension can be caused by high blood sugars. The mere presence of high blood sugar will cause water to leave tissues and enter the bloodstream, even experimentally in nondiabetics.

It is not unusual to observe a reduction in blood pressure concomitant

---

* A study of older individuals who were rotated between low-, moderate-, and high-salt diets demonstrated that those on low-salt diets experienced significantly more sleep disturbances, and had more rapid heart rates and higher serum epinephrine (adrenaline) levels. An international study called Intersalt, covering 10,079 people in 32 countries, reported in 1988 that "salt has only small importance in hypertension." More recently, another study showed that salt restriction increases insulin resistance and thus can indirectly increase blood sugar.

Large amounts of dietary salt can facilitate loss of calcium from the bones of postmenopausal women, who are already at high risk for osteoporosis (bone weakening).

with control of blood sugar. Studies have shown that many, and possibly most, hypertensive nondiabetics are insulin-resistant, and therefore have high serum insulin levels. In addition to causing elevation of serum triglycerides and reduction in serum HDL in nondiabetics, high serum insulin levels have long been known to foster salt and water retention by the kidneys. Furthermore, excessive insulin stimulates the sympathetic nervous system, which in turn speeds up the heart and constricts blood vessels, causing a further increase in blood pressure. Thus type 2 diabetics who eat lots of carbohydrate, and therefore will tend to make excessive insulin, can readily develop hypertension. Type 1 diabetics treated with the usual industrial doses of insulin to cover high-carbohydrate diets are likewise more susceptible to hypertension. One dramatic study showed that in hypertensive individuals, blood pressure is directly proportional to serum insulin level. A report from Nottingham, England, showed that a brief infusion of insulin and glucose would increase blood pressure in normal men without changing their blood sugars. A 1998 study in Glasgow, Scotland, demonstrated that salt restriction increased insulin resistance in type 2 diabetics.

Why don't all diabetics on high-carbohydrate diets or all poorly controlled diabetics have hypertension?

One reason is that the body has several very efficient systems for unloading sodium (a component of salt) and water. One of the more important of these systems is controlled by a hormone manufactured in the heart called atrial naturietic factor (ANF). When the heart is expanded by even a slight fluid overload, it produces ANF. The ANF then signals the kidneys to unload sodium and water. Hypertensive individuals, and the children of two hypertensive parents, tend to produce much lower amounts of ANF than do normal people. Nonhypertensive diabetics apparently are able to produce enough ANF to control the blood pressure effects of high blood sugars and high serum insulin levels, provided they do not have moderately advanced kidney disease. Indeed, a study, in which some of my patients participated, showed that diabetics with high blood sugars produce significantly more ANF than those with lower blood sugars (my patients).

How does all this apply to you? First, you and your physician should know if you have glomerulopathy. This is readily determined if the renal risk profile tests suggested in Chapter 2 are performed. If these tests are abnormal, your physician may advise you to reduce your salt intake because salt is much more likely to cause hypertension in people with diminished GFR.

Whether your renal risk profile is normal or abnormal, your resting blood pressure should also be measured. A proper measurement requires that you be seated in a *quiet* room, without conversation, for 15–30 minutes. Blood pressure should be measured every 5 minutes, until it drops to a low value and then starts to increase. The lowest reading is the significant one. If you get nervous in the doctor's office, then you should measure your own blood pressure at home in a similar fashion. Repeated measurements with low values just exceeding 120/70 suggest that your blood pressure is "borderline." You then may or may not benefit from dietary salt reduction. The only way to find out is to check your blood pressure while on your current salt intake, and again after following a low-salt (sodium) diet for at least two months.* Your physician can give you guidelines for such a diet, and you can consult nutritional tables such as those in the books listed on page 72. I would suggest that resting blood pressures be measured several times a day, and at the same hours each day, throughout the study. Each day's blood pressures can then be averaged, and the averages compared. If your blood pressure drops significantly on the low-salt diet, your physician may urge you to keep the salt intake down. Alternatively, he may want you to take *small* amounts of supplemental potassium, which tends to offset the effects of dietary salt on blood pressure. People with advanced kidney disease should not consume supplemental potassium. Recent studies suggest that as many as 40 percent of hypertensive patients (the so-called low-renin hypertensives) may show lower blood pressures when they take calcium supplements or increase dietary calcium consumption. Those who advocate salt restriction for all humans should read the results of the National Health and Nutrition Examination Survey, which showed that cardiovascular morbidity in obese individuals was reduced with higher salt intake (*Journal of the American Medical*

_____

* To complicate things somewhat, a 1998 report in the *Journal of Clinical Endocrinology and Metabolism* demonstrated that salt restriction in nonhypertensive type 2 diabetics reduced insulin sensitivity by 15 percent. A prior article in the *American Journal of Hypertension* found a similar effect in hypertensive individuals. Another study of rats, published in the journal *Diabetes* in 2001, found that this insulin resistance cannot be reversed by the insulin-sensitizing agent Actos.

Association, 1999; 282:2027–2034), and the 2011 studies cited earlier in this section.

WHAT ABOUT DIETARY FIBER?

"Fiber" is a general term that has come to refer to the indigestible portion of many vegetables and fruits. Some vegetable fibers, such as guar and pectin, are soluble in water. Another type of fiber, which some of us call roughage, is not water soluble. Both types appear to affect the movement of food through the gut (soluble fiber slows processing in the upper digestive tract, while insoluble fiber speeds digestion farther down). Certain insoluble fiber products, such as psyllium, have long been used as laxatives. Consumption of large amounts of dietary fiber is usually unpleasant, because both types can cause abdominal discomfort, diarrhea, and flatulence. Sources of insoluble fiber include most salad vegetables. Soluble fiber is found in many beans, such as garbanzos, and in certain fruits, such as apples.

I first learned of attempts at using fiber as an adjunct to the treatment of diabetes about thirty-five years ago. At that time, Dr. David Jenkins, in England, reported that guar gum, when added to bread, could reduce the maximum postprandial blood sugar rise from an entire meal by 36 percent in diabetic subjects. This was interesting for several reasons. First of all, the discovery occurred at a time when few new approaches to controlling blood sugar were appearing in the medical literature. Second, I missed the high-carbohydrate foods I had given up, and hoped I might possibly reinstate some. I managed to track down a supplier of powdered guar gum, and placed a considerable amount into a folded slice of bread. I knew how much a slice of bread would affect my blood sugar, and so as an experiment, I used the same amount of guar gum that Dr. Jenkins had used, and then ate the concoction on an empty stomach. The chore was difficult, because once moistened by my saliva, the guar gum stuck to my palate and was difficult to swallow. I did not find any change in the subsequent blood sugar increase. Despite the unpleasantness of choking down powdered guar gum (which is often used in commercial products such as ice cream as a thickener), I repeated this experiment on two more occasions, with the same result. When I finally met Dr. Jenkins in 2010, he explained that the guar gum should have been mixed with the flour before the bread was baked. Subsequently, some investigators have announced results similar to those of Dr. Jenkins, yet other researchers have found no effect on post-prandial blood sugar. In any event, a reduction of postprandial blood sugar increase by only 36 percent really isn't adequate for our purpose, since we're shooting for the same blood sugars as nondiabetics. This means virtually no rise after eating.

Dr. Jenkins also discovered, however, that the chronic use of guar gum resulted in a reduction of serum cholesterol levels. This is probably related to the considerable recirculation of cholesterol through the gut. The liver secretes cholesterol into bile, which is released into the upper intestine. This cholesterol is later absorbed lower in the intestines, and eventually reappears in the blood. Guar binds some of the cholesterol in the intestines, so that rather than being absorbed, it appears in the stool.

In the light of these very interesting results, other researchers studied the effect of foods (usually beans) containing other soluble forms of fiber. When beans were substituted for faster-acting forms of carbohy-drate, postprandial blood sugars in diabetics increased more slowly, and the peaks were even slightly reduced. Serum cholesterol levels were also reduced by about 15 percent. But subsequent studies, reported in 1990, have uncovered flaws in the original reports, casting serious doubt upon any direct effect of these foods upon serum lipids. In any event, post-prandial blood sugars of diabetics were never normalized by such diets.

Many popular articles and books have appeared advocating "high-fiber" diets for everyone — not just diabetics. Somehow, "fiber" came to mean all fiber, not just soluble fiber, even though the only viable studies had utilized such products as guar gum and beans. Studies discussed in the book *Trick and Treat* by Barry Groves report many adverse health effects caused by excessive fiber consumption.

In my experience, reduction of dietary carbohydrate is far more effective in preventing blood sugar increases after meals. The lower blood sugars, in turn, bring about improved lipid profiles. It is true, however, that low-carbohydrate vegetables are usually composed mostly of insoluble fiber and therefore contain far less digestible car-bohydrate than starchy vegetables. Thus if the options are either fiber or starch, there is great value in "high fiber."

Another food to join the high-fiber trend is oat bran. This has gotten a lot of play in the popular press. A patient of mine started substituting oat bran muffins for protein in her diet. Before she started, her $HgbA_{1C}$ (see page 56) was within the normal range and her ratio of total choles-terol to HDL was very low (meaning her supposed cardiac risk ratio was low). After three months on oat bran, her $HgbA_{1C}$ became elevated and her cholesterol-to-HDL ratio nearly doubled. I tried one of her tiny oat bran muffins after first injecting 3 units of rapid-acting insulin (as much as I used for an entire meal). After 3 hours, my blood sugar went up by about 100 mg/dl, to 190 mg/dl. This illustrates the adverse effect that most oat bran preparations can have upon blood sugar. This is because most such preparations contain flour. On the other hand, I find that certain bran products, such as the bran crackers listed on pages 164–165, raise blood sugar relatively little. Unlike most packaged bran products, they contain mostly bran and little flour. They therefore have very little digestible carbohydrate. You can perform similar experiments yourself. Just use your blood glucose meter.

Beware of commercial "high-fiber" products that promise cholesterol reduction. If they contain carbohydrate, they must at least be counted in your meal plan and will probably render little or no improvement in your lipid profile.

Fiber, like carbohydrate, is not essential for a healthy life. Just look at the Eskimos and other hunting populations that survive almost exclusively on protein and fat, and don't develop cardiac or circulatory diseases.*

WHAT ABOUT THE GLYCEMIC INDEX?

For a number of years, the term "glycemic index" has popped in and out of the popular press. It also has been a pet subject for many dietitians and diabetes educators. I will explain why, but I think it's important to make clear that there is simply no way to determine objectively how any given food at any given time is going to behave in any given individual, unless blood sugar is tested before and then repeatedly for

---

* As the first edition of this book was going to press, a report appeared entitled "Dietary Fiber, Glycemic Load, and Risk of Non-Insulin-Dependent Diabetes in Women" (*Journal of the American Medical Association*, 1997; 277:472–477). This study of 65,173 nurses and former nurses found a strong association between diets high in starch, flour, and sweet foods and the development of type 2 diabetes. Furthermore, consumption of minimally refined grain (such as bran without flour) lowered this risk. The combination of high glycemic foods and low intake of unrefined insoluble fiber was associated with a 2.5-fold higher incidence of diabetes. If you remember our discussion of beta cell burnout (pages 41–44), this should come as no surprise.

a number of hours after its consumption. It sounds like an elegant idea — mashed potatoes do X; table sugar does Y. As with a lot of elegant ideas, however, the reality is far more complex.

This term was, as I recall, first coined by the same Dr. Jenkins mentioned in the previous section. The concept is more complicated than the popular press would have you believe.

Imagine two graphs, each depicting a curve of a blood sugar increase over a 3-hour time span. The first curve is after eating pure glucose, the standard. The second is after eating any other food of equivalent total carbohydrate content (20 grams glucose versus 20 grams carbohydrate content of, say, rice).

Dr. Jenkins defined the glycemic index for a given food in terms of how its curve related to that of the glucose curve.

So to arrive at the index for rice, for example, the area under the 3-hour curve of blood sugar increase caused by the rice would be divided by the area under the curve for pure glucose. The measurement is usually made on a number of *nondiabetics* and then averaged, and finally expressed as a percentage. Thus, if a food generates a 3-hour area one-fifth that of glucose, its glycemic index would be 20 percent.

So what's wrong with that?

As attractive as it may seem, the concept is clearly flawed in four respects: First, diabetics show vastly higher blood sugar increases than nondiabetics. Second, digestion of the carbohydrate portion of a meal typically takes at least 5 hours (in the absence of gastroparesis), and the index ignores effects upon blood sugar that last longer than 3 hours. Third, the index is an average of values for a number of different people, and true numbers have been found to vary considerably from one person to another, from one time to another, and from one study to another. As I've pointed out, a food that makes my blood sugar rise dramatically may have little or no effect on that of one of my patients who still makes some insulin. Finally and unfortunately, many dieticians and diabetes educators still recommend foods that have been "shown" to have a "low" glycemic index in some study, and assume that an index of 40 or 50 percent is low. They may thus select apples, lima beans, and the like as appropriate for diabetics, even though consumption of typical portions of these foods will cause considerable blood sugar elevations in diabetics.

A "medium-sized" apple, according to one table of food values, contains 21 grams of carbohydrate. It will raise my own blood sugar by 105 mg/dl, and much more rapidly than I can prevent with an

injection of rapid-acting insulin. Peanuts usually have the lowest glycemic index in many studies (about 15 percent), yet 1 ounce contains
6 grams of carbohydrate and close to 1 ounce of protein. I've found
this portion to raise my blood sugar by 80 mg/dl, albeit much more
slowly than the apple. Since peanuts work so slowly (more slowly than
3 hours), I can substitute 1 ounce for 6 grams of carbohydrate and 1
ounce of protein in a meal and cover it with injected rapid-acting
insulin — but who can eat only one handful of peanuts?*

The carbohydrate foods that we recommend, salads and selected
vegetables (see Chapter 9, "The Basic Food Groups"), have glycemic
indexes much lower than peanuts and work more slowly. Furthermore, they are more filling. The issue here, though, is to understand
that such indexes are unreliable and won't help you keep your blood
sugars normalized.

WHAT DIET WILL WORK FOR YOU?

Actual results are the yardstick for an appropriate diet. We have tools
for self-monitoring of blood sugar and blood pressure. We have tests
for measuring kidney function, HgbA$_{1C}$, thrombotic risk profiles, and
lipid profiles (see Chapter 2). Under your doctor's supervision, try our
diet recommendations for at least three months. Then try any other
diet plan for three months and see what happens. The differences may
not be in the direction that the popular literature would predict.

Finally, in its most common usage, "diet" usually indicates some
sort of franchise. "The _____ Diet" (you can fill in the blank) usually
has a particular name or marketing term associated with it and often
comes with products ready for your consumption. When I use the
term, I'm referring to "diet" in the very simple sense of what you eat.
I'm not selling a brand or products, but providing guidelines so that
you can understand how foods are likely to affect you. You can then
create your own diet, one that will not only allow you to keep your
blood sugars normalized but also to satisfy yourself.

---

* By the way, natural peanut butter has a glycemic index much higher than that
of the peanuts from which it was created because it is digested more rapidly.

Don't Permit Hospitalization or Lengthy Outpatient Procedures to Impair Your Blood Sugar Control

I f ever it is necessary for you to become a hospital patient almost anywhere in the world, the chances are overwhelming that the medical and paramedical staff will give no reasonable thought to controlling your blood sugar. Most of the medical orthodoxy doesn't do it anywhere else, so why should they do it in the hospital?

The reasons for such neglect, of course, are many: lack of blood sugar control skills on the part of most hospital medical staff; unawareness of the importance of normal or near-normal blood sugars in the face of illness or surgery; and an almost pathological fear of severe hypoglycemia (and the potential for lawsuits in the United States if it occurs). Many if not most hospital dietitians have been indoctrinated by the ADA, with the result that diabetic inpatients are forced to eat high-carbohydrate foods and are deprived of protein and fat. Some of my patients tell stories of having to sneak in their own insulin and blood sugar meters, throw out hospital food, and fight tooth and nail with well-meaning but uninformed hospital personnel. This has not changed since 1980, when I wrote my first book about blood sugar control.

Many studies of hospitalized patients have demonstrated that elevated blood sugar delays surgical healing, increases risk of postsurgical morbidity and mortality, delays recovery from infections, and leaves patients open to new infections. It also has been shown to increase the death rate of patients who have been hospitalized for heart attack or stroke, and increases the likelihood of a new stroke or heart attack while in the hospital.

What can you do to help keep your blood sugars under control while in the hospital?

Most of my patients live great distances from my office, so that I am not the admitting physician or surgeon when they are hospitalized, and I am thus not in a position to write their orders, help control their diets, and directly oversee their medical care.

After sharing the frustration of my patients over the years, I've come up with a letter that has worked repeatedly for elective hospitalization, such as for surgeries planned in advance. As you will see, it relies on the prevailing fear of litigation that, when we think of what is done to diabetics, appropriately permeates the medical care system in the United States. This letter should be sent by you or your diabetologist to the admitting physician, with a copy to the hospital administrator. I've composed the letter as if you were writing it, since the odds are that you are not under the care of a diabetologist. It can, of course, be modified to suit your circumstances.

Dear Dr. _____:

I am scheduled for admission to your hospital on _____. I have type [1 or 2] diabetes and am naturally concerned about control of my blood sugars while hospitalized.

It is now generally accepted that elevated blood sugar levels impede recovery, prolong hospitalization, and increase the incidence of hospital and surgical morbidity and death. Major health problems brought about by inappropriate blood sugar elevations due to improper hospital care have justifiably led to litigation.

Since I have been successful at keeping my blood sugars essentially normal around the clock, I naturally expect equivalent care while I'm in the hands of medical professionals.

I currently take the following medications for controlling my blood sugars:

[List here doses, times, and purposes of medications: "basal insulin (or ISA) to cover the fasting state — must be given even if not eating," "pre-lunch (breakfast, supper) insulin (or ISA), to be skipped if meal is skipped." Detail also any use of insulin, glucose tablets, or liquid oral glucose for correcting off-target blood sugars, et cetera. You may also include a sample **Glucograf** sheet and request that all medications used by the hospital that may affect blood sugar be listed on it if you are not capable of listing them yourself.]

> *My hospital orders should call for a "normal diet" and not a "diabetic diet," so that I can select my own meals.*
>
> *Routine intravenous fluids should not contain caloric substances such as glucose, fructose, lactose, lactated Ringer's solution, or saline with added glucose (except for treatment of blood sugars that are below my target). All of these substances can raise my blood sugar to unacceptable levels. Normal saline solution is perfectly adequate for routine hydration. My target blood sugar is ___ mg/dl.*
>
> *If I am conscious and without cognitive impairment, I should have full responsibility for treatment of my diabetes—without outside interference.*
>
> *My blood sugar meter and blood sugar control medications, including insulin syringes, should not be confiscated by hospital personnel. This is a barbaric practice that is rapidly being abandoned in modern hospitals.* *
>
> *If I am unable to care for my own blood sugars, I expect that the hospital staff will exercise every effort to maintain my blood sugars within the range of [xx–xx].*
>
> *Sincerely,*
>
> *cc: [Hospital administrator]*
> *[Close relative or friend]*

This letter may also be of value if you are to have certain outpatient procedures, such as endoscopy, cataract surgery, hernia repair, and so on. These are frequently performed in physicians' offices or in hospitals without the requirement for staying overnight.

If you are so fortunate that you have a personal physician who supports your efforts at blood sugar control and he is on the staff of the admitting hospital, he may be able to write your medical orders, thereby saving you the effort of preparing the preceding letter.

---

* Many hospital pharmacies do not stock the products that we commonly utilize in this book, such as 25–30 unit insulin syringes with ½-unit markings; detemir (Levemir) insulin; or regular, glulisine (Apidra), lispro (Humalog), or aspart (Novolog) insulins.

Drugs That Can Affect
Blood Glucose Levels

STEPHEN FREED, RPh, Diabetes Educator
    Publisher, *Diabetes in Control* (www.diabetesincontrol.com)
    and www.diabetes911.net

DAVID JOFFE, RPh, FACA
    Editor in Chief, *Diabetes in Control* (www.diabetesincontrol.com)

GEORGE E. JACKSON, DPh

When we look at drugs that may affect glucose levels, we need to invoke some special rules. There are medicines for other diseases or aliments that can cause hypoglycemia (low blood sugar) or hyperglycemia (high blood sugar) in diabetic and nondiabetic patients. These pharmaceuticals may have an even greater effect on those with diabetes and should either be avoided or used with vigilance and with a consideration of changing the amount of the diabetes medication used.

Some medications are found to have a possible effect on the patient with diabetes but can be used more freely. Again, however, vigilance is warranted.

Whenever you start a new medication, it's important to understand if it might affect your blood sugars. It is therefore important to monitor your glucose levels carefully.

Due to the aggressive reporting requirements of the FDA, new contraindication information is constantly becoming available. Check with your pharmacist on a regular basis. And remember: If you have any questions about how your medicines can affect your blood sugars, be sure to ask your physician or pharmacist.

The effects upon blood sugar of the medications listed here will vary from one person to another, and can be anywhere from negligible to very significant. For each generic name there may be many more brand names than are listed.

GENERIC NAME (BRAND NAME)

Drugs That May Cause
Hyperglycemia (High Blood Sugar)

Abacavir (Ziagen)
Abacavir + lamivudine, zidovudine (Trizivir)
Acetazolamide (Diamox)
Acitretin (Soriatane)
Albuterol (Proventil, Ventolin)
Albuterol + ipratropium (Combivent)
Ammonium chloride
Amphotericin B (Amphocin, Fungizone)
Amphotericin B lipid formulations IV (Abelcet)
Amprenavir (Agenerase)
Anidulafungin (Eraxis)
Aripiprazole (Abilify)
Arsenic trioxide (Trisenox)
Asparaginase (Elspar)
Atazanavir (Reyataz)
Atenolol + chlorthalidone (Tenoretic)
Atorvastatin (Lipitor)
Atovaquone (Mepron)
Baclofen (Lioresal)
Benazepril + hydrochlorothiazide (Lotension)
Betamethasone topical (Alphatrex, Betatrex, Beta-Val, Diprolene,
    Diprolene AF, Diprolene Lotion, Luxiq, Maxivate)
Betamethasone +clotrimazole (Lotrisone topical)
Betaxolol Betoptic eyedrops (Kerlone oral)
Bexarotene (Targretin)
Bicalutamide (Casodex)
Bisoprolol + hydrochlorothiazide (Ziac)
Bumetanide (Bumex)
Caffeine (Caffeine in moderation may actually be beneficial in diabetes
    but in large amounts can raise blood sugar.)
Candesartan + hydrochlorothiazide (Atacand HCT)
Captopril + hydrochlorothiazide (Capozide)
Carteolol (Cartrol oral, Occupress eyedrops)
Carvedilol (Coreg)
Chlorothiazide (Diuril)
Chlorthalidone (Clorpres, Chlorthalidone tablets, Tenoretic, Thalitone)

Choline salicylate (Numerous trade names of aspirin formulations; check label)

Choline salicylate + magnesium salicylate (CMT, Tricosal, Trilisate)

Clobetasol (Clobevate, Cormax, Cormax Scalp Application, Embeline E, Olux, Temovate, Temovate E, Temovate Scalp Application)

Clozapine (Clozaril, FazaClo)

Conjugated estrogens (Cenestin, Enjuvia, Estrace, Estring, Femring, Femtrace, Gynodiol, Menest, Ogen, Premarin, Vagifem)

Conjugated estrogens + medroxyprogesterone (Premphase, Prempro)

Corticosteroids (Numerous trade names; check label)

Corticotropin

Cortisone (Numerous trade names; check label)

Cyclosporine (Gengraf, Neoral, Sandimmune)

Daclizumab (Zenapax)

Decitabine (Dacogen)

Desonide (DesOwen, Tridesilon)

Desoximetasone (Topicort)

Dexamethasone (Adrenocot, Dalalone, Decadron, Decaject, Dekasol, Dexacort, Dexasone, Dexim, Dexone, Dexamethasone Intensol, Hexadrol, Medidex, Primethasone, Solurex)

Dextromethorphan + promethazine (Phenergan with Dextromethorphan, Phen-Tuss DM)

Diazoxide (Proglycem)

Enalapril + hydrochlorothiazide (Vaseretic)

Encainide (Enkaid)

Ephedrine + guaifenesin (Primatene tablets [OTC]. This medication includes ephedrine and guaifenesin. Guaifenesin is not responsible for hyperglycemia.)

Epinephrine (EpiPen, EpiPen Jr, Primatene Mist [OTC])

Esterified estrogens, estrone, estropipate

Esterified estrogens + methyltestosterone (Estratest)

Estradiol, ethinyl estradiol (Alora, Climara, Congest, Delestrogen, Depo-Estradiol, Depogen, Estinyl, Estrace, Estraderm, Estragyn 5, Estragyn LA 5, Estrasorb, EstroGel, Estro-L.A., Gynodiol, Kestrone-5, Neo-Estrone, Menest, Menostar, Ogen, Ogen.625, Ortho-Est, Premarin, Valergen, Vivelle, Vivelle-Dot)

Estradiol + norethindrone (Activella)

Estradiol + norgestimate (Prefest)

Estramustine (Emcyt)

Ethacrynic acid (Edecrin, Sodium Edecrin)

Everolimus (Afinitor, Zortress)

Fluoxetine (Prozac, Sarafem)

Flurandrenolide (Cordran, Cordran SP, Cordran Tape)

Formoterol (Foradil Aerolizer Inhaler)

Fosamprenavir (Lexiva)

Fosinopril + hydrochlorothiazide (Monopril HCT)

Furosemide (Lasix)

Gemtuzumab ozogamicin (Mylotarg)

Glucosamine (Possible increase in insulin resistance; more likely with intravenous use.)

Hydrochlorothiazide (Aldactazide, Aldoril, Capozide, Dyazide, HydroDIURIL, Inderide, Lopressor HCT, Maxzide, Microzide, Moduretic, Timolide, Vaseretic)

Hydrochlorothiazide + irbesartan (Avalide)

Hydrochlorothiazide + lisinopril (Prinzide, Zestoretic)

Hydrochlorothiazide + losartan (Hyzaar)

Hydrochlorothiazide + metoprolol (Lopressor HCT)

Hydrochlorothiazide + moexipril (Uniretic)

Hydrochlorothiazide + quinapril (Accuretic, Quinaretic)

Hydrochlorothiazide + telmisartan (Micardis HCT)

Hydrochlorothiazide + valsartan (Diovan HCT)

Hydrocortisone (Numerous trade names of topical hydrocortisone formulations; check label)

Indapamide (Lozol)

Indinavir (Crixivan)

Interferon alfa-n1 (Alferon-N)

Interferon alfa-2a (Roferon-A)

Interferon alfa-2b (Intron-A)

Interferon alfa-2b + ribavirin (Rebetron)

Irinotecan (Camptosar)

Isoniazid (Laniazid, Nydrazid)

Isotretinoin (Accutane)

Lamivudine (Epivir, Epivir-HBV)

Levalbuterol (Xopenex, Xopenex HFA)

Levonorgestrel (Norplant System, Plan B)

Levothyroxine (Levoxyl, Synthroid)

Liothyronine (Cytomel)

Lopinavir + ritonavir (Kaletra)

Magnesium salicylate (Bayer Select Backache Pain Formula, Doan's Pills, Mobidin, Nuprin Backache Caplet)

Medroxyprogesterone (Depo-Provera, Provera)

Megestrol (Megace)

Methylprednisolone (A-methaPred, ADD-Vantage, Depo-Medrol, Medrol, Medrol Dosepak, Meprolone Unipak, Solu-Medrol)

Metolazone (Mykrox, Zaroxolyn)

Metoprolol (Lopressor, Lopressor HCT, Toprol XL)

Modafinil (Provigil)

Moxifloxacin (Avelox, Avelox I.V.)

Mycophenolate (CellCept)
Nadolol (Corgard)
Nelfinavir (Viracept)
Niacin, niacinamide (Niacor, Niaspan, Nicolar, Nicotinex, Slo-Niacin)
Nilotinib (Tasigna)
Nilutamide (Nilandron)
Nitric oxide (INOmax)
Norethindrone (Aygestin, Micronor, Nor-QD)
Norgestrel (Orvette)
Nystatin (Mycostatin, Nystat-Rx, Nystop, Pedi-Dri)
Nystatin + triamcinolone (Dermacomb, Myco II, Mycobiotic II,
    Mycogen II, Mycolog II, Myco-Triacet II, Mykacet, Mykacet II,
    Mytrex, Tristatin II)
Octreotide (Sandostatin, Sandostatin LAR)
Olanzapine (Zyprexa)
Pantoprazole (Protonix, Protonix I.V.)
Pegaspargase (Oncaspar)
Peginterferon alfa-2b (PEG-Intron)
Pentamidine (Pentam 300)
Phenylephrine* (Sudafed PE and others)
Phenytoin (Dilantin, Dilantin-125, Dilantin Infatabs, Dilantin Kapseals,
    Phenytek)
Prednisolone (AK-Pred, Blephamide, Blephamide Liquifilm, Delta Cortef,
    Econopred Plus, Inflamase Forte, Inflamase Mild, Pediapred, Poly-Pred
    Liquifilm, Pred Forte, Pred-G, Pred-G Liquifilm, Pred Mild, Prelone)
Prednisone (Prednisone Intensol, Sterapred, Sterapred DS)
Progesterone (Prometrium)
Pseudoephedrine† (Claritin D, Sudafed, and others)
Quetiapine (Seroquel)
Risperidone (Risperdal, Risperdal M-TAB)
Ritodrine (Yutopar)
Ritonavir (Norvir)
Rituximab (Rituxan)
Salmeterol (Serevent, Serevent Diskus)
Salsalate (Argesic-SA, Disalcid, Mono-Gesic, Salflex, Salsitab)
Saquinavir (Invirase)
Sodium oxybate (Xyrem)
Somatropin (Genotropin, Genotropin Miniquick, Humatrope,

---

* There are many other OTC and prescription medications that contain
phenylephrine.
† There are many other OTC and prescription medications that contain
pseudoephedrine.

Norditropin cartridges, Norditropin NordiFlex, Nutropin, Nutropin AQ, Saizen, Serostim, Zorbtive)

Sotalol (Betapace, Betapace AF, Sorine)

Streptozocin (Zanosar)

Tacrolimus (Prograf, Protopic)

Temsirolimus (Torisel)

Thyroid (Armour Thyroid, Nature-Throid)

Tipranavir (Aptivus)

Tolvaptan (Samsca)

Torsemide (Demadex, Demadex Oral)

Triamcinolone (Aristocort, Aristospan, Asthmacort, Flutex, Kenalog, Tac, Triacet)

Ursodeoxycholic acid, ursodiol (Actigall, Urso)

Valproic acid, divalproex sodium (Depacon, Depakene, Depakene Syrup, Depakote, Depakote ER, Depakote Sprinkle)

Vitamin C (ascorbic acid, ascorbate)

Vitamin E (tocopherol, tocotrienol)

Ziprasidone (Geodone)

GENERIC NAME (BRAND NAME)

Drugs That May Cause
Hypoglycemia (Low Blood Sugar)

Acebutolol (Sectral)

Acetohexamide (Dymelor)

Alcohol

Aloe (Oral herbal supplement, especially if taken with other agents such as glimepiride, glipizide, glyburide, insulin, nateglinide, or repaglinide)

Amphotericin B (Abelcet, AmBisome, Amphocin, Amphotec, Fungizone Intravenous)

Amphotericin B lipid formulations (Abelcet, AmBisome)

Asian ginseng (ginseng; *Panax ginseng*)

Aspirin (Numerous trade names; check label)

Aspirin + dipyridamole (Aggrenox)

Atenolol (Tenoretic [containing atenolol and chlorthalidone], Tenormin)

Betaxolol (Betoptic, Betoptic S eyedrops, Kerlone oral)

Bisoprolol (Zebeta)

Bisoprolol + hydrochlorothiazide (Ziac)

Bromocriptine (Cycloset)

Chloramphenicol (Chloromycetin)

Chlorpropamide (Diabinese)

Choline salicylate (Acuprin 81, Amigesic, Anacin caplets and tablets, Anacin Maximum Strength, Anaflex 750 Arthritis Pain, Ascriptin Arthritis Pain)

Choline salicylate + magnesium salicylate C (MT, Tricosal, Trilisate)

Chromium (Numerous trade names; check label)

Clarithromycin B (Biaxin Filmtab, Biaxin Granules, Biaxin XL Filmtab, Biaxin XL Pac, Prevpac)

Diazoxide (Proglycem)

Dicumarol (Coumadin, Miradon)

Diltiazem (Cardizem, Tiazac)

Disopyramide (Norpace, Norpace CR)

Dorzolamide + timolol (Cosopt)

Exenatide (Byetta)

Fluoxetine (Prozac, Sarafem)

Fosphenytoin (Cerebyx, Dilantin, Dilantin-125, Dilantin Infatabs, Dilantin Kapseals, Mesantoin, Peganone, Phenytek)

Gamma Globulin, IV only (many brands)

Glimepiride (Amaryl)

Glimepiride + rosiglitazone (Avandaryl)

Glipizide (Glucotrol, Glucotrol XL)

Glipizide + metformin (Metaglip)

Glyburide (Diabeta, Glycron, Glynase, Micronase)

Glyburide + metformin (Glucovance)

Horse chestnut (*Aesculus hippocastanum*)

Hydrochlorothiazide + metoprolol (Lopressor HCT)

Insulin (Apidra, Humalog, Humulin, Lantus, Levemir, Novolin, Novolog, NPH)

Interferon beta-1b (Betaseron)

Levofloxacin (Levaquin, Levaquin in Dextrose Injection Premix, Quixin)

Liraglutide (Victoza)

Magnesium salicylate (Bayer Select Backache Pain Formula, Doan's Pills, Mobidin, Nuprin Backache Caplet)

Metformin (Fortamet, Glucophage, Glucophage XR, Glumetza, Riomet)

Metoprolol (Lopressor, Lopressor HCT, Toprol XL)

Morphine (Kadian, MS Contin, MSIR, Roxanol)

Nadolol (Corgard)

Nateglinide (Starlix)

Nifedipine (Adalat CC, Afeditab CR, Procardia)

Octreotide (Sandostatin, Sandostatin LAR Depot)

Paloperidone (Invega)

Penicillamine (Cuprimine, Depen)

Pentamidine (Nebupent, Pentam 300)

Phenelzine (Nardil)

Phenytoin (Dilantin, Dilantin-125, Dilantin Infatabs, Dilantin Kapseals, Phenytek)

Pindolol (Visken)

Pioglitazone (Actos. Hypoglycemia usually only when in combination with other diabetic drugs such as sulfonylureas or insulin.)

Pioglitazone + glimepiride (Duetact. The glimepiride component of this drug gives it the possibility of causing hypoglycemia alone or in combination with other diabetes medicines. This is more likely to occur when one skips a regular meal or when unusual physical activities occur.)

Pioglitazone + metformin (ACTO*plus* Met, ACTO*plus* Met XR)

Pramlintide (Symlin)

Probenecid (Benemid, Probalan)

Quinine (Quinamm, Quindan, Quiphile, Q-vel, Strema)

Quinupristin + dalfopristin (Synercid)

Repaglinide (Prandin)

Repaglinide + metformin (PrandiMet)

Ritodrine (Yutopar)

Rituximab (Rituxan)

Rosiglitazone (Avandia)

Rosiglitazone + metformin (Avandamet)

Rotigotine (Neupro)

Salicylates (Numerous trade names of aspirin formulations; check label)

Salsalate (Argesic-SA, Disalcid, Mono-Gesic, Salflex, Salsitab)

Saxagliptin (Onglyza)

Selegiline (Eldepryl)

Sitagliptin (Januvia)

Sitagliptin + metformin HCL (Janumet)

Sodium ferric gluconate complex (Ferrlecit)

Somatropin (Genotropin, Genotropin Miniquick, Humatrope, Norditropin cartridges, Norditropin NordiFlex, Nutropin, Nutropin AQ, Saizen, Serostim, Zorbtive)

Sotalol (Betapace, Betapace AF, Sorine)

Streptozocin (Zanosar)

Sulfadiazine (Microsulfon)

Tacrolimus P (Prograf, Protopic)

Tetracaine (Altacaine, Pontocaine, Tetcaine)

Theophylline (Theo-24, TheoCap, Theo-Dur)

Timolol (Timoptic, Timoptic-XE)

Tolazamide (Tolinase)

Tolbutamide (Orinase)

Tranylcypromine (Parnate)

Varenicline (Chantix)

Verapamil (Calan, Calan SR, Isoptin SR, Verelan)

GENERIC NAME (BRAND NAME)

Drugs That Can Cause
Hyperglycemia or Hypoglycemia

Amphotericin B (Abelcet, AmBisome, Amphocin, Amphotec, Fungizone
  Intravenous)

Amphotericin B lipid formulations (Abelcet, AmBisome)

Betaxolol Betoptic eyedrops, (Kerlone oral)

Bisoprolol + hydrochlorothiazide (Ziac)

Choline salicylate (Numerous trade names of aspirin formulations; check
  label)

Choline salicylate + magnesium salicylate (CMT, Tricosal, Trilisate)

Darunavir (Prezista)

Diazoxide (Proglycem)

Fluoxetine (Prozac, Sarafem)

Hydrochlorothiazide + metoprolol (Lopressor HCT)

Lanreotide acetate (Somatuline)

Lithium (Eskalith, Eskalith CR, Lithobid)

Magnesium salicylate (Bayer Select Backache Pain Formula, Doan's Pills,
  Mobidin, Nuprin Backache Caplet)

Mecasermin (Increlex)

Mecasermin rinfabate (Iplex)

Metoprolol (Lopressor, Lopressor HCT, Toprol XL)

Nadolol (Corgard)

Octreotide (Sandostatin, Sandostatin LAR Depot)

Pazopanib (Votrient)

Pentamidine (Nebupent, Pentam 300)

Phenytoin (Dilantin, Dilantin-125, Dilantin Infatabs, Dilantin Kapseals,
  Phenytek)

Rifampin (Rifadin, Rimactane)

Ritodrine (Yutopar)

Rituximab (Rituxan)

Salsalate (Argesic-SA, Disalcid, Mono-Gesic, Salflex, Salsitab)

Somatropin (Genotropin, Genotropin Miniquick, Humatrope,
  Norditropin cartridges, Norditropin NordiFlex, Nutropin, Nutropin AQ,
  Saizen, Serostim, Zorbtive)

Sotalol (Betapace, Betapace AF, Sorine)

Streptozocin (Zanosar)

Sunitinib (Sutent)

Tacrolimus P (Prograf, Protopic)

GENERIC NAME (BRAND NAME)

Drugs That Can Mask* Hypoglycemia

Atenolol (Tenoretic [containing atenolol and chlorthalidone], Tenormin)
Carteolol (Cartrol oral, Occupress eyedrops)
Carvedilol (Coreg, Coreg Tiltabs)
Clonidine (Catapres, Catapres-TTS-1, Catapres-TTS-2, Catapres-TTS-3, Duraclon)
Metoprolol (Lopressor, Lopressor HCT, Toprol XL)
Nadolol (Corgard)
Nebivolol (Bystolic)
Pindolol (Visken)
Propranolol, propranolol hydrochloride (Inderal, Inderal LA, Inderide, Innopran XL, Intensol)
Timolol (Timoptic, Timoptic-XE)

Because of the constantly changing nature of the U.S. prescription and OTC drug marketplace, this list may not reflect the full range of drugs that may impact blood glucose levels. The information contained in this document is intended as an educational aid only. It is not intended as medical advice for individual conditions or treatment. It is not a substitute for a medical exam, nor does it replace the need for services provided by medical professionals. Talk to your doctor before taking any prescription or over-the-counter drugs (including any herbal medicines or supplements) or following any treatment or regimen.

---

* Recent research suggests that this may not occur.

Foot Care for Diabetics

Although not directly related to the normalization of blood sugars, this short but important section on foot care has been included because of the constant danger diabetes can present to the lower extremities.

The incidence of limb-threatening ulcerations in diabetics is very high, affecting approximately one in six to seven patients. Nonhealing "diabetic" ulcers are the major cause of leg, foot, and toe amputations in this country, after traumatic injuries such as those occurring in motor vehicle accidents. These ulcerations do not occur spontaneously; they are always preceded by gradual or sudden injury to the skin by some external factor. Preventing such injuries can prevent their sad consequences.

Virtually all diabetics who have experienced ongoing higher-than-normal blood sugars for more than five years suffer some loss of sensitivity in their feet to pain, pressure, and temperature. This is because prolonged blood sugar elevation can injure and eventually destroy all sensory nerves in the feet (sensory neuropathy). Furthermore, the nerves that control the shape of the foot are likewise injured, with a resultant deformity that includes "claw" or "hammer" toes, high arch, and prominent heads of metatarsal bones at the bases of the toes on the underside of the foot. The nerves that stimulate perspiration in the feet are also affected. This results in the classic dry, often cracked skin that we see on diabetic feet. Dry skin is both more easily damaged and slower to heal than is normal, moist skin, and cracks permit entry of infectious bacteria.

Long-term elevated blood sugar also may cause impairment of circulation in the major arteries of the legs, as well as in the minor arteries and small capillary blood vessels that supply the skin of the feet. In order to heal, injured skin can require fifty times the blood flow of normal skin. If this increase in flow is unavailable, the injury will probably deteriorate, becoming gangrenous, and facilitate an infection that spreads up the leg. This infection may not respond to antibiotics.

Blood circulation to the normal foot can readily increase a hundredfold, if necessary, in order to conduct the heat of warm objects away from the skin. Impaired circulation may make this impossible, and the resultant burn may not even cause pain.

A deformed foot with bony prominences (knuckles of toes, tips of toes, heels, and metatarsal heads at soles) may be continually rubbed or pressed by shoes. This foot is frequently unable to perceive the extent of such pressure, or shear, and may not heal readily if injured. It can be burned at relatively low temperatures. Impaired circulation likewise can prevent the warming of cold feet so that prolonged exposure to cold can cause frostbite.

The following guidelines are therefore essential for all diabetics, to prevent foot injury and the potentially grave consequences that may ensue:

- Never walk barefoot, either indoors or out.
- Purchase shoes or sneakers late in the day, when foot size is the greatest. Shoes must be comfortable at the first wearing and should not require breaking in. Pointed-toe shoes should not be worn, even if the tips are blunted. Look for shoes with a wide, deep toe box. Some dress shoes are now available in this style. A number of currently available brands of athletic shoes and walking shoes are especially accommodating and even have removable insoles so that orthotics (see below) will fit, without making the shoe too tight. If necessary, I prescribe orthopedic or custom oxfords for certain of my patients.
- Inspect the insides of your shoes daily for foreign objects, torn lining, protruding nails, or bumps. Have them repaired if you find any of these.
- Don't wear sandals with thongs between the toes.
- Try to alternate at least two different pairs of shoes every few days.
- Ideally, your feet should be examined daily for possible injury or signs of excessive rubbing or pressure from shoes—blisters, cracks or other openings in the skin, pink spots, or calluses. Be sure to check between your toes. Inspect your soles. If necessary,

use a mirror or ask another person to check them. Contact your physician immediately if any of the above signs are found.

- If the skin of your feet is dry, lubricate the entire foot. Suitable lubricants include olive oil, any vegetable oil, vitamin E oil, emu oil, mink oil, and emulsified lanolin. Many oils and lotions that contain these products as major ingredients are available commercially. Do not use petroleum jelly (Vaseline), mineral oil, or baby oil, as they are not absorbed by the skin.

- Do not smoke cigarettes. Nicotine can cause closure of the valves that permit blood to enter the small vessels that nourish the skin.

- Keep feet away from heat. Therefore no heating pads, hot water bottles, or electric blankets. Do not place feet near sources of warmth such as radiators or fireplaces. Baths and showers should feel cool—not even lukewarm. Temperature should be estimated with your hand or a bath thermometer, not with your feet. Water temperature should be less than 92°F, as even this temperature can cause burns when circulation is impaired. A bath thermometer is suggested.

- Wear warm socks and shoes of adequate size when outside in cold weather. It is wise for all diabetics to have the circulation in their feet measured every few years. If circulation is impaired, do not remain in the cold for more than 20 minutes at a time.

- Do not soak your feet in water for more than 3–4 minutes, *even if so instructed by a physician*. This causes macerated skin, which breaks down more easily and doesn't heal well. When bathing or showering, get in, get washed, and get out. Don't soak. Beware of rain, swimming pools, and any environment that may wet your feet or your shoes. If you swim regularly for exercise, before getting in the water, apply petroleum jelly (Vaseline) to your feet to protect them from the water. After leaving the water, remove the petroleum jelly with a towel.

- Do not put adhesive tape or other adhesive products like corn plasters in contact with your feet. Fragile skin might be peeled off when the tape is removed. When applying a bandage, tape should not be applied to the skin. Use roll gauze and apply tape only to the bandage.

- Do not put any medications in contact with your skin that are not prescribed by your physician. Many over-the-counter medications, such as iodine, salicylic acid, and corn-removal agents, are dangerous. Iodine products or hydrogen peroxide should never be applied to wounds *even if so directed by a physician.* Gentian violet solution is a safer and more effective antiseptic. It is especially toxic to staphylococcus aureus, the infectious agent in most skin infections.

- If the skin of your feet is dry, your cardiologist should try to avoid medicines called beta blockers for hypertension or heart disease, as these can inhibit perspiration that moistens the feet.

- Do not attempt to file down, remove, or shave calluses or corns. This is dangerous. The toughened skin of a callus is the body's way of protecting against irritation, such as by a shoe that rubs your foot. Filing it off removes that protection, and in my experience, this is the most common initial cause of foot ulcers and resultant amputations. Do not permit podiatrists, pedicurists, or anyone else to do so. If a callus is present, show it to your physician. Ask her or a podiatrist to arrange for your shoes to be stretched, prescribe special shoes, or prescribe orthotic inserts to take pressure off the callus. Your physician may instruct you in the use of a shoe stretcher or a "ball and ring," both of which can be ordered by a shoe repair shop. By eliminating the pressure on your foot, the callus should resolve over time.

- Do not trim your toenails if you cannot see them clearly. Ask a friend or relative, podiatrist, or your physician to do this for you. If the corners of your nails are pointed, you can file them with an emery board or have someone else trim them.

- If you have thickened toenails, ask your physician to have clippings tested for fungal infection. If infection is present, he should prescribe tincture of fungoid or Penlac. Tea tree oil or Vicks VapoRub may also be effective. The solutions must be applied twice daily to the nails to be effective, and must be used for about twelve months to effect a cure. It helps to first have thickened nails ground down by a podiatrist, but she must be very careful not to damage the skin or nail bed.

- Don't wear stockings or socks with elastic bands that are tight enough to cause visible depressions in the skin. Don't use garters. Don't wear socks with holes or that have been darned, have thick seams, or are so large that they bunch up.

- Phone your physician immediately if you experience any injury to your foot. I consider even a minor foot injury to be an emergency.

Procrastination can be disastrous. If your physician is uncertain about caring for a foot injury, he should refer you to a hospital-based wound care center. If he is unavailable, go there yourself without delay.

Put a copy of these instructions in your files so that you can reread them every month. Eventually, you should know them by heart.

Polycystic Ovarian Syndrome

A syndrome is not an infection, nor a specific illness, but a combination of pathologic signs or symptoms that appear in the aggregate in a single individual. Polycystic ovarian syndrome (PCOS), when it is diagnosed (and frequently it is not), usually becomes apparent at the onset of puberty in young women. Anatomically, it consists of small cysts on the tiny follicles that release egg cells at ovulation. The condition is hard to diagnose in part because the cysts are usually too small to be displayed by conventional imaging techniques, although they can sometimes be observed with transvaginal ultrasound.

The syndrome includes several menstrual characteristics that manifest more or less, depending upon the individual, such as amenorrhea (no periods whatsoever); irregular timing of periods; irregular flow during menstruation; or abnormally heavy menstrual flow. Some but not all affected individuals have hirsutism (excessive body hair)—for example, visible mustache hair that the doctor never notices because they bleach it; hair on their arms that they shave; hairy abdomen or breasts; and so on. They frequently, but not always, have a chunky, boxerlike, masculine build, but I've also seen some whose shapes are classically feminine.

Not a tremendous amount is known about the etiology or origins of PCOS. It is often a disorder of elevated levels of male sex hormones, which can cause insulin resistance in women. Usually this is caused somehow by excess serum insulin levels secondary to insulin resistance. So these people, if they're nondiabetic, may have high serum insulin levels, which bring about the high levels of male sex hormones. The precise mechanism for this is murky. Many but certainly not all of these people become diabetic, probably by the same mechanism of beta cell burnout that we see in type 2 diabetes. Most but not all of these women have difficulty losing weight. For example, I have a teenage patient who is about five and a half feet tall and came to me weighing 160 pounds. She's currently under treatment for PCOS. The best I've been able to do so far is get her weight down to about 150, but she's eating only 7 ounces of protein and 24 grams of carbohydrate per day. Her weight seems to have leveled off, and although we've instituted other measures (which we will discuss), I don't know whether she'll be able to get any more weight off without severe caloric deprivation.

A serious consequence of this condition is infertility, which affects many but not all people with this syndrome. I have one patient who had children but had to have a total hysterectomy—and it was only then that her PCOS was discovered on microscopic examination of her ovaries.

As with many syndromes, there is no single test to determine if one has PCOS, unless it can be seen on transvaginal ultrasound. The diagnosis is made either on a discovery such as the one mentioned in the preceding paragraph, or on clinical grounds, based upon a combination of signs and symptoms. One of these, as noted, is insulin resistance. But how does one diagnose insulin resistance?

One way is to experimentally determine how much 1 unit of a rapid-acting insulin will lower a person's blood sugar, assuming that the person is on a stable blood sugar control regimen and the blood sugars are not going to be dropping or increasing. For a 140-pound insulin-using type 1 diabetic, 1 unit of regular insulin would lower blood sugar about 40 mg/dl. So if you have a person of this weight and 1 unit of regular insulin lowers her blood sugar by only 20 mg/dl, that's a good indicator of insulin resistance. If the person already has abdominal obesity or generalized increase in body fat, you don't know how much of that insulin resistance is caused by the body fat and how much may be caused by the syndrome. So ultimately the diagnosis still depends upon inference from a combination of signs and symptoms.

Another way of diagnosing the syndrome is to observe the influence of the insulin-sensitizing agent Glucophage on insulin requirements and upon menses of these patients. If someone who has no periods finally starts to have periods when she's put on metformin, there's a good likelihood of a positive diagnosis. There are also some laboratory tests that can be performed to identify hormonal disturbances. The following abnormal blood tests can be costly but in combination are highly suggestive of this disorder: LH (luteinizing hormone) at least three times as high as FSH (follicle-stimulating hormone); 17-alpha-hydroxy progesterone, estronel, free estradiol, IGF-1 (insulin-like growth factor 1), and androstenodione. Perhaps the two most important hormonal indicators would be a low ratio of DHEA sulfate to free testosterone and low IGF-1 binding protein.

This condition does not necessarily lead to poor blood sugar control. One of my PCOS patients is a lovely young lady who has essentially normal blood sugars but cannot lose weight. She's distressed by that circumstance and also distressed by her failure to ovulate and have periods, which means that unless we can improve things she will not be able to have children.

There are treatments for this condition. For many years, a diuretic called spironolactone was given for female hirsutism. It was quite effective and is still being used for this element of the syndrome. When using this medication, serum potassium levels should be checked regularly, as they might increase unduly. A number of years ago, I was treating a diabetic patient who had been trying to become pregnant for at least five years. She was not obese, but she did have slightly hairy arms and some dark hair in the mustache area. Although she had quite normal blood sugars, I noticed that she had to inject considerably more insulin than I would have anticipated for someone of her weight. I therefore decided to try her on the insulin-sensitizing agent metformin (Glucophage), which lowers insulin resistance in the liver. In a few months, she had become pregnant—after years of unsuccessful visits to infertility specialists. Furthermore, her insulin requirements dropped considerably.

Several years after I made this observation, the first papers on the use of metformin to treat this particular syndrome were published. Because these women—in my practice, mostly teenagers—are so distressed by their weight problems, and because of my anticipation of their infertility, I have tried them on every medication that lowers insulin resistance that I can think of. When I learn of a blood test that will focus on a substance that causes insulin resistance, such as tumor necrosis factor alpha (TNF-alpha), I test these patients, and indeed, I have seen very high levels of this substance in some—but again, not all—of them. When I find TNF-alpha elevated, I may prescribe several substances that have been shown to lower the blood levels or to reduce its action. Some TNF-alpha inhibitors that came up on an Internet search include the NSAID sulindac; EGCG, the main constituent of green tea; 1,25 dihydroxy vitamin D-3 (calcitriol), which is sold only by prescription and whose dosage must be carefully regulated to prevent hypercalcemia; quercetin, a widely marketed dietary supplement (most often made from the skins of onions and garlic); circumin; and Trental (pentoxifylline). This last medication has been used for many years, with only limited success, for intermittent claudication, a condition caused by poor circulation in the legs. I save Trental as something of a last resort, because it must be taken at the end of a meal, and if a person mistakenly takes it on an empty stomach, it can cause considerable gastric distress.

I refer likely PCOS patients to specialized physicians called reproductive endocrinologists for confirmation of my diagnosis and for prescription of sex hormone replacement therapy (birth control pills). I continue to address their blood sugar problems myself.

When treating PCOS, I usually begin with metformin, starting with timing to cover that time of day when basal insulin doses are greatest. For example, I may use the timed-release Glucophage XR at bedtime to help lower bedtime doses of Levemir insulin. I may also try Actos, an insulin-sensitizing agent that reduces the insulin resistance of fat and muscle cells.

Next I might add a medication called ramipril, which has also been shown to lower insulin resistance. Ramipril is used commonly to treat hypertension and diabetic kidney disease. It is an ACE inhibitor but differs from other such medications in that it affects more tissues. It can, however, cause a dry cough in some users that resolves when it is discontinued.

I also may use some of the supplements recommended in Chapter 15 for the amelioration of insulin resistance.

For several years I have been following the development of a medication that has been shown to ameliorate some of the consequences of PCOS. Its chemical name is d-chiro inositol. It has been shown to lower blood levels in women of the male sex hormone testosterone—both in the free and protein-bound forms. According to a study of PCOS patients published in the April 29, 1999, issue of the *New England Journal of Medicine,* its use increased the rate of ovulation from 27 percent in those taking a placebo to 86 percent in those taking the drug. As with other agents that lower insulin resistance, it lowered serum cholesterol and triglyceride levels as well as blood pressure.

It also lowered serum DHEA sulfate, a precursor of male sex hormones. An appropriate dose would be 1,200 mg daily.

Since my patients suffering from PCOS are very distressed by their inability to lose weight, even after we have gotten them to ovulate, I searched the Internet for sources of d-chiro inositol. I found the product already being sold in the United States and manufactured in New Zealand. It is distributed through several retailers by Humanetics Corporation of Eden Prairie, Minnesota, under the brand name Inzitol. They can be found on the Web at www.humaneticsingredients.com. Internet sources for a version product called d-Pinitol 600 include www.rockwellnutrition.com and www.drhoffman.com.

I suspect that the problem of PCOS is more common than most physicians realize, simply because usually it can only be diagnosed inferentially.

Glossary

Adrenaline: See **Epinephrine.**

Aerobic exercise: Activity that is mild enough to permit muscles to function for extended periods without developing an oxygen deficit. Examples include jogging, casual biking, slow swimming, walking, dancing. See also **anaerobic exercise.**

Alpha cells: The cells of the pancreas that produce **glucagon.**

Amino acids: The "building blocks" of proteins. Protein molecules are strings of amino acids bound together in various sequences and patterns. Amino acids can be partially converted to glucose very slowly by the liver and, to a lesser degree, by the kidneys and intestines.

Amylin: A hormone made by the beta cells of the pancreas that causes satiety, slows stomach-emptying, and reduces the blood sugar increase caused by **glucagon.** See **Symlin.**

Anaerobic exercise: Strenuous activity that causes a temporary oxygen deficit in the muscles being exercised. Such exercise can be performed only briefly before you run out of breath or the muscle fatigues. Anaerobic exercise utilizes nineteen times as much glucose as aerobic exercise for a given amount of work. It tends to build muscle mass and thereby reduce insulin resistance. Examples include sprinting, uphill biking, push-ups, speed-swimming, and repetitive lifting of heavy weights. See also **aerobic exercise.**

Analog insulin: A synthetic insulin whose molecular structure differs slightly from that of human insulin, usually in order to make it act more rapidly or much more slowly than human insulin. Analog insulins include lispro (Humalog), glulisine (Apidra), aspart (Novolog), glargine (Lantus), and detemir (Levemir).

Apidra: A more-rapid-acting clear insulin similar to **Novolog.** Known generically as glulisine.

Aspart insulin: A clear, more-rapid-acting analog insulin, slower than lispro but more rapid than regular insulin. Brand name: Novolog.

Atherosclerosis: Injury to or plaque deposits on the lining of any large artery. This can eventually lead to total blockage of the artery and death of the tissues or organs to which it supplies blood. Also called arteriosclerosis or macrovascular disease.

Autonomic neuropathy: Damage to autonomic nerves, usually by chronically elevated blood sugars. Autonomic nerves direct bodily functions that are not consciously controlled—such as heart rate, digestion, sweating, erections of the penis, blood pressure, bladder tone, and dilation and constriction of the pupils of the eyes.

Basal: In discussions of blood sugar control, refers to the fasting state. Basal insulin refers to long-acting insulins administered in just the right doses to prevent blood sugar rise while fasting. Basal doses of oral blood sugar–lowering agents are the exact doses of long-acting pills that will prevent blood sugar rise while fasting.

Beta blockers: Medications used for the treatment of high blood pressure or angina (heart pain) that tend to slow the rate and contractility of the heart.

Beta cell burnout: Destruction of pancreatic beta cells caused by over-stimulation of insulin production or by toxic effects of high blood sugars.

Beta cells: Cells located in the pancreas that produce and store insulin and another hormone, amylin, and release them into the bloodstream.

Blood glucose: Blood sugar.

Blood glucose profile: A record of blood sugars (glucose) measured a number of times daily for a period of several days or weeks. Often accompanied by related data covering meals, medications, exercise, infection or illness, and any other events that may affect blood sugar levels.

Blood glucose self-monitoring: The act of measuring and recording your own blood sugars, usually utilizing a single drop of finger-stick blood and a blood glucose meter.

Bolus insulin: An injection of rapid-acting insulin used to prevent blood sugar elevation by a meal or to lower an elevated blood sugar. See also **coverage.**

Byetta: An injectable **GLP-1** analog **incretin mimetic** that stimulates **amylin** and insulin production, while also duplicating some of the effects of amylin. Known generically as exenatide.

Carbohydrate: One of the three basic sources (protein, fat, carbohydrate) of calories or energy in foods. Carbohydrate molecules are usually chains of sugars strung together like beads on a necklace. Of the three basic caloric foods, carbohydrate raises blood sugar the most.

cc: Cubic centimeter. A measure of volume; 1/1,000 of a liter or quart. Also called milliliter (ml).

Complex carbohydrate: Made from longer, more complex chains of sugars, some are digested more slowly and raise blood sugar less rapidly than simple sugars.

Complications of diabetes: The long-term destructive effects of elevated blood sugars on most of the tissues and organs of the body.

Counterregulatory hormones: Hormones produced by the body, often in times of stress or illness, that bring about an increase in blood sugar. These include **glucagon, epinephrine,** cortisol, and growth hormone.

Coverage: The practice of injecting rapid-acting insulin to lower an elevated blood sugar. Coverage may also refer to the use of a rapid-acting insulin or oral hypoglycemic agent to cover a meal, thereby preventing a postprandial blood sugar rise. See also **bolus insulin.**

C-peptide: A by-product of insulin production by the pancreas, which when measured in the blood indicates how much insulin was recently made. People who make no insulin make no C-peptide.

Creatinine clearance: A kidney function test that estimates the **glomerular filtration rate.** It requires a 24-hour urine collection and a small sample of blood.

Crystalline insulin: See **regular insulin.**

Cystatin-C: A substance measured in the blood that is inversely related to the **glomerular filtration rate (GFR)** and doesn't require collection of a 24-hour urine for GFR estimation.

Dawn phenomenon: An apparent reduction in the effectiveness of insulin in lowering or maintaining blood sugar due to rapid clearance of insulin from the bloodstream by the liver. It may begin about an hour before arising in the morning and continue for 2–3 hours after awakening.

Delayed stomach-emptying: See **gastroparesis.**

Detemir insulin: A long-acting analog insulin. Brand name: Levemir.

DKA: Diabetic ketoacidosis. See **ketoacidosis.**

DPP-4 antagonist: A medication that inhibits the enzyme (DPP-4) that destroys **GLP-1,** thereby increasing blood levels of GLP-1. See **Januvia** and **Onglyza.**

Dyslipidemia: Any abnormality in the **lipid profile.**

Epinephrine: A hormone produced by the adrenal glands in response to stresses such as extreme exercise, pain, fright, anger, and hypoglycemia. Elevated blood levels of epinephrine can cause tremors, sweating, and increases of heart rate and blood sugar. Also called adrenaline.

Essential amino acids: Amino acids that the body cannot manufacture and therefore must, for survival, be provided by protein in the diet.

Essential fatty acids: Fatty acids that the body cannot manufacture and therefore must, for survival, be provided by fat in the diet. See also **fatty acid** and **triglycerides.**

Fasting blood glucose, fasting blood sugar: Blood sugar value when measured before the first meal of the day, usually at least 8 hours after any prior consumption of food.

Fat: One of the three basic sources (protein, fat, carbohydrate) of calories or energy in foods. It can be found in milk, cheese, egg yolks, meat, fish, fowl, nuts, oils, and some vegetables. Consumption of pure fat does not directly affect blood sugar.

Fatty acid: A chain of carbon and hydrogen atoms that is one of the building blocks of fat. See also **triglycerides.**

Fibrinogen: A precursor of fibrin, which is the structural element of blood clots. Elevated levels of fibrinogen in the blood can be caused by high blood sugars and are associated with increased risk for heart attacks, strokes, retinopathy, kidney damage, and other complications of diabetes.

Fructose: A sugar occurring especially in fruits, fruit juices, and honey.

Gastroparesis: A neuropathy caused by years of blood sugar elevation, which can severely impair the muscular and secretory activities of the stomach. Gastrointestinal discomfort may sometimes be present after meals. Blood sugars after meals may be unpredictable because of a random effect upon the rate of stomach-emptying. Also called delayed stomach-emptying and gastroparesis diabeticorum.

Glargine insulin: A clear, long-acting analog insulin that the author no longer prescribes. Brand name: Lantus.

Glomerular filtration rate (GFR): The kidneys filter blood and produce urine by means of about 1 million microscopic glomeruli. The GFR is a measure of how much filtering the kidneys perform in a given time period. See also **glomerulus.**

Glomerulopathy: The condition of damaged glomeruli.

Glomerulus: The microscopic filtering unit of the kidneys that removes water and other substances from blood, thereby creating urine.

GLP-1 (glucagon-like peptide-1): An **incretin** hormone made by the intestines when distended by food. It signals the pancreas to produce **insulin, glucagon,** and **amylin.** It may also independently cause satiety and other effects.

Glucagon: A hormone produced by the alpha cells of the pancreas that raises blood sugar by causing the liver and muscles to break down proteins and stored glycogen to glucose.

GLUCOGRAF III data sheet: A preprinted form used by diabetics for recording blood sugar measurements, medications, exercise, and meals. Illustrated on page 89.

Gluconeogenesis: The conversion of amino acids (the building blocks of proteins) to glucose by the liver and to a lesser degree by the intestines and the kidneys.

Glucophage: The preferred brand of **metformin.**

Glucose: A naturally occurring sugar, which when measured in the blood is called blood sugar. Glucose is the building block of most carbohydrates and of **glycogen.**

Glucose challenge: An event, such as a high-carbohydrate meal, that can raise blood sugar significantly.

Glucose transporters: Specialized protein molecules that insulin causes to migrate from inside a cell to the surface. They protrude from the surface and bring blood glucose into the cell.

Glulisine insulin: A rapid-acting analog insulin. Brand name: Apidra.

Glycated hemoglobin: By measuring the glycation of hemoglobin, the principal protein of red blood cells, we can estimate one's average blood sugar over the prior four months. See also **glycation.**

Glycation: The permanent binding of glucose to proteins of blood or body tissues. Glycation of proteins can adversely affect their structure and function, leading to many of the complications of diabetes.

Glycemic index: A crude index that attempts to compare the blood sugar–raising effect of a food to that of pure glucose.

Glycogen: A starchy substance formed from glucose that is stored in the liver and muscles. It can be rapidly converted back to glucose by the action of certain counterregulatory hormones.

Glycosylation: The reversible binding of glucose to proteins of blood or body tissues. If a protein is glycosylated for more than 24 hours, a rearrangement of the attachment renders it permanent. See also **glycation.**

HDL: Abbreviation for high-density lipoprotein, a submicroscopic particle found in the blood that transports cholesterol and triglycerides from arterial walls to the liver. Also known as the "good" cholesterol. High blood levels of HDL are believed to offer protection from coronary artery disease, peripheral vascular disease, and stroke. See also **LDL.**

Hemoglobin A$_{1C}$ (HgbA$_{1C}$): The most commonly measured indicator of glycated hemoglobin.

High-density lipoprotein: See **HDL.**

Homocysteine: A substance found in the blood that can increase risk of kidney disease or heart attack. May be elevated when vitamin B-6, vitamin B-12, and folate levels are low.

Humalog: Brand name for a clear, more-rapid insulin. Also known generically as lispro.

Human insulin: Any insulin whose molecular structure is identical to that of human insulin. The only human insulins currently on the market in the United States are regular and NPH.

Hyperglycemia: Abnormally high blood sugar.

Hyperinsulinemia: Abnormally high blood insulin level.

Hyperlipidemia: A vague term that commonly refers to any of a number of abnormalities of fatty substances in the blood. These may include elevated triglycerides, elevated LDL (the "bad" cholesterol), or low levels of HDL (the "good" cholesterol). More properly called **dyslipidemia.**

Hyperosmolar coma: A frequently fatal dehydrated condition with loss of consciousness, caused by extremely high blood sugars in diabetics who make enough insulin to prevent **ketoacidosis.** Usually affects elderly type 2 diabetics.

Hypertension: High blood pressure.

Hypoglycemia: Abnormally low blood sugar.

Hypoglycemia unawareness: Inability to experience or perceive the physical symptoms of low blood sugar.

Hypotension: Abnormally low blood pressure.

IDDM: Abbreviation for insulin-dependent diabetes mellitus; see **type 1 diabetes.**

Impaired glucose tolerance (IGT): A mild or early form of diabetes that can slowly cause many of the long-term complications of "full-blown" diabetes. Frequently precedes the onset of diabetes. A treatable disorder.

Incretin mimetics (IMs): Prescription drugs that either act like the hormone amylin (Symlin) or stimulate the production of amylin by surviving beta cells (Byetta, Victoza, Onglyza, Tradjenta, and Januvia). Amylin plays a role in fine-tuning postprandial blood sugars and in causing satiety.

Incretins: Hormones secreted into the bloodstream by the intestines in response to food, signaling the pancreas that food is being digested. The principal effect is caused by **GLP-1.**

Insulin: A hormone produced by the beta cells of the pancreas gland that facilitates the entry of glucose into most cells of the body. Insulin is also the principal fat-building hormone. See also **analog insulin** and **human insulin.**

Insulin-mimetic agent: An oral agent (pill) that lowers blood sugar by acting like insulin but without causing fat storage.

Insulin receptors: Protein molecules on the surface of most cells of the body that bind circulating insulin. It is the binding of insulin by a cell that indirectly facilitates the entry of glucose into the cell.

Insulin resistance: Reduced sensitivity of the body to the effect of insulin on blood sugar.

Insulin-sensitizing agent (ISA): An oral agent (pill) that helps control blood sugar by lowering **insulin resistance.**

Intramuscular (IM): Used to describe an injection (as of rapid-acting insulin) into muscle in order to speed up its action.

Januvia: An oral **DPP-4 antagonist** that is usually taken once daily. Similar to **Onglyza** and **Tradjenta.** Known generically as liragliptin.

Ketoacidosis: An acute, life-threatening condition caused by the combination of very high blood sugars and dehydration. It involves high blood levels of **ketones,** including acetone, and an acidification of the blood.

Ketones: By-products of fat metabolism that include acetone, the principal component of nail polish remover. May be present in the blood when a person is fasting or losing weight, or when blood sugars are very high in people who don't make insulin. See also **ketoacidosis.**

Lactose: A sugar found in milk and some cheeses that is converted to glucose by the liver.

LDL: Abbreviation for low-density lipoprotein, a particle in the blood that deposits cholesterol and triglycerides in arterial walls. Also known as the "bad" cholesterol. Elevated LDL is claimed to be a risk factor for coronary artery disease and peripheral vascular disease. More important as a measure of disease risk than the LDL value itself is the ratio of LDL to HDL. For accurate measurement, a "direct LDL" or "real LDL" test must be ordered. LDL is harmful only when it is oxidized or glycated or in the form of small, dense particles, all of which are caused by elevated blood sugars. See also **HDL.**

Levemir: A clear, long-acting insulin recommended in this book. Known generically as detemir.

Lipid profile: A battery of measurements of fatty substances in the blood. It may include **LDL, total cholesterol, triglycerides, HDL,** and **lipoprotein(a).**

Lipoprotein: Submicroscopic particle that carries fatty substances such as cholesterol and triglycerides through the bloodstream. Examples of lipoproteins include HDL, LDL, apolipoproteins, and lipoprotein(a).

Lipoprotein(a): A **lipoprotein** that increases risk of heart attack by interfering with the body's mechanism for dissolving blood clots. Abbreviated Lp(a).

Lispro: See **Humalog.**

Low-density lipoprotein: See **LDL.**

Lower esophageal sphincter (LES): A muscular band near the lower end of the esophagus, a tube connecting the throat to the stomach. Normal contraction of this band after swallowing prevents regurgitation of stomach contents.

Macrovascular: Relating to large blood vessels.

Maltodextrin: A mixture of sugars derived from corn syrup; used as a sweetener in many packaged foods. Should be avoided by diabetics.

Maturity-onset diabetes: See **type 2 diabetes.**

Metformin: Sold generically and under the brand name Glucophage, this **insulin-sensitizing agent** is one of the most effective that we have. Rather than increasing insulin production and "burning out" pancreatic beta cells, it increases the body's sensitivity to its own or injected insulin. In my experience, not all generic metformins match the efficacy of the original or extended-release Glucophage.

mg/dl: Milligrams per deciliter. The unit of blood sugar measurement in the United States. See also **mmol/l.**

Microaneurysms: Ballooning of microscopic blood vessels, caused by destruction of cells (pericytes) that line the outer walls of these vessels. Microaneurysms are often found in the retinas of the eyes of diabetics who have had elevated blood sugars for prolonged periods.

Microangiopathy: Injury to small blood vessels, commonly found in long-standing poorly controlled diabetes. A major cause of blindness and kidney disease in diabetics.

Microvascular: Relating to small blood vessels.

mmol/l: Millimoles per liter. The international unit of blood sugar measurement. See also **mg/dl** (1 mmol/l = 18 mg/dl).

Monounsaturated fats: Fats whose molecules contain fatty acids that are missing one pair of hydrogen atoms. These fats are believed by some to offer protection from vascular disease because their consumption may lower serum LDL and raise HDL in some high-risk individuals.

Nephropathy: Damage to kidneys. In this book, the term is limited to damage caused by high blood sugars.

Neuroglycopenia: A blood sugar so low that inadequate glucose is getting into the brain. As a result, cognition, coordination, and level of consciousness may become severely impaired. A severe form of **hypoglycemia.**

Neuropathy: Damage to nerves. In this book, the term is limited to damage caused by high blood sugars.

Neurotransmitters: The chemical "messengers" of the central and peripheral nervous systems.

NIDDM: Abbreviation for non-insulin-dependent diabetes mellitus. Not entirely accurately used interchangeably with the term type 2 diabetes, or maturity-onset diabetes. See **type 2 diabetes.**

Novolog: See **Aspart insulin.**

NPH insulin: A cloudy, intermediate-acting human insulin that lowers or maintains blood sugar for a period of about 12 hours after injection when used in **physiologic doses.**

Onglyza: An oral **DPP-4 antagonist** that is usually taken once daily. Similar to **Januvia** and **Tradjenta.** Known generically as saxagliptin.

Oral hypoglycemic agent (OHA): A pill used to lower blood sugar in type 2 diabetics by stimulating the pancreas to produce more insulin. Also used to designate insulin sensitizing agents.

Pancreas: A large abdominal organ that manufactures insulin, glucagon, amylin, and other hormones, secreting them into the bloodstream. The pancreas also produces digestive enzymes and bicarbonate, which are secreted into the upper gastrointestinal tract, beyond the stomach.

Phase I insulin response: A sudden release of insulin by the pancreas in response to a **glucose challenge,** such as a meal. This may represent the release of stored insulin granules. Usually impaired in early diabetes.

Phase II insulin response: The continued slower release of (probably newly manufactured) insulin from the pancreas that occurs after the phase I insulin response.

Physiologic doses of insulin: Doses of injected insulin calculated to approximate the amounts made in the body by nondiabetics. These relatively small doses are in contrast to the large, "industrial" doses usually prescribed by physicians who do not follow the methods of this book.

Platelets: Small particles in the blood that play a major role in causing blood to clot.

Polyunsaturated fats: Fats made from fatty acids that are missing more than one pair of hydrogen atoms. Dietary consumption may reduce elevated serum **LDL** levels for some individuals. These fats are unstable and readily oxidized.

Postprandial: After a meal.

Postural hypotension: A sudden drop in blood pressure upon standing.

Preprandial: Before a meal.

Progressive exercise: A planned exercise program wherein the work required per session becomes greater and greater over a period of weeks, months, or years.

Protein: One of the three basic sources (protein, fat, carbohydrate) of calories or energy in foods. The principal nutritional component of fish, poultry, meat, cheese, and egg white, it is also present in other foods in lesser amounts. The major component of most human tissues other than fat and water.

Pyloric valve (pylorus): A muscular band at the exit of the stomach that relaxes to permit stomach-emptying in normal individuals. In people with diabetic **gastroparesis,** the pyloric valve may be randomly in spasm and thereby delay stomach-emptying.

Regular insulin: Also called simply **regular.** A commonly used clear, rapid-acting human insulin. Not as rapid-acting as analog insulins such as Humalog, Apidra, and Novolog. Also called crystalline insulin.

Renal: Relating to the kidney.

Renal risk profile: A series of tests that can reflect damage suffered by the kidneys.

Retinopathy: Injury to the retina, or light-sensing surface, in the rear of the eye. Usually caused by chronically high blood sugars in diabetics.

R-R interval study: A quantitative, objective test for **autonomic neuropathy.** The test is similar to an electrocardiogram, but the patient breathes deeply while the test is under way.

Stevia: A sugarless herbal sweetener, sold as liquid or powder in health food stores. Brands that contain **maltodextrin** should not be used.

Subcutaneous: Below the skin but above muscle, as in a subcutaneous injection.

Sucrose: Table sugar. The sucrose molecule consists of one glucose molecule bound to one fructose molecule.

Sugars: A group of chemical compounds consisting of six carbon atoms bound to hydrogen and oxygen atoms. Most sugars taste sweet and can be converted to glucose (blood sugar) by the body. Some sugars are formed by the joining together of two other sugars. Sugars are the simplest **carbohydrates.**

Sulfonylureas: A class of oral hypoglycemic agents that are chemically related to sulfa drugs. They lower blood sugar by stimulating pancreatic beta cells to make more insulin, and carry with them a danger of "burning out" those cells.

Symlin: An injectable analog of human **amylin.** Known generically as pramlintide.

Thiazolidinediones: A class of drugs that lower insulin resistance, principally in fat and muscle cells. They also inhibit renal deterioration from high blood sugars independently of their effect upon blood sugar. They have also been found to delay or prevent the onset of diabetes in some high-risk individuals. The thiazolidinediones available in the United States are rosiglitazone (Avandia) and pioglitazone (Actos). The use of Avandia is restricted by the FDA.

Thrombotic risk profile: A group of blood tests that can reflect the tendency of blood to clot inappropriately, thereby increasing the risk for heart attacks, poor circulation, kidney impairment, and certain types of stroke. These tests include fibrinogen, lipoprotein(a), and C-reactive protein.

Total cholesterol: The sum of serum **HDL** plus serum **LDL** plus approximately one-fifth of serum **triglycerides.**

Tradjenta: An oral DPP-4 **antagonist** that is usually taken once daily. Similar to **Onglyza** and **Januvia.** Known generically as liragliptin.

Triglycerides: Substances found in blood and fatty tissues comprising the storage form of fat. Each triglyceride molecule consists of three fatty acid molecules bound to a glycerol molecule. Serum triglyceride is frequently elevated when blood sugar is high. Elevated levels can be a risk factor for cardiac and vascular disease.

Truncal obesity: A form of obesity, also called central or visceral obesity, in which the circumference of the waist is greater than the circumference of the hips in males or greater than 80 percent of the hip circumference in females.

Type 1 diabetes: A type of diabetes, usually appearing before the age of forty-five, that involves total or near total loss of the capacity to produce insulin. Also called insulin-dependent diabetes mellitus (IDDM), autoimmune diabetes, or juvenile-onset diabetes.

Type 2 diabetes: The type of diabetes that usually appears after the age of forty-five and is commonly associated with obesity. It involves partial loss of insulin-producing capability, diminished non-insulin-mediated glucose transport, and resistance to the glucose transport effects of insulin. Also not quite accurately called non-insulin-dependent diabetes mellitus (NIDDM), insulin-resistant diabetes, or maturity-onset diabetes. Now found to appear in many obese children.

Unit: A measure of the biological effectiveness of insulin at reducing blood sugar. The lines on the scale of an insulin syringe frequently measure increments of 1 unit. The lines on some newer syringes represent increments of ½ unit.

Vagus nerve: The largest nerve in the body, and the main neural component of the part of the nervous system that regulates the parasympathetic autonomic (involuntary) functions of the body, including heart rate, blood pressure, breathing, penile erections, and digestion.

Vascular: Relating to blood vessels.

Victoza: An injectable **GLP-1** agonist used once daily. Especially effective for appetite suppression. Known generically as liraglutide.

Visceral obesity: See **truncal obesity.**

Recipe Index

General Index

dehydration
dangers of, 364–365
exercise and, 230, 364
fluid replacement, 369–371, 370n, 371n, 483
frequent urination and, 39, 363–364, 365
insulin resistance and, 100, 363, 365, 365n
medications and, 365, 365n, 368
supplies for, 71, 74
urgency of, 362, 373
vicious circle of, 363–364
delayed stomach-emptying. *See* gastroparesis (delayed stomach-emptying)
De Loach, Stan, 122n
dementia. *See* memory, short-term
Denmark study, 470
dental infections, 105–106, 256, 374–375
depression, 37
desserts. *See also* Jell-O brand gelatin desserts
checking labels and, 152
"fat-free," 172
as "no-no" food, 160
very low-carbohydrate desserts, 170
detemir insulin (D, Levemir)
action time of, 274, 284, 285–286, 287
care of, 281, 282
dosage of, 239, 294–295, 502
hospital pharmacies and, 483
supplies, 72, 77
Dex4 bits, 71, 73, 75, 233n, 342, 343
Dex4 gel, 73, 77–78, 348–349
Dex4 Liquid Blast, 73, 75, 78, 235, 396–397
Dex4 tablets, 71, 73, 75, 232, 233, 342
dextrin, 151
Dextro Energen, 71, 75, 343
Dextro Energy, 71, 75
dextrose, 149, 151, 154, 160
diabetes. *See also* tests; treatment plans
"brittle," 7, 26
"chemical," 9
complications from, xiii–xv, xvii, 10, 12, 22, 45, 46, 48, 55, 119–120, 120n, 137, 463
imbalanced self-regulating systems and, 37
latent autoimmune diabetes (LADA), 41
mortality risk and, 467
myths of, xiii
statistics on, 35, 41
diabetes, type 1 (insulin-dependent diabetes mellitus [IDDM], juvenile-onset)
blood sugar normalization and, 40–41
complications of, xiii, 36–37, 108
dawn phenomenon and, 98
exercise and, 224, 228, 229, 232
gluconeogenesis and, 96
growth stunted from, xiv, 407–408
honeymoon period, 103–104
hypoglycemia and, 360–361
incretin mimetics and, 216–217
insulin and, 38–40
insulin dosage and, 112
insulin-producing ability and, 39, 40
insulin resistance and, 100–101
life expectancy and, xv

overeating and, 206
parental fears, xiii–xiv
target BG and, 124
treatment plans for, 115–116
diabetes, type 2 (non-insulin-dependent diabetes mellitus [NIDDM], maturity-onset)
blood sugar levels and, 46
cause of, 42
dawn phenomenon and, 98
exercise and, 225, 227, 228, 238
gluconeogenesis and, 96–97
incidence of, 35–36, 41
insulin injections and, 265
as insulin-resistant diabetes, 36n, 42, 106, 199
ISAs and, 253
obesity and, 41–42, 193, 196
onset of, 44
overeating and, 206
postprandial levels of glucose and, 140–141
small, frequent meals, 114, 182
stress and, 100
target BG and, 123–124
treatment plans for, 115
Diabetes Care, 66, 122n, 123, 466, 472n, 473
Diabetes Center, 73, 81, 117–118, 362
Diabetes Control and Complication Trial (DCCT), 40–41, 301
Diabetes Diet, The (Bernstein), 170, 171, 183, 186, 413
Diabetes (journal), 466, 467n, 475n
Diabetes: The Glucograf Method for Normalizing Blood Sugar (Bernstein), xxi
Diabetic Nephropathy, 470
diabetic supplies and tools
advances in, xiii–xiv, xix
for all diabetics, 71–77
for insulin-using diabetics only, 72–73, 77–78
ordering, 70
treatment plans and, 119
Diabinese, 9
diarrhea
dehydration and, 363, 364, 371–372
fluid replacement and, 371
insulin dosage and, 367–368
supplies for, 71, 74
Diastix, 72, 76, 147–148, 153, 162, 166
diet. *See also* carbohydrate (CHO); fat, dietary; protein (PRO); snacking; vitamins and vitamin supplements; *and individual food items*
acceptable foods, 157–159, 162–171
awareness of food contents, 171–172
basic rules, 146–147
breakfast, 46, 47, 48, 50–51, 178, 178n, 183–185, 190–192, 308–311
carbohydrate estimation and, 110
consistency in, 147
diet foods, 150–151, 160
eating out, 147–148, 290, 305–306
eliminating simple sugars, 146–157
exchange diet, 12, 177
gastroparesis and, 146, 392–395
importance of, 5, 7, 17, 19, 20–21, 24–25, 145–147
lunch, 178, 185–186, 190–192, 308–311

General Index